Straight A's

in

Medical-Surgical Nursing

Second Edition

Wolters Kluwer | Lippincott Williams & Wilkins
Health

Philadelphia · Baltimore · New York · London
Buenos Aires · Hong Kong · Sydney · Tokyo

STAFF

Executive Publisher
Judith A. Schilling McCann, RN, MSN

Editorial Director
David Moreau

Clinical Director
Joan M. Robinson, RN, MSN

Art Director
Mary Ludwicki

Electronic Project Manager
John Macalino

Clinical Project Manager
Kate Stout, RN, MSN, CCRN

Editor
Karen C. Comerford

Copy Editors
Kimberly Bilotta (supervisor),
Scotti Cohn, Jeannine Fielding,
Amy Furman, Shana Harrington,
Dona Perkins, Lisa Stockslager,
Dorothy P. Terry

Designer
Matie A. Patterson

Digital Composition Services
Diane Paluba (manager),
Joyce Rossi Biletz, Donald Knauss,
Donna S. Morris

Associate Manufacturing Manager
Beth J. Welsh

Editorial Assistants
Karen J. Kirk, Jeri O'Shea,
Linda K. Ruhf

Indexer
Karen C. Comerford

STRMS2E011107

**Library of Congress
Cataloging-in-Publication Data**

Straight A's in medical-surgical nursing. — 2nd ed.
    p. ; cm.
Includes bibliographical references and index.
    1. Nursing—Outlines, syllabi, etc. 2. Nursing—Examinations, questions, etc. 3. Surgical nursing—Outlines, syllabi, etc. 4. Surgical nursing—Examinations, questions, etc. I. Lippincott Williams & Wilkins. II. Title: Medical-surgical nursing.
    [DNLM: 1. Nursing Care—Examination Questions. 2. Perioperative Nursing—Examination Questions. WY 100 S896 2007]
    RT52.S77 2008
    617'.0231076—dc22
ISBN-13: 978-1-58255-694-9 (alk. paper)
ISBN-10: 1-58255-694-6 (alk. paper)   2007032105

Contents

Advisory board

Contributors and consultants

Helen Ballestas, RN, MSN, CRRN
Instructor
New York Institute of Technology
Old Westbury

Michele R. Bunning, RN, MSN
Associate Professor
Good Samaritan College of Nursing and Health Science
Cincinnati

Susan K. Callen, RN, MSN
Teaching Specialist
UPMC Shadyside School of Nursing
Pittsburgh

Marsha Conroy, RN, MSN, APN
Nurse Educator
Cuyahoga Community College
Cleveland

Kim Cooper, RN, MSN
Nursing Department Program Chair
Ivy Tech Community College
Terre Haute, Ind.

Sally L. Gaines, RN, MSN
Nursing Instructor
West Texas A&M University
Canyon

April N. Hart, RN, MSN, FNP, BC
Assistant Professor
Bethel College
Mishawaka, Ind.

Donna Headrick, RN, MSN, FNP
Professor
Bakersfield (Calif.) College

Lajuana B. Jordan, RN, MSN, GNP
Nursing Instructor
Danville (Va.) Regional Medical Center
School of Health Professions, Nursing Program

Kathy J. Keister, RN, PhD
Assistant Professor
Miami University
Middletown, Ohio

Jennifer M. Lee, RN, BSN, CCRN
Staff Nurse
AnMed Health
Anderson, S.C.
Graduate Teaching Assistant
Clemson (S.C.) University

Juanita Manning-Walsh, RN, PhD
Assistant Professor
Western Michigan University
Kalamazoo

Kimberly Smith, RN, BSN, LNC
Legal Nurse Consultant/Healthcare Advocate
Nursing Analysis & Review
Byron, Minn.

Lisa A. Streeter, RN, BS
Master Instructor
Madison Oneida BOCES
Utica, N.Y.

Allison J. Terry, RN, PhD
Director of Community Certification
Department of Mental Health, Mental Retardation Division
Montgomery, Ala.

Sheryl Thomas, RN, MSN
Nursing Instructor
Wayne County Community College
Detroit

Reginald Williams, RN, BSN
Adjunct Practical Nurse Instructor
Microtech Training Center
Jersey City, N.J.

How to use this book

Straight A's is a multivolume study guide series developed especially for nursing students. Each volume provides essential course material in a unique two-column design. The easy-to-read interior outline format offers a succinct review of key facts as presented in leading textbooks on the subject. The bulleted exterior columns provide only the most crucial information, allowing for quick, efficient review right before an important quiz or test.

Special features appear in every chapter to make information accessible and easy to remember. The Pretest helps the student identify topic areas that may require more study. Learning objectives encourage the student to evaluate knowledge before and after study. The Chapter overview highlights the chapter's major concepts. The NCLEX checks at the end of each chapter offer additional opportunities to review material and assess knowledge gained before moving on to new information.

Other features appear throughout the book to facilitate learning. Clinical alerts appear in color to bring the reader's attention to important, potentially life-threatening considerations that could affect patient care. Time-out for teaching highlights key areas to address when teaching patients. Go with the flow charts promote critical thinking. Finally, a Windows-based software program (see CD-ROM on inside back cover) poses more than 250 multiple-choice and alternate-format NCLEX-style questions to assess student knowledge.

The Straight A's volumes are designed as learning tools, not as primary information sources. When read conscientiously as a supplement to class attendance and textbook reading, Straight A's can enhance understanding and help improve test scores and final grades.

Foreword

Faculty who teach prelicensure nursing students are often anxious about which content to emphasize in their programs' medical-surgical courses. Again and again they discuss how to divide the information across courses, how much detail to share with students, and how many facts and critical thinking skills to evaluate in tests. Whether they teach two, three, or more medical-surgical courses in the curriculum, they take into account that the NCLEX-RN exam tests a large amount of this multifaceted and pertinent area of nursing.

This concern about how best to teach students inspires medical-surgical nursing faculty to choose different strategies that they think will help students learn the basics of various disorders that affect adult patients. Faculty often use a case study approach in which complex patient stories are described and students are challenged to actively participate in each lesson and absorb the most knowledge possible during each teaching-learning episode. Faculty hope that the stories will anchor students' memory to important information. No matter the focus of lectures, whether outlined in study guides, online postings, or PowerPoint slides or specified in exam blueprints or test maps, students struggle to retain facts and principles and successfully pass medical-surgical courses. They must bring the knowledge accumulated from previous science and medical-surgical and other nursing courses to subsequent courses. Nursing faculty expect students to come "up to speed" quickly by bringing formerly learned information to mind.

The purpose of this book is to improve student performance while in school and ultimately to ensure success on the NCLEX-RN. The outline approach helps students to improve comprehension of medical-surgical nursing. The book functions as a total learning approach since it covers essential areas. It serves as an advanced organizer that students can use before reading more detailed textbook sections and attending lectures on corresponding topics. The elements of different body systems are presented, with pretest questions and end-of-chapter posttests; NCLEX-style questions demarcate each chapter. Students can test their understanding before and after reviewing chapters. They will benefit first from reading chapter headings to gain an overview of the structure and content of each body system covered. Using the book as a self-paced approach to learning medical-surgical nursing, students can prepare for upcoming classes, review material in preparation for clinical assignments and tests, and reinforce previous learning as they enroll in successive medical-surgical nursing courses. The outline structure of the book allows students to work as independent learners.

As an advance organizer, this book defines and yet limits the scope of medical-surgical nursing practice by including critical material and eliminating "nice to know" content. Ten chapters are presented. Anatomy and physiology and assessment findings are detailed in succinct form, encouraging students to remember concepts, principles, and facts from prior courses. Students' recall of content is reinforced using outlines, tables, and illustrations. They study newer content using common headings used throughout the text. Nursing interventions are framed by disease causation, pathophysiology, assessment and diagnostic test findings, medical and surgical management, and other relevant topics. Straight A's in Medical-Surgical Nursing, Second edition, provides students with a structure for learning complex content and many opportunities to reflect on how new information fits with what they have already learned.

Zane Robinson Wolf, RN, PhD, FAAN
Dean and Professor, School of Nursing and Health Sciences
La Salle University
Philadelphia

Cardiovascular system

PRETEST

1. A client complains of crushing chest pain that radiates to his left arm. He should be presented with the following treatment:

- ☒ 1. Aspirin, oxygen, nitroglycerin, and morphine
- ☐ 2. Aspirin, oxygen, nitroglycerin, and codeine
- ☐ 3. Oxygen, nitroglycerin, meperidine, and thrombolytics
- ☐ 4. Aspirin, oxygen, nitroprusside, and morphine

CORRECT ANSWER: 1

2. Which lifestyle changes should a client diagnosed with coronary artery disease consider?

- ☐ 1. Smoking cessation
- ☐ 2. Establishing a regular exercise routine
- ☐ 3. Weight reduction
- ☒ 4. All of the above

CORRECT ANSWER: 4

3. A client's cardiac monitor alarm sounds, indicating ventricular tachycardia. The nurse should:

- ☐ 1. perform immediate defibrillation.
- ☒ 2. assess the client.
- ☐ 3. call the physician.
- ☐ 4. administer a precordial thump.

CORRECT ANSWER: 2

4. A complication of peripheral vascular disease may be:

☒ 1. stasis ulcer.

☐ 2. pressure ulcer.

☐ 3. gastric ulcer.

☐ 4. duodenal ulcer.

CORRECT ANSWER: 1

5. A key diagnostic test for heart failure is:

☐ 1. serum potassium.

☒ 2. B-type natriuretic peptide.

☐ 3. troponin I.

☐ 4. cardiac enzymes.

CORRECT ANSWER: 2

LEARNING OBJECTIVES

After studying this chapter, you should be able to:

● Describe the psychosocial impact of cardiovascular disorders.

● Differentiate between modifiable and nonmodifiable risk factors in the development of a cardiovascular disorder.

● List three probable and three possible nursing diagnoses for a patient with a cardiovascular disorder.

● Identify nursing interventions for a patient with a cardiovascular disorder.

● Write three teaching goals for a patient with a cardiovascular disorder.

CHAPTER OVERVIEW

Caring for the patient with a cardiovascular disorder requires a thorough understanding of cardiovascular anatomy and physiology as well as hemodynamic function. A comprehensive assessment is essential for planning and implementing appropriate patient care. The assessment includes a complete history, physical examination, diagnostic testing, identification of modifiable and nonmodifiable risk factors, and information related to the psychosocial impact of the disorder on the patient.

Nursing diagnoses focus primarily on ineffective tissue perfusion and decreased cardiac output. Nursing interventions are designed to decrease the cardiac workload and increase blood supply, thereby improving tissue perfusion. Patient teaching—a crucial nursing activity—involves information about the specific disorder, diagnostic testing and procedures, treatment plan, medication regimens, signs and symptoms of possible complications, stress management, smoking cessation, medical or surgical follow-up, and reduction of modifiable risk factors through weight control, activity, and diet modifications.

ANATOMY AND PHYSIOLOGY REVIEW

● **Cardiac structures**
  - The heart is a muscular organ composed of two atria and two ventricles
  - It's surrounded by a pericardial sac that consists of two layers
    – Visceral (inner) layer
    – Parietal (outer) layer
  - The heart wall has three layers
    – Epicardium (visceral pericardium)
    – Myocardium
    – Endocardium
  - The heart has four valves
    – Tricuspid (atrioventricular [AV] valve)
    – Mitral (AV valve)
    – Pulmonic (semilunar valve)
    – Aortic (semilunar valve)

● **Myocardial blood supply**
  - The left coronary artery (LCA) branches into the left anterior descending (LAD) artery and the circumflex artery
    – The LAD artery supplies blood to the anterior wall of the left ventricle, the anterior ventricular septum, and the bundle branches
    – The circumflex artery provides blood to the lateral and posterior portions of the left ventricle
  - The right coronary artery (RCA) fills the groove between the atria and ventricles and gives rise to the acute marginal artery, ending as the posterior descending artery
    – The RCA sends blood to the sinus and atrioventricular nodes and to the right atrium

Layers of the heart's wall

- Epicardium (visceral pericardium)
- Myocardium
- Endocardium

Valves of the heart

- Tricuspid (AV valve)
- Mitral (AV valve)
- Pulmonic (semilunar valve)
- Aortic (semilunar valve)

Main arteries of the heart

- LCA
- RCA

Key facts about circulation through the heart

- Inferior and superior venae cavae to right atrium
- Through tricuspid valve to right ventricle
- Through pulmonic valve to pulmonary artery
- To lungs
- Through pulmonary veins to left atrium
- Through mitral valve to left ventricle
- Through aortic valve to aorta
- To systemic circulation

Components of the cardiac conduction system

- SA node
- Intra-atrial tracts
- AV junction
- Bundle of His
- Right and left bundle branches
- Purkinje fibers

Key facts about electrical conduction

- Heart's muscle fibers generate and conduct electrical impulses
- Impulses follow a right-to-left, top-to-bottom path
- Initiated at the SA node
- Impulse moves through the conduction system to the ventricles

Normal cardiac conduction

Each electrical impulse travels from the sinoatrial node (1) through the intra-atrial tracts (2), producing atrial contraction. The impulse slows momentarily as it passes through the atrioventricular junction (3) to the bundle of His (4). It then descends the left and right bundle branches (5) and reaches the Purkinje fibers (6), stimulating ventricular contraction.

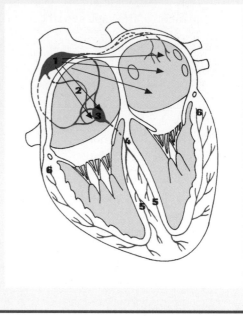

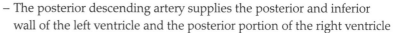

    – The posterior descending artery supplies the posterior and inferior wall of the left ventricle and the posterior portion of the right ventricle
- Coronary arteries receive blood primarily during ventricular relaxation (diastole)
- Blood is pumped out to systemic circulation during contraction of the ventricles (systole)

● Circulation

- Blood flows from the inferior and superior venae cavae to the right atrium
- Through the tricuspid valve to the right ventricle
- Through the pulmonic valve to the pulmonary artery, to the lungs where blood is oxygenated, through the pulmonary veins to the left atrium
- Through the mitral valve to the left ventricle
- Through the aortic valve to the aorta and systemic circulation

● Electrical conduction

- The heart contains specialized muscle fibers that generate and conduct their own electrical impulses spontaneously
- The sinoatrial (SA) node, internodal tracts, AV node, bundle of His, right and left bundle branches, and Purkinje fibers make up the system that conducts electrical impulses and coordinates chamber contraction (see *Normal cardiac conduction*)
- Impulses follow a right-to-left, top-to-bottom path
- A normal electrical impulse is initiated at the SA node, the heart's intrinsic pacemaker

- Once generated, the normal impulse must move forward through the conduction system to the ventricles
- Numerous events occur almost simultaneously in the following order after initiation of the impulse at the SA node
  - Atrial depolarization
  - Atrial contraction
  - Impulse transmission to the AV node
  - Impulse transmission to the bundle of His, bundle branches, and Purkinje fibers
  - Ventricular depolarization
  - Ventricular contraction
  - Ventricular repolarization

● **Cardiac function**
  - Cardiac output (CO) is the total amount of blood ejected per minute
  - Stroke volume (SV) is the amount of blood ejected with each beat
  - Cardiac output equals stroke volume times heart rate (HR) (CO = SV × HR)
  - Alterations in CO affect every body system
  - Ejection fraction is the percent of left ventricular end-diastolic volume ejected during systole (normally 60% to 70%)

● **Blood vessels**
  - Arteries are three-layered vessels (intima, media, adventitia) that carry oxygenated blood from the heart to the tissues
  - Arterioles are small-resistance vessels that feed into capillaries
  - Capillaries join arterioles to venules (larger, lower-pressured vessels than arterioles), where nutrients and wastes are exchanged
  - Venules join capillaries to veins
  - Veins are large-capacity, low-pressure vessels that return unoxygenated blood to the heart

PHYSICAL ASSESSMENT FINDINGS

● **History**
  - Dyspnea
  - Paroxysmal nocturnal dyspnea
  - Orthopnea
  - Chest pain or pain in jaw, shoulder, neck, back, or one or both arms (see *Patterns of cardiac pain*, page 6)
  - Fatigue and weakness
  - Cough
  - Syncope
  - Palpitations
  - Leg pain

● **Physical examination**
  - Blood pressure changes
  - Pulse changes including rate, rhythm, and quality

Key facts about cardiac function

- CO is the total amount of blood ejected per minute.
- SV is the amount of blood ejected with each beat.
- CO = SV × HR.

Key characteristics of blood vessels

Arteries
- Three-layered vessels
- Carry oxygenated blood from the heart to the tissues

Veins
- Large capacity, low-pressure vessels
- Return unoxygenated blood to the heart

Key signs and symptoms of cardiovascular disorders

- Dyspnea
- Chest pain
- Syncope
- Pulse and blood pressure changes
- Edema
- Arrhythmias

Patterns of cardiac pain

- Pericarditis: sudden onset of mild ache to severe pain, deep or superficial; "stabbing," "knife-like"; continuous pain lasting for several days; residual soreness
- Angina: gradual or sudden onset of mild-to-moderate pressure; deep sensation; varied pattern of attacks; "tightness," "squeezing," "crushing," "pressure"; pain usually lasts less than 15 minutes and not more than 30 minutes (average: 3 minutes)
- Myocardial infarction: sudden onset of persistent, severe pressure; deep sensation; "crushing," "squeezing," "heavy," "oppressive"; pain lasts 30 minutes to 2 hours; waxes and wanes; residual soreness 1 to 3 days

Patterns of cardiac pain

PERICARDITIS
Onset and duration
- Sudden onset; continuous pain lasting for days; residual soreness

Location and radiation
- Substernal pain to left of midline; radiation to back or subclavicular area

Quality and intensity
- Mild ache to severe pain, deep or superficial; "stabbing," "knifelike"

Signs and symptoms
- Precordial friction rub; increased pain with movement, inspiration, laughing, coughing; decreased pain with sitting or leaning forward (sitting up pulls the heart away from the diaphragm)

Precipitating factors
- Myocardial infarction or upper respiratory tract infection; invasive cardiac trauma

ANGINA
Onset and duration
- Gradual or sudden onset; pain usually lasts less than 15 minutes and not more than 30 minutes (average: 3 minutes)

Location and radiation
- Substernal or anterior chest pain, not sharply localized; radiation to back, neck, arms, jaws, upper abdomen, or fingers

Quality and intensity
- Mild-to-moderate pressure; deep sensation; varied pattern of attacks; "tightness," "squeezing," "crushing," "pressure"

Signs and symptoms
- Dyspnea; diaphoresis; nausea; urge to void; belching; apprehension

Precipitating factors
- Exertion; stress; eating; cold or hot and humid weather

MYOCARDIAL INFARCTION
Onset and duration
- Sudden onset; pain lasts 30 minutes to 2 hours; waxes and wanes; residual soreness 1 to 3 days

Location and radiation
- Substernal, midline, or anterior chest pain; radiation to jaws, neck, back, shoulders, or one or both arms

Quality and intensity
- Persistent, severe pressure; deep sensation; "crushing," "squeezing," "heavy," "oppressive"

Signs and symptoms
- Nausea; vomiting; apprehension; dyspnea; diaphoresis; increased or decreased blood pressure; gallop heart sound; "sensation of impending doom"

Precipitating factors
- Occurrence at rest or during physical exertion or emotional stress

- Clammy skin or diaphoresis
- Pallor
- Abnormal heart sounds
- Edema
- Arrhythmias
- Jugular vein distention
- Respiratory distress

- Vascular bruits
- Point of maximal impulse alterations
- Pruritus

DIAGNOSTIC TESTS AND PROCEDURES

- **Electrocardiography**
  - Definition and purpose
    - Noninvasive test of the heart
    - Graphical representation of the heart's electrical activity
  - Nursing interventions
    - Explain the procedure and its purpose
    - Determine the patient's ability to lie still
    - Reassure the patient that electrical shock won't occur
    - Interpret electrocardiogram (ECG) for changes, such as life-threatening arrhythmias

- **Ambulatory electrocardiography (Holter monitoring)**
  - Definition and purpose
    - Noninvasive test of the heart
    - Recording of the heart's electrical activity and cardiac events for 24 hours
  - Nursing interventions
    - Explain the procedure and its purpose
    - Instruct the patient to keep an activity and event diary
    - Advise the patient not to bathe, shower, operate machinery, or use a microwave oven or an electric shaver while wearing the monitor

- **Cardiac catheterization**
  - Definition and purpose
    - Fluoroscopic procedure using a radiopaque dye
    - Examination of the intracardiac structures, pressures, oxygenation, and cardiac output after the dye is injected
  - Nursing interventions before the procedure
    - Explain the procedure and its purpose
    - Withhold the patient's food and fluids after midnight
    - Take baseline vital signs and palpate peripheral pulses
    - Place obtained written informed consent in the patient's chart
    - Inform the patient about possible nausea, chest pain, flushing of the face, or throat irritation from the injection of radiopaque dye
    - Note the patient's allergies to seafood, iodine, or radiopaque dyes
    - Shave and scrub the insertion site, as ordered
    - Mark peripheral pulses with an "X"
    - Administer sedation, as prescribed
    - Remove all jewelry and prosthetic devices
    - Ensure patent I.V. access
  - Nursing interventions after the procedure

Key facts about electrocardiography

- Noninvasive test
- Graphical representation of the heart's electrical activity
- Intervention: interpret ECG for changes

Key facts about ambulatory electrocardiography

- Noninvasive test
- Records the heart's electrical activity and cardiac events for 24 hours
- Intervention: advise the patient on activity limitations while wearing monitor

Key facts about cardiac catheterization

- Invasive, fluoroscopic procedure
- Examines intracardiac structures, pressures, oxygenation, and cardiac output
- Intervention
- Note the patient's allergies before testing
- Monitor insertion site and pulses after the procedure

Key facts about coronary arteriography

- Invasive, fluoroscopic procedure
- Examines the coronary artery
- Intervention
- Note the patient's allergies before the test and monitor his vital signs
- Monitor insertion site and pulses after the procedure

– Monitor vital signs, peripheral pulses, and the insertion site for bleeding
– Maintain a pressure dressing and bed rest for 4 to 8 hours, or as ordered
– Increase fluid intake unless contraindicated
– Allay the patient's anxiety
– **Monitor for complaints of chest pain, a possible sign of myocardial infarction (MI)—a serious complication of cardiac catheterization—and report immediately**
– Keep affected leg extended
– Assess peripheral pulses in both legs and compare to baseline
– Monitor urinary output
– Monitor for delayed reaction to radiopaque dye

● **Coronary arteriography**
- Definition and purpose
  – Fluoroscopic procedure using a radiopaque dye
  – Examination of the coronary arteries
- Nursing interventions before the procedure
  – Explain the procedure and its purpose
  – Place obtained written informed consent in the patient's chart
  – **Note the patient's allergies to iodine, seafood, or radiopaque dyes**
  – Monitor the patient's vital signs
  – Allay the patient's anxiety
  – Inform the patient about possible flushing of the face or throat irritation from the injection
- Nursing interventions after the procedure
  – Check the insertion site for bleeding
  – Assess peripheral pulses
  – Maintain a pressure dressing and bed rest

● **Digital subtraction angiography**
- Definition and purpose
  – Invasive procedure using a computer system and fluoroscopy with an image intensifier
  – Complete visualization of the arterial blood supply to a specific area, especially the carotid and cerebral arteries
- Nursing interventions before the procedure
  – Explain the procedure and its purpose
  – Place obtained written informed consent in the patient's chart
  – Monitor the patient's vital signs
  – Remove all jewelry in the area to be imaged
  – Perform a baseline neurologic examination before cerebral angiography
  – Administer sedation, as ordered
- Nursing interventions after the procedure
  – Check the insertion site for bleeding

Key facts about digital subtraction angiography

- Invasive, fluoroscopic procedure
- Allows for complete visualization of the arterial blood supply to a specific area (especially the carotid and cerebral arteries)
- Intervention
- Perform a baseline neurologic examination before cerebral angiography
- Monitor the insertion site after the procedure

– Instruct the patient to drink at least 1 qt (1 L) of fluid

– Monitor for delayed reaction to radiopaque dye

Echocardiography

- Definition and purpose
  – Noninvasive examination of the heart
  – Uses echoes from sound waves to visualize intracardiac structures and direction of blood flow
- Nursing interventions
  – Explain the procedure and its purpose
  – Determine the patient's ability to lie still

Exercise testing (stress)

- Definition and purpose
  – Noninvasive test of the heart
  – Study of the heart's electrical activity and ischemic events during prescribed levels of exercise
- Nursing interventions
  – Explain the procedure and its purpose
  – Withhold food and fluids, especially those that contain caffeine, for 1 hour before the test
  – Instruct the patient to wear loose-fitting clothing and supportive shoes

Nuclear cardiology

- Definition and purpose
  – Visual examination of the heart using radioisotopes
  – Imaging of myocardial perfusion and contractility after I.V. injection of isotopes
- Nursing interventions
  – Explain the procedure and its purpose
  – Allay the patient's anxiety
  – Determine the patient's ability to lie still during the procedure

Hemodynamic monitoring (single procedure or continuous monitoring)

- Definition and purpose
  – Invasive procedure placing a balloon-tipped, flow-directed catheter in the pulmonary artery
  – Examination of intracardiac pressures and cardiac output
- Nursing interventions before the procedure
  – Explain the procedure and its purpose
  – Place obtained written informed consent in the patient's chart
- Nursing interventions after the procedure
  – Check the insertion site for signs of infection
  – Monitor the pressure tracings and record readings (see *Putting hemodynamic monitoring to use,* page 10)

Chest X-ray

- Definition and purpose
  – Noninvasive examination of the heart and lungs

Key facts about echocardiography

- Noninvasive test
- Visualizes intracardiac structures and direction of blood flow
- Intervention: determine the patient's ability to lie still

Key facts about exercise testing

- Noninvasive test
- Study of the heart's electrical activity and ischemic events during prescribed levels of exercise
- Intervention: withhold food and fluids for 1 hour before the test

Key facts about nuclear cardiology

- Noninvasive test
- Allows for visual examination of the heart
- Intervention: determine the patient's ability to lie still

Key facts about hemodynamic monitoring

- Invasive procedure involving catheter placed in pulmonary artery
- Allows for examination of intracardiac pressures and cardiac output
- Intervention: monitor the pressure tracings and record readings

Key facts about chest X-ray

- Noninvasive test
- Provides radiographic picture of the heart and lungs
- Intervention: ensure that the patient removes jewelry before test

Normal values in hemodynamic monitoring

- RAP or CVP — 1 to 6 mm Hg (1.34 to 8 cm H_2O)
- RVP — systolic: 15 to 25 mm Hg; diastolic: 0 to 8 mm Hg
- PAP — systolic: 15 to 25 mm Hg; diastolic: 8 to 15 mm Hg; mean: 10 to 20 mm Hg
- PAWP — mean pressure: 6 to 12 mm Hg
- LAP — 6 to 12 mm Hg
- CO — 4 to 8 L

What hemodynamic monitoring measures

- RAP or CVP
- RVP
- PAP
- PAWP
- LAP
- CO

Putting hemodynamic monitoring to use

Hemodynamic monitoring provides information on intracardiac pressures and cardiac output. To understand intracardiac pressures, picture the cardiovascular system as a continuous loop with constantly changing pressure gradients that keep the blood moving.

RIGHT ATRIAL PRESSURE (RAP), OR CENTRAL VENOUS PRESSURE (CVP)

The RAP reflects right atrial, or right heart, function and end-diastolic pressure.

- **Normal:** 1 to 6 mm Hg (1.34 to 8 cm H_2O). (To convert mm Hg to cm H_2O, multiply mm Hg by 1.34)
- **Elevated value suggests:** right-sided heart failure, volume overload, tricuspid valve stenosis or insufficiency, constrictive pericarditis, pulmonary hypertension, cardiac tamponade, or right ventricular infarction.
- **Low value suggests:** reduced circulating blood volume.

RIGHT VENTRICULAR PRESSURE (RVP)

Right ventricular (RV) systolic pressure normally equals pulmonary artery systolic pressure; RV end-diastolic pressure, which equals RAP, reflects RV function.

- **Normal:** systolic, 15 to 25 mm Hg; diastolic, 0 to 8 mm Hg.
- **Elevated value suggests:** mitral stenosis or insufficiency; pulmonary disease; hypoxemia; constrictive pericarditis; chronic heart failure; atrial and ventricular septal defects; and patent ductus arteriosus.

PULMONARY ARTERY PRESSURE (PAP)

Pulmonary artery systolic pressure reflects right ventricular function and pulmonary circulation pressures. Pulmonary artery diastolic pressure reflects left ventricular pressures, specifically left ventricular end-diastolic pressure.

- **Normal:** Systolic, 15 to 25 mm Hg; diastolic, 8 to 15 mm Hg; mean, 10 to 20 mm Hg.

- **Elevated value suggests:** left-sided heart failure, increased pulmonary blood flow (left or right shunting, as in atrial or ventricular septal defects), and any condition causing increased pulmonary arteriolar resistance.

PULMONARY ARTERY WEDGE PRESSURE (PAWP)

PAWP reflects left atrial and left ventricular pressures unless the patient has mitral stenosis. Changes in PAWP reflect changes in left ventricular filling pressure. The heart momentarily relaxes during diastole as it fills with blood from the pulmonary veins; this permits the pulmonary vasculature, left atrium, and left ventricle to act as a single chamber.

- **Normal:** mean pressure, 6 to 12 mm Hg.
- **Elevated value suggests:** left-sided heart failure, mitral stenosis or insufficiency, pericardial tamponade, fluid overload.
- **Low value suggests:** hypovolemia.

LEFT ATRIAL PRESSURE (LAP)

This value reflects left ventricular end-diastolic pressure in patients without mitral valve disease.

- **Normal:** 6 to 12 mm Hg.

CARDIAC OUTPUT (CO)

Cardiac output is the amount of blood ejected by the heart each minute.

- **Normal:** 4 to 8 L; varies with a patient's weight, height, and body surface area. Adjusting the cardiac output to the patient's size yields a measurement called the *cardiac index*.

- Radiographic picture of the heart and lungs
- Nursing interventions
  - Explain the procedure and its purpose
  - Determine the patient's ability to hold his breath
  - Ensure that the patient removes jewelry

Blood chemistries

- Definition and purpose
  - Laboratory test of a blood sample
  - Analysis for sodium, potassium, magnesium, calcium, glucose, phosphorus, cholesterol, triglycerides, uric acid, bicarbonate, creatine, blood urea nitrogen (BUN), bilirubin, creatine kinase (CK), CK isoenzymes, lactate dehydrogenase (LD), LD isoenzymes, troponin I, troponin T, aspartate aminotransferase (AST), and alanine aminotransferase
- Nursing interventions
  - Explain the procedure and its purpose
  - Note any drugs that may alter test results
  - Restrict the patient's exercise before the blood sample is drawn
  - Withhold I.M. injections or note the time of the injection on the laboratory slip (alter CK levels)
  - Withhold food and fluids, as ordered
  - Assess the venipuncture site for bleeding after the procedure

Hematologic studies

- Definition and purpose
  - Laboratory test of a blood sample
  - Analysis for red blood cells (RBCs), white blood cells (WBCs), erythrocyte sedimentation rate (ESR), prothrombin time (PT), partial thromboplastin time (PTT), platelets, hemoglobin (Hb), and hematocrit (HCT)
- Nursing interventions
  - Explain the procedure and its purpose
  - Note any drugs that might alter test results before the procedure
  - Assess the venipuncture site for bleeding after the procedure

Arterial blood gas (ABG) analysis

- Definition and purpose
  - Test of arterial blood
  - Assessment of tissue oxygenation, ventilation, and acid-base status
- Nursing interventions before the procedure
  - Explain the procedure and its purpose
  - Document the patient's temperature
  - Note supplemental oxygen or mechanical ventilation the patient is receiving
  - Perform Allen's test prior to performing a radial puncture
  - Avoid using a limb with an arteriovenous shunt, or on affected side following mastectomy

- Nursing interventions after the procedure
  - Maintain pressure to the site for at least 5 minutes, or longer if bleeding continues
  - Check the site for bleeding
  - Check peripheral pulses in the affected limb

● **Doppler ultrasound**
- Definition and purpose
  - Noninvasive procedure that transforms echoes from sound waves into audible sounds
  - Examination of blood flow in peripheral circulation
- Nursing interventions
  - Explain the procedure and its purpose
  - Determine the patient's ability to lie still

● **Venography**
- Definition and purpose
  - Visualization of the veins after I.V. injection of a dye
  - Diagnosis of deep vein thrombosis or incompetent valves
- Nursing interventions before the procedure
  - Explain the procedure and its purpose
  - Withhold food and fluids after midnight
  - Record the patient's baseline vital signs and peripheral pulses
  - Place obtained written informed consent in the patient's chart
  - Note the patient's allergies to seafood, iodine, or radiopaque dyes
  - Inform the patient about possible flushing of the face or throat irritation from the injection
  - Ensure the patient is adequately hydrated
- Nursing interventions after the procedure
  - Check the injection site for bleeding and hematoma
  - Force fluids unless contraindicated
  - Evaluate for signs of delayed reaction to radiopaque dye
  - Assess vital signs and compare to baseline

● **Pulse oximetry**
- Definition and purpose
  - Noninvasive procedure using infrared light to measure arterial oxygen saturation in the blood
  - Continuous measurement of oxygen saturation assists in pulmonary assessment of patient and weaning patient from a ventilator
- Nursing interventions
  - Explain the procedure and its purpose
  - Avoid placing the sensor on an extremity that has impeded blood flow
  - Protect the sensor from bright light
  - Attach the monitoring sensor to a fingertip, ear lobe, or toe
  - Consider using the earlobe if the patient has artificial nails, nail tips, or nail polish, as these may interfere with light transmission

(some sensors can accurately read through these as long as polish is removed, but this isn't recommended)

PSYCHOSOCIAL IMPACT OF CARDIOVASCULAR DISORDERS

● **Developmental impact**
- Fear of rejection
- Lowered self-esteem
- Fear of dying
- Role conflict

● **Economic impact**
- Disruption or loss of employment
- Cost of hospitalization, medications, and special diets

● **Occupational and recreational impact**
- Restrictions in work activity
- Changes in leisure activity
- Restrictions in physical activity (walking, climbing stairs)
- Restrictions in activity related to environmental temperature; for example, hot or cold weather may interfere with the patient's ability to take walks or go outside

● **Social impact**
- Changes in dietary habits such as dining out
- Changes in sexual function and habits
- Changes in role performance, including work and family roles
- Social isolation

RISK FACTORS

● **Modifiable risk factors**
- Smoking
- Diet
- Hypertension
- Hypercholesterolemia
- Obesity
- Physical inactivity
- Emotional stress

● **Nonmodifiable risk factors**
- Gender
- Family history of cardiovascular illness
- Personal history of cardiovascular illness
- Ethnicity
- Race
- Age

Key psychosocial impact of a cardiovascular disorder
- Fear of dying
- Financial issues related to loss of wages and medical costs
- Restrictions in activity
- Changes in role performance

Modifiable risk factors
- Smoking
- Diet
- Hypertension
- Hypercholesterolemia
- Obesity
- Physical inactivity
- Emotional stress

Nonmodifiable risk factors
- Gender
- Family history of cardiovascular illness
- Personal history of cardiovascular illness
- Ethnicity
- Race
- Age

Key cardiovascular nursing diagnoses

- Decreased cardiac output
- Chronic pain
- Ineffective tissue perfusion: Cardiopulmonary
- Ineffective tissue perfusion: Peripheral
- Ineffective tissue perfusion: Cerebral
- Risk for peripheral neurovascular dysfunction

NURSING DIAGNOSES

● Probable nursing diagnoses
- Decreased cardiac output
- Acute pain
- Chronic pain
- Ineffective tissue perfusion: Cardiopulmonary
- Impaired gas exchange
- Anxiety
- Fear
- Ineffective tissue perfusion: Peripheral
- Ineffective tissue perfusion: Cerebral
- Risk for peripheral neurovascular dysfunction

● Possible nursing diagnoses
- Excess fluid volume
- Activity intolerance
- Ineffective coping
- Disabled family coping
- Situational low self-esteem
- Ineffective role performance
- Disturbed body image
- Sexual dysfunction
- Noncompliance
- Chronic low self-esteem
- Risk for situational low self-esteem
- Fatigue

CARDIAC SURGERY

● Description
- Coronary artery bypass graft (CABG)—surgical revascularization of the coronary arteries using the saphenous veins or the internal mammary artery to bypass an obstruction caused by atherosclerosis
- Valve replacement—surgical replacement of stenotic or incompetent valves with a mechanical or bioprosthetic valve, such as Starr-Edwards "ball-in-cage" valves, porcine valves, or Bjork-Shiley "tilting disk" valves
- Valvular annuloplasty—surgical repair or reconstruction of the leaflets and annulus of the valve
- Mitral valve commissurotomy—surgical opening of the fused portion of the mitral valve leaflets, using a dilator
- Valvuloplasty—surgical repair or reconstruction of the valve
- Percutaneous transluminal valvuloplasty—dilation of calcified and stenotic valvular leaflets, using a balloon catheter
- Percutaneous transluminal coronary angioplasty (PTCA)—dilation of a coronary artery using a balloon-tipped catheter to compress plaque against the vessel wall (see *Relieving occlusions with angioplasty*)

Key cardiac surgery options

- CABG
- Valve replacement
- Valvular annuloplasty
- Mitral valve commissurotomy
- Percutaneous transluminal coronary angioplasty
- PTCA

Relieving occlusions with angioplasty

Percutaneous transluminal coronary angioplasty can open an occluded coronary artery without opening the chest—an important advantage over bypass surgery. Initially, coronary angiography must confirm the presence and location of the arterial occlusion. Next, the cardiologist threads a guide catheter through the patient's femoral artery into the coronary artery under fluoroscopic guidance, as shown at right.

When angiography shows the guide catheter positioned at the occlusion site, the cardiologist carefully inserts a smaller double-lumen balloon catheter through the guide catheter and directs the balloon through the occlusion (lower left).

A marked pressure gradient will be obvious.

The cardiologist alternately inflates and deflates the balloon until an angiogram verifies successful arterial dilation (lower right) and the pressure gradient has decreased.

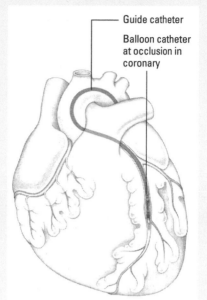

Guide catheter

Balloon catheter at occlusion in coronary

Key facts about angioplasty

- Invasive procedure to open an occluded artery without surgery
- Performed under fluoroscopy by a cardiologist
- A balloon catheter is guided through the occlusion
- The balloon is inflated to flatten plaque and dilate the artery's diameter

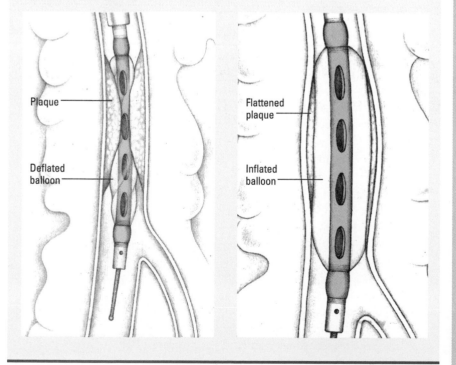

Plaque

Deflated balloon

Flattened plaque

Inflated balloon

Key interventions before cardiac surgery

- Demonstrate postoperative turning, coughing, and deep breathing; splinting; and ROM exercises.
- Explain the postoperative need for drainage tubes, surgical dressings, oxygen therapy, I.V. therapy, and pain control.

Key monitoring parameters after surgery

- Cardiac, respiratory, and neurologic status
- Vital signs
- Pain level
- I/O
- Laboratory studies
- Cardiac rhythm and ECG
- Hemodynamic variables
- Daily weight
- Pulse oximetry
- Water-seal chest drainage system for chest tubes
- I.V. fluids and medication infusions
- Position and patency of drainage tubes and catheters

● **Preoperative nursing interventions**
- Complete patient and family preoperative teaching
  - Explain the procedure and its purpose
  - Describe the operating room, postanesthesia care unit (PACU), and preoperative and postoperative routines
  - Demonstrate postoperative turning, coughing, deep breathing, splinting; incentive spirometry, and range-of-motion (ROM) exercises
  - Explain the postoperative need for drainage tubes, surgical dressings, oxygen therapy, I.V. therapy, and pain control
- Answer all questions to allay the patient's and family's anxiety about surgery
- Document the patient's history and physical assessment database
- Obtain baseline hemodynamic variables, ECG readings, and ABG studies
- Complete a preoperative checklist
- Administer preoperative medications

● **Postoperative nursing interventions**
- Monitor cardiac, respiratory, and neurologic status
- Assess pain level, administer analgesics as prescribed, and evaluate effects
- Administer oxygen by endotracheal (ET) tube, nasal canulla, or mask, as indicated
- Monitor vital signs, intake and output (I/O), laboratory studies, cardiac rhythm and ECG, hemodynamic variables, daily weight, and pulse oximetry
- Monitor and maintain the water-seal chest drainage system for mediastinal and pleural chest tubes
- Monitor and maintain the position and patency of drainage tubes and catheters, such as a nasogastric (NG) tube, indwelling urinary catheter, and wound drainage and chest tubes
- Administer I.V. fluids, medication infusions, and transfusion therapy, as prescribed
- Inspect and change the surgical dressing, as ordered
- Provide incentive spirometry after extubation
- Reinforce turning, coughing, and deep breathing, and splinting of the incision
- Administer antiarrhythmics, anticoagulants, vasopressors, beta-adrenergic blockers, diuretics, or cardiac glycosides, as prescribed
- Observe the cardiac monitor for arrhythmias
- Check peripheral circulation: color, temperature, pulses, and complaints of abnormal sensations, such as numbness or tingling
- Insulate epicardial pacing wires; have temporary pacemaker available
- Administer antibiotics, as prescribed
- Assess for return of peristalsis
- Provide the prescribed diet, as tolerated
- Assist the patient with active and passive ROM and isometric exercises, as tolerated
- Allay the patient's anxiety

- Encourage the patient to express feelings about changes in body image or a fear of dying
- Provide information about support groups such as Mended Hearts
- Individualize home care instructions
  - Avoid driving and heavy lifting for 6 weeks
  - Complete incision care daily
  - Elevate the leg with the saphenous graft when seated
  - Wear antiembolism stockings
  - Follow a low-sodium, low-fat diet
  - Comply with medical follow-up

● **Possible surgical complications**
  - Bleeding from the mediastinal tube
  - MI
  - Decreased cardiac output
  - Cardiac arrhythmias
  - Cardiac tamponade
  - Heart block
  - Embolism
  - Valve malfunction
  - Respiratory failure

PACEMAKER THERAPY

● **Description**
  - Electronic device that stimulates the heart to contract when the intrinsic pacemaker or conduction system fails
  - May be temporary or permanent, based on emergent need or underlying cause

● **Types of pacemakers**
  - Demand (synchronous, noncompetitive)—pacemaker fires when inherent heart rate falls below predetermined set rate
  - Fixed rate (asynchronous, competitive)—pacemaker fires at a constant, preset rate
  - Temporary—pulse generator is attached to pacemaker wires that are inserted temporarily
    - Transvenous
    - Epicardial
    - Transcutaneous
  - Permanent—pulse generator implanted in subcutaneous tissue in right or left pectoral area or abdomen

● **Pacemaker components**
  - Pulse generator—power source of pacemaker, which is controlled electronically
    - Plutonium—lasts 20+ years
    - Lithium—lasts 10 years

– Mercury-zinc—lasts 3 to 4 years
- Lead—insulated wire implanted in the heart and connected to pulse generator to transmit electrical impulses from the pulse generator to the heart
- Controls
  – Sensitivity
  – Rate
  – Output

● **Classification system—International Pacemaker Code** (see *Pacemaker codes*)

● **Preoperative nursing interventions**
- Complete patient and family preoperative teaching
  – Explain the procedure and its purpose
  – Describe the operating room, PACU, and preoperative and postoperative routines
  – Demonstrate postoperative turning, coughing, deep breathing, splinting, and ROM exercises
  – Explain the postoperative procedure for surgical dressings, oxygen therapy, I.V. therapy, activity restrictions, and pain control
- Complete a preoperative checklist
- Administer preoperative medications, as prescribed
- Answer all questions to allay the patient's and family's anxiety about surgery
- Document the patient's history and physical assessment database
- Obtain a baseline assessment of heart rhythm and rate and peripheral circulation
- Administer antibiotics, as prescribed

● **Postoperative nursing interventions**
- Assess cardiac status: heart sounds, rhythm
- Assess pain level, administer analgesics as prescribed, and evaluate effects
- Monitor vital signs, I/O, neurovascular checks, and pulse oximetry
- Obtain a 12-lead ECG as ordered
- Protect control settings if temporary pacer
- Change dressing as ordered
- Monitor insertion site for signs of infection
- Immobilize upper extremity, as ordered
- Individualize home care instructions
  – **Recognize signs of pacemaker malfunction**
  – Carry a pacemaker identification card at all times
  – Perform active ROM to upper extremity on side of insertion
  – Check pulse daily
  – Avoid physical contact sports
  – Recognize signs of electrical interference
  – Comply with pacemaker checks and follow-up care per cardiologist's orders
  – Know the rate and battery life of the pacemaker

Key steps before pacemaker insertion
- Obtain a baseline of heart rhythm and rate and peripheral circulation.
- Complete patient and family preoperative teaching.

Key steps after pacemaker insertion
- Obtain a 12-lead ECG as ordered.
- Protect control settings if temporary pacer.
- Monitor vital signs and cardiac rhythm.

Key home care instructions after pacemaker insertion
- Recognize signs of pacemaker malfunction.
- Carry a pacemaker identification card at all times.
- Check pulse daily.

Pacemaker codes

CHAMBER PACED	CHAMBER SENSED	RESPONSE TO SENSING	PROGRAMMABLE FUNCTIONS AND RATE MODULATION	ANTITACHY-ARRHYTHMIA FUNCTIONS
V (ventricle)	V (ventricle)	T (triggers pacing)	P (programmable rate, output, or both)	P (pacing)
A (atrium)	A (atrium)	I (inhibits pacing)	M (multiprogrammable rate, output, sensitivity)	S (shock)
D (dual, A + V)	D (dual, A + V)	D (dual, T + I)	C (communicating functions, such as telemetry)	D (dual, P + S)
O (none)	O (none)	O (none)	R (rate modulation) O (none)	O (none)

– Understand that firing of implantable-cardioverter-defibrillator, if inserted, needs immediate follow-up

● **Possible surgical complications**
  • Pneumothorax
  • Perforation of heart
  • Infection
  • Breakage of a lead
  • Migration of a lead

ABDOMINAL ANEURYSM RESECTION

● **Description**
  • Surgical removal of a portion of weakened arterial wall with an end-to-end anastomosis using a prosthetic graft

● **Preoperative nursing interventions**
  • Complete patient and family preoperative teaching
    – Explain the procedure and its purpose
    – Describe the operating room, PACU, and preoperative and postoperative routines
    – Demonstrate postoperative turning, coughing, deep breathing, splinting, incentive spirometry, and ROM exercises
    – Explain the postoperative need for drainage tubes, surgical dressings, oxygen therapy, I.V. therapy, and pain control
  • Complete a preoperative checklist
  • Administer preoperative medications, as prescribed
  • Answer all questions to allay the patient's and family's anxiety about surgery

- Document the patient's history and physical assessment database
- Assess renal status and I/O

● **Postoperative nursing interventions**
- Monitor cardiac, respiratory, neurologic, and renal status
- Assess fluid balance
- Assess pain level, administer analgesics as prescribed, and evaluate effects
- Administer I.V. fluids, medication infusions, and transfusion therapy, as prescribed
- Administer oxygen and maintain an ET tube to the ventilator
- Encourage incentive spirometry after extubation
- Reinforce turning, coughing, and deep breathing, and splinting of the incision
- Monitor vital signs, I/O, laboratory studies, cardiac rhythm and ECG, hemodynamic variables, and pulse oximetry
- Monitor and maintain the position and patency of NG tubes and indwelling urinary catheters
- Administer antibiotics, as prescribed
- Assess for scrotal and retroperitoneal bleeding
- Check peripheral circulation: color, temperature, complaints of abnormal sensation, and pulses in extremities
- Inspect and change the surgical dressing, as directed
- Reposition every 2 hours
- Assist the patient with active and passive ROM and isometric exercises, as tolerated
- Assess for return of peristalsis
- Provide the prescribed diet, as tolerated
- **Measure and record the patient's abdominal girth**
- Provide emotional support to allay the patient's anxiety
- Individualize home care instructions
    - Avoid lifting, bending, and driving for 6 weeks or as the surgeon allows
    - Monitor blood pressure daily
    - Identify ways to reduce stress
    - Complete incision care daily; note signs and symptoms of infection
    - Comply with medical follow-up

● **Possible surgical complications**
- Renal failure
- Graft hemorrhage
- Retroperitoneal rupture
- Infection

VASCULAR GRAFTING

● **Description**
- Surgical revascularization of an artery
- Uses a synthetic or autogenous graft
- Bypasses or resects the diseased segment

Key monitoring parameters after abdominal aneurysm resection

- Cardiac, respiratory, renal, and neurologic status
- Vital signs
- I/O
- Laboratory studies
- ECG
- Hemodynamic variables
- Pulse oximetry
- Abdominal girth

Key complications after abdominal aneurysm repair

- Renal failure
- Retroperitoneal rupture
- Infection

Key facts about vascular grafting

- Surgical revascularization of an artery
- Uses a graft
- Bypasses or resects the diseased segment
- Types include femoropopliteal, aortofemoral, aortoiliac, femorofemoral, and axillofemoral

● **Types of revascularization**
- Femoropopliteal
- Aortofemoral
- Aortoiliac
- Femorofemoral
- Axillofemoral

● **Preoperative nursing interventions**
- Complete patient and family preoperative teaching
  - Explain the procedure and its purpose
  - Describe the operating room, PACU, and preoperative and postoperative routines
  - Demonstrate postoperative turning, coughing, deep breathing, splinting, incentive spirometry, and ROM exercises
  - Explain the postoperative need for drainage tubes, surgical dressings, oxygen therapy, I.V. therapy, and pain control
- Complete a preoperative checklist
- Administer preoperative medications, as prescribed
- Answer any questions to allay the patient's and family's anxiety about surgery
- Document the patient's history and physical assessment database
- Obtain a baseline assessment of peripheral circulation; mark pulses in affected area
- Administer antibiotics, as prescribed

● **Postoperative nursing interventions**
- Monitor cardiac and neurovascular status
- Assess pain level, administer analgesics as prescribed, and evaluate effects
- Administer I.V. fluids and transfusion therapy, as prescribed
- Monitor vital signs, I/O, laboratory studies, neurovascular checks, and pulse oximetry
- Monitor and maintain the position and patency of NG tubes and indwelling urinary catheters
- Administer anticoagulants, as prescribed, and monitor coagulation studies
- Inspect and change the surgical dressing, as directed
- **Keep the patient in semi-Fowler's position; avoid positioning on or flexion of the graft site**
- Provide a bed cradle
- Monitor peripheral circulation: temperature, color, pulses, and complaints of abnormal sensations in extremities distal to the graft site
- Measure and record the patient's ankle, calf, and thigh circumferences
- Reinforce turning, coughing, and deep breathing and splinting of the incision, and encourage incentive spirometry
- Assess for return of peristalsis
- Provide the prescribed diet, as tolerated
- Assist the patient with active and passive ROM and isometric exercises, as tolerated
- Provide emotional support to allay the patient's anxiety

Key complications after vascular grafting

- Thrombosis
- Embolism
- Hemorrhage

Key facts about hypertension

- Normal: SBP less than 120 mm Hg/DBP less than 80 mm Hg
- Prehypertension: SBP 120 to 139 mm Hg or DBP 80 to 89 mm Hg
- Stage 1: SBP 140 to 159 mm Hg or DBP 90 to 99 mm Hg
- Stage 2: SBP greater than or equal to 160 mm Hg or DBP greater than or equal to 100 mm Hg

Common causes of hypertension

- Primary—unknown
- Secondary—results from another disorder

How hypertension happens

- Narrowing of the arterioles
- Increased force needed to circulate blood

- Encourage the patient to express feelings about changes in body image
- Increase ambulation, as tolerated
- Individualize home care instructions
    - Avoid pressure or flexion of the graft site
    - Avoid wearing constrictive clothing
    - Complete incision care daily
    - Check pulses distal to the graft site daily
    - Adhere to long-term anticoagulant therapy
    - Provide proper foot care daily
    - Comply with medical follow-up

● **Possible surgical complications**
  - Thrombosis
  - Embolism
  - Graft rejection
  - Hemorrhage
  - Infection

HYPERTENSION

● **Definition**
  - High blood pressure
  - Classifications
    - Normal: less than 120 mm Hg/less than 80 mm Hg
    - Prehypertension: systolic blood pressure (SBP) 120 to 139 mm Hg or diastolic blood pressure (DBP) 80 to 89 mm Hg
    - Stage 1: SBP 140 to 159 mm Hg or DBP 90 to 99 mm Hg
    - Stage 2: SBP greater than or equal to 160 mm Hg or DBP greater than or equal to 100 mm Hg

● **Causes**
  - Primary hypertension—unknown etiology
  - Secondary hypertension—results from another disorder
    - Renal disease
    - Pheochromocytoma
    - Cushing's disease
    - Diabetes mellitus
    - Coronary artery disease

● **Pathophysiology**
  - Blood pressure = Cardiac output $\times$ peripheral resistance
  - Narrowing of the arterioles, which increases peripheral resistance
  - Increased force needed to circulate blood, which elevates blood pressure (see *Understanding blood pressure regulation*)

● **Assessment findings**
  - Asymptomatic
  - Elevated blood pressure reading
  - Headache
  - Vision disturbances

Understanding blood pressure regulation

Hypertension may result from a disturbance in one of these intrinsic mechanisms.

RENIN-ANGIOTENSIN SYSTEM

The renin-angiotensin system acts to increase blood pressure through these mechanisms:

- sodium depletion, reduced blood pressure, and dehydration stimulate renin release
- renin reacts with angiotensin, a liver enzyme, and converts it to angiotensin I, which increases preload and afterload
- angiotensin I converts to angiotensin II in the lungs; angiotensin II is a potent vasoconstrictor that targets the arterioles
- circulating angiotensin II works to increase preload and afterload by stimulating the adrenal cortex to secrete aldosterone; this increases blood volume by conserving sodium and water.

AUTOREGULATION

Several intrinsic mechanisms work to change an artery's diameter to maintain tissue and organ perfusion despite fluctuations in systemic blood pressure. These mechanisms include stress relaxation and capillary fluid shifts.

- In stress relaxation, blood vessels gradually dilate when blood pressure rises to reduce peripheral resistance.
- In capillary fluid shift, plasma moves between vessels and extravascular spaces to maintain intravascular volume.

SYMPATHETIC NERVOUS SYSTEM

When blood pressure drops, baroreceptors in the aortic arch and carotid sinuses decrease their inhibition of the medulla's vasomotor center. The consequent increases in sympathetic stimulation of the heart by norepinephrine increases cardiac output by strengthening the contractile force, raising the heart rate, and augmenting peripheral resistance by vasoconstriction. Stress can also stimulate the sympathetic nervous system to increase cardiac output and peripheral vascular resistance.

ANTIDIURETIC HORMONE

The release of antidiuretic hormone can regulate hypotension by increasing reabsorption of water by the kidney. With reabsorption, blood plasma volume increases, thus raising blood pressure.

Intrinsic blood pressure regulators

- Renin-angiotensin system
- Autoregulation
- Sympathetic nervous system
- Antidiuretic hormone

Key signs and symptoms of hypertension

- Asymptomatic
- Elevated blood pressure reading
- Dizziness
- Headache
- Vision disturbances

- Left ventricular hypertrophy
- Renal failure
- Dizziness
- Papilledema
- Heart failure
- Cerebral ischemia

● **Diagnostic test findings**

- Blood pressure: sustained readings greater than 140/90 mm Hg
- ECG: left ventricular hypertrophy
- Chest X-ray: cardiomegaly
- Ophthalmoscopic examination: retinal changes, such as severe vasoconstriction, papilledema, and retinopathy

Diagnosing hypertension

- Sustained blood pressure readings greater than 140/90 mm Hg

Treating hypertension

- Low-sodium, low-calorie, low-cholesterol, low-fat diet
- Increased activity
- Smoking cessation
- Medications
- – Diuretics
- – Antihypertensives
- – Vasodilators
- – Calcium channel blockers
- – Beta-adrenergic blockers
- – ACE inhibitors
- – ARBs

Key nursing interventions for a patient with hypertension

- Assess cardiovascular status.
- Monitor and record vital signs, I/O, laboratory studies, and daily weight.
- Take an average of two or more blood pressure readings rather than relying on one single abnormal reading.
- Administer medications, as prescribed, and evaluate effects.

Key complications of hypertension

- CAD
- Stroke
- Renal failure
- Hypertensive crisis

● Medical management

- Diet: low-sodium, low-calorie, low-cholesterol, and low-fat; restrict alcohol and caffeine
- Weight reduction
- Activity: as tolerated
- Smoking cessation
- Monitoring: vital signs, ECG, and I/O
- Laboratory studies: sodium, potassium, and cholesterol
- Thiazide diuretics: chlorothiazide (Diuril), hydrochlorothiazide (HydroDIURIL)
- Loop diuretics: furosemide (Lasix), bumetanide (Bumex)
- Potassium-sparing diuretic: spironolactone (Aldactone)
- Antihypertensives: methyldopa (Aldomet), hydralazine (Apresoline), prazosin (Minipress), doxazosin (Cardura)
- Calcium channel blockers: amlodipine (Norvasc), nifedipine (Procardia), verapamil (Calan), diltiazem (Cardizem), nicardipine (Cardene)
- Beta-adrenergic blockers: propranolol (Inderal), metoprolol (Lopressor), carteolol (Cartrol), labetolol (Normodyne)
- Angiotensin-converting enzyme (ACE) inhibitors: captopril (Capoten), enalapril (Vasotec), lisinopril (Prinivil)
- Angiotensin II receptor blockers (ARBs): candesartan (Atacand), irbesartan (Avapro), losartan (Cozaar), valsartan (Diovan)
- Vasodilator: nitroprusside (Nipride), used for hypertensive crisis

● Nursing interventions

- Assess cardiovascular status
- Monitor and record vital signs, I/O, laboratory studies, and daily weight
- Administer medications, as prescribed, and evaluate effects
- Maintain the patient's prescribed diet
- Encourage the patient to express feelings about daily stress
- Maintain a quiet environment
- Provide information about the American Heart Association
- Take an average of two or more blood pressure readings rather than relying on one single abnormal reading
- Individualize home care instructions (for more information about teaching, see *Patients with cardiovascular disorders*)
  - – Take blood pressure daily
  - – Modify diet and lose weight, if indicated
  - – Start an exercise program
  - – Follow instructions for medication use
  - – Comply with medical follow-up
- Provide information about the disorder and its implications

● Complications

- Coronary artery disease (CAD)
- Transient ischemic attack (TIA)
- MI
- Stroke

![icon] **TIME-OUT FOR TEACHING**

Patients with cardiovascular disorders

Be sure to include these topics when teaching patients with cardiovascular disorders.

- Smoking cessation
- Regular exercise
- Optimal weight maintenance
- Medication therapy, including the action, adverse effects, and scheduling
- Dietary recommendations and restrictions
- Managing blood glucose levels
- Stress reduction
- Rest and activity patterns
- Frequent blood pressure monitoring
- Risk factor modification

- Vision changes
- Renal failure
- Heart failure
- Hypertensive crisis

● **Possible surgical interventions**
- None

CORONARY ARTERY DISEASE

● **Definitions**
- Arteriosclerosis—loss of elasticity of the arteries' intimal layer (sometimes called hardening of the arteries)
- Atherosclerosis—accumulation in the arteries of fatty plaque made of lipids

● **Causes**
- Aging
- Stress
- Genetics
- Depletion of estrogen after menopause
- High-fat, high-cholesterol diet
- Use of tobacco and alcohol
- Hypertension
- Diabetes mellitus
- Overweight or obesity
- Inactivity

● **Pathophysiology**
- Narrowing or obstruction of the coronary arteries by an embolus, vasospasm, or accumulated plaque (see *Atherosclerotic plaque development*, page 26)
- Decreased perfusion and inadequate myocardial oxygen supply

● **Assessment findings**
- Elevated blood pressure

Key facts about CAD

- Arteriosclerosis: loss of elasticity in the artery wall
- Atherosclerosis: accumulation of fatty plaque in the arteries

Common causes of CAD

- Use of tobacco and alcohol
- Hypertension
- Diabetes mellitus
- Overweight or obesity

How CAD happens

- Narrowing or obstruction of the coronary arteries
- Decreased perfusion
- Inadequate myocardial oxygen supply

Key facts about atherosclerotic plaque development

- Stiffening and loss of dilatory response leads to fatty deposits in the vessel.
- Fibrous plaque and lipids progressively narrow the lumen and impede blood flow to the myocardium.
- Plaque continues to grow, and in advanced stages, may become a calcified lesion that may rupture.

Key signs and symptoms of CAD

- Angina
- Elevated blood pressure

Diagnosing CAD

- Coronary arteriography: plaque formation
- ECG or Holter monitoring: ST depression, T-wave inversion

Atherosclerotic plaque development

The illustrations below show how plaque develops in coronary arteries, eventually leading to calcification and rupture of lesions if left untreated.

1. The coronary arteries are made of three layers: intima (the innermost layer, media (the middle layer), and adventitia (the outermost layer).

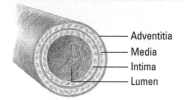

3. Fibrous plaque and lipids progressively narrow the lumen and impede blood flow to the myocardium.

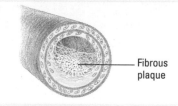

2. Stiffening and loss of dilatory response leads to fatty deposits in the vessel.

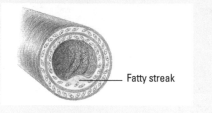

4. The plaque continues to grow and, in advanced stages, may become a complicated calcified lesion that may rupture.

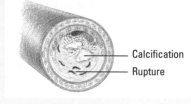

- History of angina
- Dyspnea
- Peripheral edema
- Fatigue

● **Diagnostic test findings**
- ECG or Holter monitoring: ST depression, T-wave inversion
- Stress test: elevated ST segment, multiple premature ventricular contractions on ECG, chest pain
- Coronary arteriography: plaque formation
- Blood chemistry: increased cholesterol (decreased high-density lipoproteins, increased low-density lipoproteins)
- Cardiac enzymes and proteins: monitor for increase in CK, CK-MB, LD, LD isoenzymes, troponin I, and troponin T

● **Medical management**
- Diet: low-calorie, low-sodium, low-cholesterol, and low-fat; increased dietary fiber
- Weight reduction
- Oxygen therapy

- Monitoring: vital signs, ECG, hemodynamic variables, I/O, and neuro-vascular checks
- Laboratory studies: sodium, potassium, cholesterol, CK, LD, AST, CK isoenzymes, LD isoenzymes, troponin I, and ABGs
- Smoking cessation
- Monitoring blood glucose levels (for patients with diabetes mellitus)
- Monitoring blood pressure
- Antiplatelet agents: aspirin, clopidogrel (Plavix)
- Nitrates: nitroglycerin (Nitro-Bid), isosorbide dinitrate (Isordil)
- Antilipemic agents: cholestyramine (Questran), atorvastatin (Lipitor), simvastatin (Zocor), ezetimibe (Zetia), nicotinic acid (Niacin), gemfibrozil (Lopid), colestipol (Colestid)
- Analgesic: morphine (I.V.)
- Beta-adrenergic blockers: propranolol (Inderal), nadolol (Corgard)
- Calcium channel blockers: nifedipine (Procardia), verapamil (Calan), diltiazem (Cardizem)
- ACE inhibitors:
    - enalapril (Vasotec)
    - lisinopril (Zestril)
- Antianxiety agent: diazepam (Valium)
- Laser angioplasty
- Atherectomy

● Nursing interventions

- Assess cardiovascular status
- Administer oxygen and medications, as prescribed
- Monitor and record vital signs, hemodynamic variables, I/O, ECG, and laboratory studies
- Obtain ECG during anginal episodes
- Maintain the patient's prescribed diet
- Encourage the patient to express anxiety, fears, or concerns
- Provide information about the American Heart Association
- Individualize home care instructions
- Follow the disorder and treatment plan
    - Follow instructions for medication use
    - Comply with medical follow-up
    - Adhere to activity limitations
    - Limit dietary fat and alcohol intake

● Complications

- Angina
- MI
- Heart failure
- Arrhythmias
- Stroke

● Possible surgical intervention

- CABG
- PTCA

Treating CAD

- Low-calorie, low-sodium, low-cholesterol, and low-fat diet; increased dietary fiber
- Weight reduction
- Smoking cessation
- Monitoring blood glucose levels
- Medication
- Aspirin
- Cholesterol-lowering agents
- Nitrates
- Beta-adrenergic blockers
- Calcium channel blockers
- Analgesics
- Antianxiety agents

Key nursing interventions for a patient with CAD

- Assess cardiovascular status.
- Monitor and record vital signs, hemodynamic variables, I/O, ECG, and laboratory studies.
- Obtain ECG during anginal episodes.
- Administer oxygen and medications, as prescribed.

Key complications of CAD

- Angina
- MI
- Stroke

Key facts about angina

- Chest pain caused by inadequate myocardial oxygen supply
- Four types: classical effort (exertional angina, chronic stable angina), unstable or acute angina, Prinzmetal or variant angina, and microvascular angina

Common causes of angina

- Atherosclerosis or CAD
- Vasospasm

How angina happens

- Plaque accumulation causes narrowing of the coronary arteries
- Obstruction of blood flow diminishes myocardial oxygen supply

Key signs and symptoms of angina

- Substernal, crushing, compressing pain:
- May radiate to the arms
- Usually lasts 3 to 5 minutes
- Usually occurs after exertion, emotional excitement, or exposure to cold but also can develop when the patient is at rest
- Dyspnea

Diagnosing acute anginal pain

- ECG: ST depression, T-wave inversion

ANGINA

Definition
- Angina is chest pain caused by inadequate myocardial oxygen supply
  - Classical effort (exertional angina, chronic stable angina)—consistent symptoms with pain relieved by rest
  - Unstable or acute angina—increase in severity, duration, and frequency of pain which is eventually relieved by nitroglycerin
  - Prinzmetal or variant angina—pain that occurs at rest
  - Microvascular angina—impairment of vasodilator reserve causes angina-like chest pain in a patient with normal coronary arteries
- Complaints of chest pain have increased significance in a patient with a peripheral vascular problem

Causes
- Atherosclerosis or CAD
- Vasospasm
- Aortic stenosis
- Activity or disease that increases metabolic demands

Pathophysiology
- Narrowing of the coronary arteries, which results from plaque accumulation in the intimal lining
- Obstruction of blood flow, which diminishes myocardial oxygen supply

Assessment findings
- Substernal, crushing, compressing pain
  - May radiate to the arms
  - Usually lasts 3 to 5 minutes
  - Usually occurs after exertion, emotional excitement, or exposure to cold but also can develop when the patient is at rest
- Dyspnea
- Palpitations
- Epigastric distress
- Tachycardia
- Diaphoresis
- Anxiety

Diagnostic test findings
- ECG: ST depression, T-wave inversion during acute pain
- Stress test: abnormal ECG, chest pain
- Coronary arteriography: plaque accumulation
- Blood chemistry: increased low-density lipoproteins, decreased high-density lipoproteins
- Cardiac enzymes: within normal limits, depending on severity and type of angina
- Holter monitoring: ST depression, T-wave inversion

Medical management
- Diet: low-calorie, low-sodium, and low-cholesterol

- Oxygen therapy
- Monitoring: vital signs, ECG, hemodynamic variables, I/O, and neurovascular checks
- Laboratory studies: ABGs, sodium, potassium, CK with isoenzymes, LD with isoenzymes, troponin I, troponin T, and AST
- PTCA
- Nitrates: nitroglycerin (Nitrostat), isosorbide dinitrate (Isordil)
- Analgesics: morphine, meperidine (Demerol)
- Beta-adrenergic blockers: propranolol (Inderal), nadolol (Corgard), atenolol (Tenormin), metoprolol (Lopressor)
- Calcium channel blockers: verapamil (Calan), diltiazem (Cardizem), nifedipine (Procardia), nicardipine (Cardene)
- ACE inhibitors: captopril (Capoten), enalapril (Vasotec), lisinopril (Prinivil), quinapril (Accupril)
- Cardiac glycoside: digoxin (Lanoxin)
- Antiarrhythmics: amiodarone (Cordarone), procainamide (Pronestyl), adenosine (Adenocard)

● **Nursing interventions**
- Assess pain level
- Assess cardiovascular status
- Monitor and record vital signs, hemodynamic variables, I/O, and laboratory studies
- Administer oxygen and medications, as prescribed
- Obtain an ECG reading during anginal episodes
- Encourage the patient to express anxiety, fears, or concerns
- Advise the patient to rest if pain begins
- Keep the patient in semi-Fowler's position
- Maintain the patient's prescribed diet
- Provide information about the American Heart Association
- Individualize home care instructions
- Follow the disorder and treatment plan
    - Follow instructions for medication use
    - Comply with medical follow-up
    - Know the difference between angina and MI
    - Avoid activities or situations that cause angina, such as exertion, heavy meals, emotional upsets, and exposure to cold
    - Seek medical attention if pain lasts longer than 20 minutes
- Discuss medication use and possible adverse effects

● **Complications**
- Arrhythmias
- Heart failure
- MI

● **Possible surgical intervention**
- CABG

Treating angina
- Oxygen therapy
- PTCA
- Analgesics
- Nitrates
- Beta-adrenergic blockers
- Calcium channel blockers
- ACE inhibitors

Key nursing interventions for a patient with angina
- Assess cardiovascular status.
- Assess for chest pain.
- Obtain an ECG reading during anginal episodes.
- Administer oxygen and medications, as prescribed.

Key complications of angina
- MI
- Arrhythmias

MYOCARDIAL INFARCTION

Key facts about MI

- Death of myocardial muscle cells
- Result of inadequate perfusion and oxygenation

Common causes of MI

- Atherosclerosis
- Embolism or thrombus

How MI happens

- Plaque accumulation narrows and obstructs the coronary arteries
- Lack of oxygen causes death of a portion of the myocardial muscle cells

Key signs and symptoms of MI

- Crushing, burning, tightness, or squeezing substernal pain:
- May radiate to the jaw, back, arms, neck, ears, or shoulders
- Lasts longer than anginal pain, usually longer than 30 minutes
- Unrelieved by rest or nitroglycerin
- May not be present (asymptomatic or "silent" MI)
- Dyspnea

Diagnosing MI

- ECG: enlarged Q wave, elevated ST segment and T-wave inversion
- Elevated myoglobin and troponin I, and positive CK-MB fraction

● **Definition**
- Death of a portion of the myocardial muscle cells caused by a lack of oxygen from inadequate perfusion

● **Causes**
- Atherosclerosis
- Inadequate perfusion to meet metabolic demands
- Embolism or thrombus
- Coronary artery spasm

● **Pathophysiology**
- Narrowing and eventual obstruction of the coronary arteries from plaque accumulation
- Death of the myocardial cells from inadequate perfusion and oxygenation

● **Assessment findings**
- Crushing, burning, tightness, or squeezing substernal pain
  - May radiate to the jaw, back, arms, neck, ears, or shoulders
  - Lasts longer than anginal pain, usually longer than 30 minutes
  - Is unrelieved by rest or nitroglycerin
  - May not be present (asymptomatic or "silent" MI)
- Dyspnea, tachypnea, crackles, and frothy sputum
- Nausea and vomiting
- Anxiety
- Restlessness, confusion, agitation
- Fatigue (especially in women)
- Diaphoresis
- Pallor
- Arrhythmias
- Elevated temperature

● **Diagnostic test findings**
- ECG: enlarged Q wave, elevated ST segment, T-wave inversion (see *Pinpointing MI*)
- Blood chemistry: increased CK, LD, lipids; positive CK-MB fraction; flipped LD_1 (LD_1 levels exceed LD_2 levels, the reversal of their normal patterns), and elevated myoglobin, troponin I, and troponin T
- Hematology: increased WBC count

● **Medical management**
- Aspirin (preferably chewed)
- Nitrates: nitroglycerin (I.V.), sublingual, translingual
- Oxygen at 2 to 4 L via nasal cannula
- Analgesics: morphine, meperidine (Demerol)
- Thrombolytic therapy: anistreplase (Eminase), anisoylated plasminogen-streptokinase activator complex, streptokinase (Streptase)
- Monitoring: vital signs, I/O, ECG, and hemodynamic variables

Pinpointing MI

Myocardial infarction (MI) has a central area of necrosis surrounded by a zone of injury that may recover if revascularization occurs. This zone of injury is surrounded by an outer ring of reversible ischemia. Characteristic electrocardiographic changes are associated with each zone.

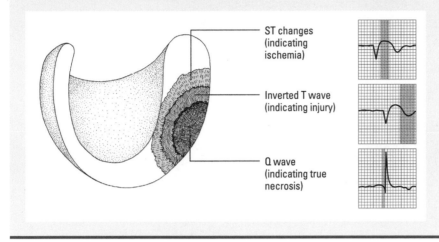

ST changes (indicating ischemia)

Inverted T wave (indicating injury)

Q wave (indicating true necrosis)

- Laboratory studies: ABGs, CK, CK isoenzymes, LD, LD isoenzymes, myoglobin, troponin I, troponin T, PTT, WBC, sodium, potassium, and glucose
- Antiarrhythmics: amiodarone (Cordarone), procainamide (Pronestyl)
- Antiplatelet agents: aspirin; ticlopidine (Ticlid) if unable to tolerate aspirin
- Anticoagulant: heparin
- Electrolyte replacement: magnesium sulfate
- Antihypertensives: hydralazine (Apresoline), methyldopa (Aldomet)
- ACE inhibitors: captopril (Capoten), enalaprilat (Vasotec)
- Beta-adrenergic blockers: propranolol (Inderal), atenolol (Tenormin); beta-adrenergic blockers are contraindicated if the patient also has heart failure, hypotension, or bronchospasm
- Calcium channel blockers: verapamil (Calan), diltiazem (Cardizem), nifedipine (Procardia), nicardipine (Cardene)
- Intra-aortic balloon pump (IABP)
- Left ventricular assist device
- Diet: low-calorie, low-cholesterol, low-fat
- PTCA
- Laser angioplasty
- Vascular stents
- Atherectomy
- **Nursing interventions**
  - Assess pain level and administer oxygen and medications, as prescribed
  - Assess cardiovascular and respiratory status
  - **Obtain an ECG reading during acute pain**

Key facts about MI changes and zones

- ST changes (indicate ischemia)
- Inverted T wave (indicates injury)
- Q wave (indicates true necrosis)

Treating MI

- Antiarrhythmics
- Antiplatelet agents
- Anticoagulants
- Analgesics
- Antihypertensives
- ACE inhibitors
- Nitrates
- Beta-adrenergic blockers
- Calcium channel blockers

Key nursing interventions for a patient with MI

- Assess cardiovascular and respiratory status.
- Monitor and record vital signs, I/O, hemodynamic variables, laboratory studies, and ECG results.
- Obtain an ECG reading during acute pain.
- Administer oxygen and medications, as prescribed.

- Monitor and record vital signs, I/O, hemodynamic variables, laboratory studies, and ECG results
- Maintain bed rest
- Provide emotional support to allay the patient's anxiety
- Maintain the patient's prescribed diet
- Provide information about the American Heart Association
- Individualize home care instructions
- Follow the disorder and treatment plan
  - Follow instructions for medication use
  - Comply with medical follow-up
  - Participate in a cardiac rehabilitation program
  - Maintain a low-cholesterol, low-fat, low-sodium diet
  - Know the difference between the pain of angina and MI
  - Alternate rest periods with activity

● Complications

- Arrhythmias
- Cardiogenic shock
- Heart failure
- Papillary muscle rupture
- Pericarditis
- Thromboembolism
- Death

● Possible surgical intervention

- CABG

HEART FAILURE: LEFT-SIDED

● Definition

- Failure of the left side of the heart to pump enough blood to meet metabolic demands

● Causes

- Atherosclerosis or CAD
- Fluid overload
- MI
- Valvular stenosis
- Valvular insufficiency
- Hypertension
- Cardiac conduction defects
- Cardiomyopathy
- Infection
- Immune and connective disorder
- Endocrine imbalance

Key complications of MI

- Arrhythmias
- Heart failure
- Cardiogenic shock
- Death

Key facts about left-sided heart failure

- The left side of the heart fails to pump enough blood to meet metabolic demands
- Fluid overload occurs

Common causes of left-sided heart failure

- Atherosclerosis
- Fluid overload
- MI
- Valvular stenosis

Pathophysiology

- Decreased myocardial contractility or increased myocardial workload, either of which increases left ventricular pressure and left atrial pressure and reduces cardiac output
- Impaired oxygenation and respiratory manifestations of fluid overload

Assessment findings

- Dyspnea
- Paroxysmal nocturnal dyspnea
- Crackles, wheezes, rhonchi
- Cough
- Hemoptysis
- Gallop rhythm: S_3, S_4
- Arrhythmias
- Fatigue
- Anxiety
- Orthopnea
- Tachycardia
- Tachypnea
- Diaphoresis
- Decreased pulse oximetry readings

Diagnostic test findings

- Chest X-ray: increased pulmonary congestion, left ventricular hypertrophy
- B-type natriuretic peptid (BNP): elevated
- Echocardiography: increased size of cardiac chambers and decreased wall motion
- Hemodynamic monitoring: increased pulmonary artery wedge pressure (PAWP), central venous pressure (CVP), and pulmonary artery pressure (PAP), and decreased cardiac output
- ABGs: hypoxemia, hypercapnia
- ECG: left ventricular hypertrophy, ST-T wave changes
- Blood chemistry: decreased potassium, sodium; increased BUN, creatinine, decreased myoglobin
- Urinalysis: proteinuria, RBCs, casts

Medical management

- Oxygen therapy
- Monitoring: vital signs, I/O, ECG, pulse oximetry, and hemodynamic variables
- Diuretics: furosemide (Lasix), bumetanide (Bumex), metolazone (Zaroxolyn), spironolactone (Aldactone), acetazolamide (Diamox)
- Nesiritide (Natrecor)
- Position: semi-Fowler's
- Activity: bed rest, active ROM and isometric exercises
- I.V. therapy: electrolyte replacement
- Laboratory studies: ABGs, sodium, potassium, BUN, creatinine, cardiac enzymes, and BNP
- Indwelling urinary catheter

How left-sided heart failure happens

- Myocardial contractility or increased myocardial workload increases left ventricular pressure and left atrial pressure.
- Cardiac output is reduced.

Key signs and symptoms of left-sided heart failure

- Dyspnea
- Crackles, wheezes, rhonchi
- Decreased pulse oximetry readings

Diagnosing left-sided heart failure

- Chest X-ray:
- Increased pulmonary congestion, left ventricular hypertrophy
- BNP: elevated

Treating left-sided heart failure

- Oxygen therapy
- Monitoring: vital signs, I/O, ECG, hemodynamic variables, pulse oximetry
- Diuretics
- Nesiritide (Natricor)
- Low-sodium diet; limit fluids
- Semi-Fowler's position

- IABP
- Left ventricular assist device
- Analgesic: morphine (I.V.)
- Vasodilator: nitroprusside (Nipride)
- Cardiac inotropes: dopamine (Intropin), dobutamine (Dobutrex)
- Cardiac glycoside: digoxin (Lanoxin)
- Nitrates: isosorbide dinitrate (Isordil), nitroglycerin (Nitro-Bid)
- ACE inhibitors: captopril (Capoten), enalapril (Vasotec), lisinopril (Prinivil)
- Phosphodiesterase inhibitor: inamrinone (Inocor)
- Diet: low-sodium; limit fluids

● **Nursing interventions**
- Assess cardiovascular and respiratory status
- Monitor and record vital signs, CVP, hemodynamic variables, I/O, and laboratory studies, and pulse oximetry
- Administer I.V. fluids, oxygen, and medications, as prescribed
- Keep the patient in semi-Fowler's position
- Restrict oral fluids
- Maintain the patient's prescribed diet
- Provide suctioning, turning, coughing, and deep breathing
- Weigh the patient daily
- Assess peripheral edema
- Provide information about the American Heart Association
- Individualize home care instructions
- Follow the disorder and treatment plan
  - Follow instructions for medication use
  - Comply with medical follow-up
  - Restrict fluids, as directed
  - Monitor daily weight and report gain of 2 lb (0.9 kg) or more if it occurs within 1 to 2 days
  - Limit sodium intake
  - Supplement the diet with foods high in potassium
  - Recognize the signs and symptoms of fluid overload

● **Complications**
- Respiratory failure
- Digoxin toxicity
- Cardiogenic shock
- Pulmonary edema
- Hypokalemia

● **Possible surgical interventions**
- Implantable left ventricular device
- CABG
- Heart valve replacement
- Heart transplant (if severe heart failure)

Key nursing interventions for a patient with left-sided heart failure

- Administer oxygen and monitor pulse oximetry readings.
- Monitor vital signs, I/O, and laboratory studies.
- Administer medications, as prescribed.
- Restrict oral fluids.
- Weigh the patient daily.

Key complications of left-sided heart failure

- Respiratory failure
- Pulmonary edema

HEART FAILURE: RIGHT-SIDED

- **Definition**
  - Failure of the right side of the heart to pump enough blood to meet metabolic demands

- **Causes**
  - Atherosclerosis
  - Left-sided heart failure
  - Chronic obstructive pulmonary disease
  - Valvular stenosis
  - Valvular insufficiency
  - Pulmonary hypertension

- **Pathophysiology**
  - Increased pressure from left-sided heart failure
  - Increased venous congestion in the systemic circulation with fluid overload
  - Increased resistance in lungs

- **Assessment findings**
  - Jugular vein distention
  - Anorexia
  - Nausea, vomiting
  - Abdominal distention
  - Ascites
  - Hepatomegaly
  - Dependent edema, peripheral edema
  - Weight gain
  - Signs of left-sided heart failure
  - Gallop rhythm: S_3, S_4
  - Tachycardia
  - Fatigue
  - Nocturia
  - Decreased pulse oximetry readings

- **Diagnostic test findings**
  - Chest X-ray: pulmonary congestion, cardiomegaly, pleural effusions
  - Echocardiogram: increased size of chambers, decrease in wall motion
  - Hemodynamic monitoring: increased PAWP, PAP, CVP; decreased cardiac output
  - ABGs: hypoxemia
  - ECG: left and right ventricular hypertrophy
  - Blood chemistry: decreased sodium, potassium; increased BUN, creatinine
  - BNP: elevated

- **Medical management**
  - Oxygen therapy
  - Monitoring: vital signs, I/O, ECG, and hemodynamic variables

Key facts about right-sided heart failure
- Right side of the heart fails to pump enough blood to meet metabolic demands
- Fluid overload occurs

Common causes of right-sided heart failure
- Atherosclerosis
- Left-sided heart failure

How right-sided heart failure happens
- Increased pressure from left-sided heart failure
- Increased venous congestion
- Increased resistance in lungs

Key signs and symptoms of right-sided heart failure
- Signs of left-sided heart failure
- Jugular vein distention
- Dependent edema, peripheral edema
- Weight gain

Diagnosing right-sided heart failure
- Chest X-ray:
  - Pulmonary congestion, cardiomegaly, pleural effusions
- BNP: elevated

Treating right-sided heart failure

- Oxygen therapy
- Vital signs, I/O, ECG, and hemodynamic variables monitoring
- Diuretics
- Nesiritide (Natrecor)
- Semi-Fowler's position
- Low-sodium diet; limit fluids
- Analgesics

Key nursing interventions for a patient with right-sided heart failure

- Assess cardiovascular and respiratory systems.
- Provide oxygen and monitor pulse oximetry.
- Monitor and record vital signs, I/O, hemodynamic variables, and laboratory studies.
- Administer medications.
- Keep the patient in semi-Fowler's position.
- Assess peripheral edema.
- Restrict oral fluids.
- Weigh the patient daily.

Key complications of right-sided heart failure

- Respiratory failure
- Pulmonary edema
- Cardiogenic shock

- Diuretics: furosemide (Lasix), bumetanide (Bumex), metolazone (Zaroxolyn), spironolactone (Aldactone), acetazolamide (Diamox)
- Nesiritide (Natrecor)
- Position: semi-Fowler's
- Activity: bed rest, active ROM and isometric exercises
- Diet: low-sodium; limit fluids
- I.V. therapy: electrolyte replacement
- Laboratory studies: ABGs, sodium, potassium, BUN, and creatinine
- Indwelling urinary catheter
- Analgesic: morphine (I.V.)
- Vasodilator: nitroprusside (Nipride)
- Cardiac inotropes: dopamine (Intropin), dobutamine (Dobutrex)
- Cardiac glycoside: digoxin (Lanoxin)
- Nitrates: isosorbide dinitrate (Isordil), nitroglycerin (Nitro-Bid)
- IABP
- Thoracentesis
- Paracentesis

● **Nursing interventions**
- Assess cardiovascular and respiratory status
- Monitor and record vital signs, I/O, hemodynamic variables, pulse oximetry, and laboratory studies
- Administer oxygen, I.V. fluids, and medications, as prescribed
- Keep the patient in semi-Fowler's position
- Restrict oral fluids
- Maintain the patient's prescribed diet (low-sodium, low-cholesterol, no caffeine)
- Provide suctioning, turning, coughing, and deep breathing
- Assess peripheral edema
- Weigh the patient daily
- Measure and record the patient's abdominal girth
- Individualize home care instructions
- Follow the disorder and treatment plan
    - Follow instructions for medication use
    - Comply with medical follow-up
    - Restrict fluids
    - Elevate the legs when seated
    - Limit sodium intake
    - Supplement the diet with foods high in potassium
    - Recognize the signs and symptoms of fluid overload

● **Complications**
- Respiratory failure
- Digoxin toxicity
- Cardiogenic shock
- Pulmonary edema
- Hypokalemia
- Hypernatremia

- **Possible surgical interventions**
  - Implantable left ventricular device
  - CABG
  - Heart valve replacement
  - Heart transplant (for severe heart failure)

ACUTE PULMONARY EDEMA

- **Definition**
  - Complication of left-sided heart failure; results in increased pressure in the capillaries of the lungs and acute transudation of fluid
- **Causes**
  - Atherosclerosis
  - MI
  - Myocarditis
  - Valvular disease
  - Smoke inhalation
  - Drug overdose: heroin, barbiturates, morphine
  - Overload of I.V. fluids
  - Heart failure
  - Acute respiratory distress syndrome
- **Pathophysiology**
  - PAWP exceeds intravascular osmotic pressure
  - Alveolar and interstitial edema result from the heart's failure to pump adequately
  - Impaired oxygenation and hypoxia result
- **Assessment findings**
  - Dyspnea
  - Paroxysmal cough
  - Blood-tinged, frothy sputum
  - Orthopnea
  - Tachypnea
  - Agitation
  - Anxiety
  - Restlessness
  - Intense fear
  - Chest pain
  - Syncope
  - Tachycardia
  - Cold, clammy skin
  - Diaphoresis
  - Decreased pulse oximetry readings
  - Gallop rhythm: S_3, S_4
  - Jugular vein distention
- **Diagnostic test findings**
  - Chest X-ray: interstitial edema

Key facts about acute pulmonary edema

- Complication of left-sided heart failure
- Results in acute transudation of fluid

Common causes of pulmonary edema

- Heart failure
- Atherosclerosis
- Valvular disease

How acute pulmonary edema happens

- Edema results from heart's inability to pump adequately
- Results in impaired oxygenation and hypoxia

Key signs and symptoms of acute pulmonary edema

- Dyspnea
- Paroxysmal cough
- Blood-tinged, frothy sputum
- Tachypnea
- Restlessness
- Chest pain

Diagnosing acute pulmonary edema

- Chest X-ray—interstitial edema
- ABGs—respiratory alkalosis or acidosis

Treating acute pulmonary edema

- Oxygen therapy
- Vital signs, I/O, ECG, and hemo-dynamic variables monitoring
- High Fowler's position
- Diuretics
- Pulse oximetry
- Low-sodium diet; limit fluids
- Analgesics
- Cardiac inotropes
- Bronchodilators

Key nursing interventions for a patient with acute pulmonary edema

- Assess cardiovascular and res-piratory status.
- Administer oxygen and monitor pulse oximetry.
- Provide suctioning, turning, coughing, and deep breathing.
- Keep the patient in high Fowler's position.
- Allay the patient's anxiety.
- Note the color, amount, and consistency of sputum.

Key complications of acute pulmonary edema

- Respiratory failure
- Pulmonary embolism

- ABGs: respiratory alkalosis or acidosis
- ECG: tachycardia, ventricular enlargement
- Hemodynamic monitoring: increased PAWP, CVP, PAP; decreased cardiac output

● **Medical management**
- Oxygen therapy with possible endotracheal intubation and mechanical ventilation
- Monitoring: vital signs, I/O, ECG, and hemodynamic variables, and pulse oximetry
- Diuretics: furosemide (Lasix), bumetanide (Bumex), metolazone (Zaroxolyn)
- Position: high Fowler's
- Activity: bed rest; active ROM and isometric exercises
- Diet: low-sodium; limit fluids
- I.V. therapy: electrolyte replacement
- Laboratory studies: sodium, potassium, ABGs, BUN, and creatinine
- Indwelling urinary catheter
- ET tube suctioning
- Analgesic: morphine (I.V.)
- Vasodilator: nitroprusside (Nipride)
- Cardiac inotropes: dopamine (Intropin), dobutamine (Dobutrex)
- Cardiac glycoside: digoxin (Lanoxin)
- Nitrates: isosorbide dinitrate (Isordil), nitroglycerin (Nitro-Bid)
- Bronchodilator: aminophylline (Somophyllin)

● **Nursing interventions**
- Assess cardiovascular and respiratory status
- Monitor and record vital signs, I/O, hemodynamic variables, laboratory studies, and daily weight
- Administer oxygen and monitor pulse oximetry; assist with ET intu-bation, if indicated
- Keep the patient in high Fowler's position
- Withhold food and fluids, as directed
- Administer I.V. fluids and medications, as prescribed
- Provide suctioning, turning, coughing, and deep breathing
- Provide emotional support to allay the patient's anxiety
- Encourage the patient to express his feelings such as a fear of suffocation
- Note the color, amount, and consistency of sputum
- Individualize home care instructions
- Follow the disorder and treatment plan
  - Follow instructions for medication use
  - Comply with medical follow-up
  - Weigh daily
  - Recognize the signs of fluid overload
  - Sleep with the head of the bed elevated
  - Supplement the diet with foods high in potassium

● **Complications**
- Respiratory failure

- Digoxin toxicity
- Pulmonary embolism
- Hypokalemia
- Hypernatremia

● **Possible surgical interventions**
- None

CARDIOGENIC SHOCK

● **Definition**
- Failure of the heart to pump adequately, thereby reducing cardiac output and compromising tissue perfusion

● **Causes**
- MI
- Myocarditis
- Advanced heart block
- Heart failure
- Metabolic abnormalities
- Cardiac tamponade
- Pulmonary embolus

● **Pathophysiology**
- Decreased stroke volume and cardiac output; increased left ventricular volume, increased peripheral resistance due to increased sympathetic nervous system activity (see *What happens in cardiogenic shock,* page 40)
- Compensatory increases in heart rate and contractility, which raise the demand for myocardial oxygen
- Imbalance between oxygen supply and demand, which increases myocardial ischemia and further compromises the heart's pumping action

● **Assessment findings**
- Hypotension (systolic pressure of less than 90 mm Hg)
- Oliguria (urine output of less than 30 ml/hour)
- Cold, clammy, pale skin
- Decreased level of consciousness
- Tachycardia
- Chest pain
- Restlessness
- Decreased pulse oximetry readings
- Tachypnea
- Chest pain
- Anxiety
- Arrhythmias and ECG changes
- Disorientation and confusion
- Jugular vein distention

● **Diagnostic test findings**
- ABGs: metabolic acidosis, hypoxemia

Key facts about cardiogenic shock

- Decreased stroke volume and cardiac output cause compensatory changes in heart rate and contractility
- Imbalance between oxygen supply and demand causes failure of the heart to pump adequately
- Cardiac output is reduced and tissue perfusion is compromised

Most common cause of cardiogenic shock

- MI

Key signs and symptoms of cardiogenic shock

- Hypotension
- Oliguria
- Cold, clammy, pale skin
- Tachycardia
- Restlessness

Diagnosing cardiogenic shock

- ABGs: metabolic acidosis, hypoxemia
- ECG: MI (enlarged Q wave, ST elevation)

How cardiogenic shock happens

- Decreased myocardial contractility results in inadequate cardiac output
- Stroke volume decreases, leading to an increased heart rate and decreased left ventricular emptying
- Preload increases and coronary artery perfusion and collateral blood flow decrease
- Pulmonary congestion and myocardial hypoxia result
- Compensatory mechanisms are triggered to prevent decompensation and death

 GO WITH THE FLOW

What happens in cardiogenic shock

When the myocardium can't contract sufficiently to maintain adequate cardiac output, stroke volume decreases and the heart can't eject an adequate volume of blood with each contraction. The blood backs up behind the weakened left ventricle, increasing preload and causing pulmonary congestion. In addition, to compensate for the drop in stroke volume, the heart rate increases in an attempt to maintain cardiac output. As a result of the diminished stroke volume, coronary artery perfusion and collateral blood flow decrease. All of these mechanisms increase the workload of the heart and enhance left-sided heart failure. The result is myocardial hypoxia, further decreased cardiac output, and a triggering of compensatory mechanisms to prevent decompensation and death.

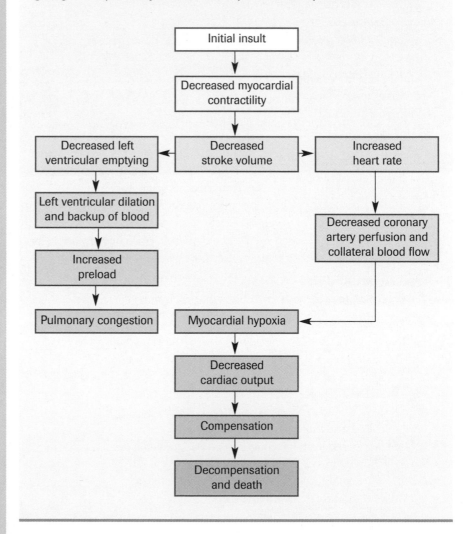

- ECG: MI (enlarged Q wave, ST elevation)
- Blood chemistry: increased BUN, creatinine, hyperglycemia, hypernatremia, hypokalemia, elevated cardiac enzymes, elevated troponin
- Echocardiogram may identify cause of shock
- Chest X-ray: may show signs of left ventricular failure
- Hemodynamic monitoring: decreased stroke volume, mixed venous oxygen saturation, and cardiac output; increased PAWP, CVP, PAP, and systemic vascular resistance

● Medical management

- Oxygen therapy with endotracheal intubation and mechanical ventilation
- Monitoring: vital signs, I/O, ECG, hemodynamic variables, and level of consciousness
- Diet: withhold food and fluids
- I.V. therapy: electrolyte replacement, fluids as needed
- Position: semi-Fowler's
- Activity: bed rest; passive ROM and isometric exercises
- Laboratory studies: potassium, sodium, BUN, creatinine, and ABGs
- Indwelling urinary catheter
- ET tube suctioning
- IABP
- Diuretics: furosemide (Lasix), bumetanide (Bumex), metolazone (Zaroxolyn)
- Vasodilator: nitroglycerin (Nitro-Bid)
- Cardiac inotropes: dobutamine (Dobutrex), inamrinone (Inocor)
- Cardiac glycoside: digoxin (Lanoxin)
- Vasopressor: norepinephrine (Levophed), dopamine (Intropin)
- Adrenergic agent: epinephrine (Adrenalin)
- Analgesics: morphine (Duramorph)
- Hemopump
- Pulse oximetry
- Thrombolytic therapy

● Nursing interventions

- Assess cardiovascular status, respiratory status, and fluid balance
- Administer oxygen and assist with endotracheal intubation
- Monitor and record vital signs, I/O, hemodynamic variables, level of consciousness (LOC), pulse oximetry, and laboratory studies
- Administer I.V. fluids and medications, as prescribed
- Withhold food and fluids, as directed
- Provide suctioning, turning, coughing, and deep breathing
- Keep the patient in semi-Fowler's position
- Provide emotional support to allay the patient's anxiety
- Individualize home care instructions
  - Follow instructions for medication use
  - Comply with medical follow-up
  - Recognize the signs and symptoms of fluid overload
  - Adhere to activity limitations

Treating cardiogenic shock

- Oxygen therapy
- Semi-Fowler's position
- IABP
- Diuretics
- Vasodilators
- Cardiac inotropes
- Cardiac glycosides
- Vasopressors
- Adrenergic agents

Key nursing interventions for a patient with cardiogenic shock

- Administer I.V. fluids, oxygen, and medications, as prescribed.
- Assess cardiovascular status, respiratory status, and fluid balance.
- Monitor and record vital signs, I/O, hemodynamic variables, LOC, and laboratory studies.

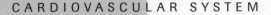
Key complications of cardiogenic shock

- Arrhythmia
- Cardiac arrest

Key facts about mitral stenosis

- Narrowing of the mitral valve opening
- Limited blood flow from the left atrium to the left ventricle occurs

Common causes of mitral stenosis

- Rheumatic fever
- Infective endocarditis
- Congenital

How mitral stenosis happens

- Thickening and calcification of valvular tissue occur
- Pressure in the left atrium is increased
- Pulmonary hypertension and left atrial hypertrophy occur
- Right ventricular failure results

Key signs and symptoms of mitral stenosis

- Fatigue
- Dyspnea on exertion
- Peripheral edema
- Orthopnea

– Alternate rest periods with activity
– Maintain low-fat, low-sodium diet

- **Complications**
  - Arrhythmias
  - Cardiac arrest
  - Infection
  - Death

- **Possible surgical interventions**
  - CABG
  - Heart transplantation
  - PTCA
  - Left ventricular access device

MITRAL STENOSIS

- **Definition**
  - Narrowing of the mitral valve opening

- **Causes**
  - Rheumatic fever
  - Congenital
  - Carcinoid syndrome
  - Infective endocarditis
  - Systemic lupus erythematosus

- **Pathophysiology**
  - Thickening and calcification of valvular tissue, thereby narrowing the mitral valve opening and limiting blood flow from the left atrium to the left ventricle
  - Increased pressure in the left atrium, leading to pulmonary hypertension and left atrial hypertrophy
  - Right ventricular failure, producing pulmonary congestion

- **Assessment findings**
  - Fatigue
  - Low cardiac output
  - Dyspnea on exertion
  - Right-sided heart failure
  - Cough
  - Peripheral edema
  - Atrial fibrillation
  - Orthopnea
  - Jugular vein distention
  - Tachycardia
  - Paroxysmal nocturnal dyspnea
  - Hemoptysis
  - Murmurs, clicks

Diagnostic test findings
- Chest X-ray: enlargement of the left atrium and right ventricle; pulmonary congestion
- Echocardiogram: thickening of the mitral valve and left atrial enlargement
- Cardiac catheterization: increased left atrial pressure, PAWP; decreased cardiac output
- Angiography: mitral stenosis

Medical management
- Oxygen therapy
- Monitoring: vital signs, I/O, ECG, and hemodynamic variables
- Activity: bed rest; active ROM and isometric exercises
- Laboratory studies: sodium, potassium, PT, PTT, and ABGs
- Diet: low-sodium; limit fluids
- Position: semi-Fowler's
- Indwelling urinary catheter
- Cardiac glycoside: digoxin (Lanoxin)
- Nitrates: isosorbide dinitrate (Isordil), nitroglycerin (Nitro-Bid)
- Diuretics: furosemide (Lasix), bumetanide (Bumex)
- Antiarrhythmics: amiodarone (Cordarone), procainamide (Pronestyl)
- Anticoagulants: warfarin (Coumadin)
- Antibiotics: penicillin G potassium (Pentids)
- Percutaneous transluminal valvuloplasty

Nursing interventions
- Assess cardiovascular and respiratory status
- Monitor and record vital signs, I/O, hemodynamic variables, laboratory studies, and ECG and pulse oximetry readings
- Administer I.V. fluids, oxygen, and medications, as prescribed
- Maintain the patient's prescribed diet; restrict oral fluids
- Keep the patient in semi-Fowler's position
- Assess pain level
- Provide emotional support to allay the patient's anxiety
- Assess peripheral edema
- Individualize home care instructions
- Follow the disorder and treatment plan
  - Follow instructions for medication use
  - Comply with medical follow-up
  - Recognize the signs and symptoms of heart failure
  - Adhere to activity limitations; alternate rest periods with activity
  - Monitor for infection, avoid exposure to people with infections, and seek treatment if infection develops
  - Test stools for occult blood

Complications
- Thrombosis
- Embolism
- Heart failure
- Atrial fibrillation

Diagnosing mitral stenosis
- Chest X-ray: enlargement of the left atrium and right ventricle; pulmonary congestion
- Echocardiogram: thickening of the mitral valve and left atrial enlargement

Treating mitral stenosis
- Low-sodium diet; fluid restrictions
- Semi-Fowler's position
- Cardiac glycosides
- Nitrates
- Diuretics
- Antiarrhythmics
- Anticoagulants
- Antibiotics

Key nursing interventions for a patient with mitral stenosis
- Administer I.V. fluids, oxygen, and medications, as prescribed.
- Assess cardiovascular and respiratory response.
- Monitor and record vital signs, I/O, hemodynamic variables, laboratory studies, and ECG readings.
- Individualize home care instructions
  - Recognize the signs and symptoms of heart failure.
  - Adhere to activity limitations.
  - Monitor for infection, avoid exposure to people with infections, and seek treatment if infection develops.
  - Test stools for occult blood.

Key complications of mitral stenosis
- Thrombosis
- Embolism
- Atrial fibrillation

Key facts about mitral insufficiency

- An incomplete closure of the mitral valve
- Backflow of blood to the left atrium occurs

Common causes of mitral insufficiency

- Rheumatic fever
- Myxomatous degeneration

How mitral insufficiency happens

- Valvular incompetence
- Increased left atrial pressure, pulmonary hypertension and left atrial hypertrophy results

Key signs and symptoms of mitral insufficiency

- Fatigue
- Dyspnea on exertion
- Peripheral edema
- Angina pectoris
- Orthopnea

Diagnosing mitral insufficiency

- Echocardiogram: enlarged left atrium, abnormal movement of the mitral valve
- Cardiac catheterization: increased left atrial pressure and increased left ventricular pressure

Treating mitral insufficiency

- Semi-Fowler's position
- Low-sodium diet; fluid restrictions
- Cardiac glycosides
- Nitrates
- Diuretics
- Antiarrhythmics
- Anticoagulants

● **Possible surgical interventions**
- Valve replacement
- Open mitral commissurotomy

MITRAL INSUFFICIENCY

● **Definition**
- Incomplete closure of the mitral valve
- Also known as *mitral regurgitation*

● **Causes**
- Rheumatic fever
- Myxomatous degeneration
- Ruptured chorae tendineae
- Collagen-vascular disease

● **Pathophysiology**
- Valvular incompetence
- Backflow of blood to the left atrium
- Increased left atrial pressure, pulmonary hypertension, and left atrial hypertrophy

● **Assessment findings**
- Shortness of breath
- Cough
- Fatigue
- Dyspnea on exertion
- Peripheral edema
- Atrial fibrillation
- Angina pectoris
- Orthopnea
- Hemoptysis
- Murmurs and clicks
- S_3

● **Diagnostic test findings**
- Chest X-ray: enlargement of the left atrium and the left ventricle
- ECG: atrial fibrillation, left atrial hypertension, and left ventricular hypertrophy
- Echocardiogram: enlargement of the left atrium, abnormal movement of the mitral valve
- Cardiac catheterization: increased left atrial and left ventricular pressure
- Cardiac angiography: insufficiency

● **Medical management**
- Oxygen therapy
- Monitoring: vital signs, I/O, ECG, and hemodynamic variables
- Position: semi-Fowler's
- Diet: low-sodium; limit fluids
- Laboratory studies: sodium, potassium, BUN, creatinine, and ABGs

- Indwelling urinary catheter
- Cardiac glycoside: digoxin (Lanoxin)
- Nitrates: isosorbide (Isordil), nitroglycerin (Nitro-Bid)
- Diuretics: furosemide (Lasix), bumetanide (Bumex)
- Antiarrhythmics: quinidine (Cardioquin), procainamide (Pronestyl)
- Anticoagulants: warfarin (Coumadin)

● **Nursing interventions**
- Assess cardiovascular and respiratory status
- Monitor and record vital signs, I/O, hemodynamic variables, laboratory studies, and ECG readings
- Administer I.V. fluids, oxygen, and medications, as prescribed
- Keep the patient in semi-Fowler's position
- Maintain the patient's prescribed diet; limit oral fluids
- Assess pain level
- Assess peripheral edema
- Provide emotional support to allay the patient's anxiety
- Provide information about the American Heart Association
- Individualize home care instructions
- Follow the disorder and treatment plan
  - Follow instructions for medication use
  - Comply with medical follow-up
  - Test stools for occult blood
  - Adhere to activity limitations; alternate rest periods with activity
  - Monitor for infection, avoid exposure to people with infections, and seek treatment if infection develops

● **Complications**
- Embolism
- Thrombosis
- Heart failure
- Ruptured papillary muscle
- Pulmonary edema
- Arrhythmias

● **Possible surgical interventions**
- Mitral valve replacement
- Valvuloplasty

AORTIC STENOSIS

● **Definition**
- Narrowing of the aortic valve

● **Causes**
- Syphilis
- Rheumatic fever
- Atherosclerosis
- Congenital malformations

Key nursing interventions for a patient with mitral insufficiency

- Maintain the patient's prescribed diet; limit oral fluids.
- Keep the patient in semi-Fowler's position.
- Assess peripheral edema.

Key complications of mitral insufficiency

- Heart failure
- Pulmonary edema
- Arrhythmias

Key facts about aortic stenosis

- Narrowing of the aortic valve
- Lower cardiac output causes increased congestion in the lungs, resulting in right-sided heart failure

Common causes of aortic stenosis

- Congenital malformations
- Rheumatic fever

How aortic stenosis happens

- Fibrosis and calcification of valvular tissue narrows valve opening
- Blood flow is limited
- Left ventricular pressure increases
- Left ventricular hypertrophy and right-sided heart failure result

Key signs and symptoms of aortic stenosis

- Anginal episodes
- Pulmonary hypertension
- Left-sided heart failure
- Orthopnea

Diagnosing aortic stenosis

- ECG: left bundle-branch block, first-degree heart block, left ventricular hypertrophy
- Echocardiogram: thickened left ventricular wall, thickened aortic valve that moves abnormally

Treating aortic stenosis

- Low-sodium diet; fluid restrictions
- Monitoring laboratory studies
- Cardiac glycosides
- Nitrates
- Diuretics
- Percutaneous transluminal valvuloplasty

Key nursing interventions for a patient with aortic stenosis

- Maintain the patient's prescribed diet; limit fluids.
- Assess cardiovascular and respiratory status.
- Monitor and record vital signs, I/O, hemodynamic variables, laboratory studies, and ECG readings.

● Pathophysiology

- Fibrosis and calcification of valvular tissue, which narrows the valve opening and limits blood flow
- Increased left ventricular pressure, which causes hypertrophy of the left ventricle and lowers cardiac output
- Increased congestion in the lungs, which results in right-sided heart failure

● Assessment findings

- Anginal episodes
- Syncope
- Signs and symptoms of pulmonary hypertension
- Signs and symptoms of left-sided heart failure
- Fatigue
- Orthopnea
- Paroxysmal nocturnal dyspnea
- Murmurs and clicks

● Diagnostic test findings

- Chest X-ray: aortic valve calcification, left ventricular enlargement
- ECG: left bundle-branch block, first-degree heart block, left ventricular hypertrophy
- Echocardiogram: thickened left ventricular wall, thickened aortic valve that moves abnormally
- Cardiac catheterization: increased left ventricular pressure

● Medical management

- Monitoring: vital signs, I/O, ECG, and hemodynamic variables
- Laboratory studies: sodium, potassium, BUN, creatinine, and ABGs
- Diet: low-sodium; limit fluids
- Cardiac glycoside: digoxin (Lanoxin)
- Nitrates: isosorbide (Isordil), nitroglycerin (Nitro-Bid)
- Diuretics: furosemide (Lasix), bumetanide (Bumex)
- Percutaneous transluminal valvuloplasty

● Nursing interventions

- Assess cardiovascular and respiratory status
- Monitor and record vital signs, I/O, hemodynamic variables, laboratory studies, and ECG readings
- Administer I.V. therapy and medications, as prescribed
- Maintain the patient's prescribed diet; limit fluids
- Assess pain level
- Provide emotional support to allay the patient's anxiety
- Provide information about the American Heart Association
- Individualize home care instructions
- Follow the disorder and treatment plan
  - Follow instructions for medication use
  - Comply with medical follow-up
  - Recognize the signs and symptoms of heart failure
  - Adhere to activity limitations; alternate rest periods with activity

– Follow dietary restrictions and recommendations

- **Complications**
  - Heart failure
  - Pulmonary edema
  - Left ventricular hypertrophy
  - Endocarditis
  - Arrhythmias
- **Possible surgical interventions**
  - Aortic valve replacement
  - Commissurotomy

AORTIC INSUFFICIENCY

- **Definition**
  - Incomplete closure of the aortic valve
  - Also known as *aortic regurgitation*
- **Causes**
  - Rheumatic fever
  - Infective endocarditis
  - Syphilis
  - Atherosclerosis
  - Congenital defect
  - Hypertension
- **Pathophysiology**
  - Widening of the left ventricle of the heart occurs
  - Retrograde flow of blood from the aorta to the left ventricle
  - Left ventricular hypertrophy
- **Assessment findings**
  - Signs of left-sided heart failure
  - Dyspnea on exertion
  - Dizziness
  - Neck pain
  - Orthopnea
  - Anginal episodes
  - Tachycardia
  - Paroxysmal nocturnal dyspnea
  - Murmurs and clicks
- **Diagnostic test findings**
  - Chest X-ray: enlarged left ventricle, aortic valve calcification
  - ECG: left ventricular hypertrophy, sinus tachycardia
  - Echocardiogram: left ventricular enlargement, abnormal valve movement
  - Cardiac catheterization: increased left atrial and left ventricular pressures, insufficiency

Key complications of aortic stenosis
- Left ventricular hypertrophy
- Heart failure

Key facts about aortic insufficiency
- Retrograde flow of blood from the aorta to the left ventricle
- An incomplete closure of the aortic valve

Common causes of aortic insufficiency
- Hypertension
- Congenital defect
- Infective endocarditis

How aortic insufficiency happens
- Widening of left ventricle occurs
- Retrograde blood from aorta to left ventricle results in left ventricular hypertrophy

Key signs and symptoms of aortic insufficiency
- Signs of left-sided heart failure
- Dyspnea on exertion
- Dizziness
- Anginal episodes

Diagnosing aortic insufficiency
- Chest X-ray: enlarged left ventricle, aortic valve calcification
- Echocardiogram: left ventricular enlargement, abnormal valve movement

Treating aortic insufficiency

- Low-sodium diet; limit fluids
- Antibiotics
- Cardiac glycosides
- Nitrates
- Diuretics
- Vasodilators
- ACE inhibitors

Key nursing interventions for a patient with aortic insufficiency

- Maintain the patient's prescribed diet; restrict oral fluids.
- Administer I.V. fluids and medications, as necessary.
- Assess cardiovascular and respiratory status.
- Monitor and record vital signs, I/O, hemodynamic variables, and laboratory studies.

Key complications of aortic insufficiency

- Heart failure
- Left ventricular hypertrophy

Key facts about PVD

- Chronic inadequate blood flow in the lower extremities
- Three types: arteriosclerosis obliterans, Raynaud's phenomenon, and Buerger's disease

● Medical management

- Monitoring: vital signs, I/O, ECG, and hemodynamic variables
- Laboratory studies: ABGs, sodium, potassium, BUN, and creatinine
- Diet: low-sodium; limit fluids
- Antibiotic: penicillin G potassium (Pentids)
- Cardiac glycoside: digoxin (Lanoxin)
- Nitrates: isosorbide (Isordil), nitroglycerin (Nitro-Bid)
- Diuretics: furosemide (Lasix), bumetanide (Bumex)
- Vasodilators: hydralazine (Apresoline), nifedipine (Procardia)
- ACE inhibitors: captopril (Capoten), enalapril (Vasotec), lisinopril (Prinivil)

● Nursing interventions

- Assess cardiovascular and respiratory status
- Monitor and record vital signs, I/O, hemodynamic variables, and laboratory studies
- Assess pain level
- Administer I.V. fluids and medications, as prescribed
- Maintain the patient's prescribed diet; restrict oral fluids
- Provide emotional support to allay the patient's anxiety
- Provide information about the American Heart Association
- Individualize home care instructions
- Follow the disorder and treatment plan
  - Follow instructions for medication use
  - Comply with medical follow-up
  - Recognize the signs and symptoms of heart failure
  - Adhere to activity limitations; alternate rest periods with activity
  - Monitor for infection

● Complications

- Heart failure
- Thrombosis
- Embolism
- Infection
- Left ventricular hypertrophy

● Possible surgical interventions

- Valvuloplasty
- Valve replacement

PERIPHERAL VASCULAR DISEASE (PVD)

● Definition

- Chronic inadequate blood flow in the lower extremities

● Types

- Arteriosclerosis obliterans—sclerosis of arterioles resulting in thickening of the walls and occlusion
- Raynaud's phenomenon—intermittent vasoconstriction and ischemia of fingers and toes accompanied by pallor and cyanosis

- Buerger's disease (thromboangiitis obliterans)—inflammation of blood vessels resulting in occlusion of the vessel

● **Causes**
- Atherosclerosis
- Vasospasm
- Inflammation

● **Pathophysiology**
- Arterial thickening and loss of elasticity, narrowing the diameter of the artery
- Decreased perfusion and blood clot formation, causing arterial blockage and ischemia (common sites are the femoral, popliteal, and iliac arteries and the aorta)

● **Assessment findings**
- Intermittent claudication
- Pain in extremities at rest
- Trophic changes: thickened nails, absence of hair, and taut, shiny skin
- Diminished or absent pulses in extremities (a unilateral finding has greater significance than bilateral findings) (see *Managing diminished or absent pulse*, pages 50 and 51)
- Temperature changes in extremities
- Color changes in extremities: rubor, cyanosis, pallor
- Ulcerations in extremities

● **Diagnostic test findings**
- Arteriography: location of obstructing plaque
- Doppler studies: decreased blood flow and arterial pressure
- Blood chemistry: increased lipids

● **Medical management**
- Monitoring: vital signs, I/O, and neurovascular checks
- Activity: active ROM and isometric exercises, as tolerated
- Laboratory studies: serum lipids, PTT, and PT
- Diet: low-fat, low-calorie
- Bed cradle
- Antiplatelet agent: aspirin
- Vasodilator: pentoxifylline (Trental)
- Anticoagulant: warfarin (Coumadin)
- Antilipemics: cholestyramine (Questran), lovastatin (Mevacor)
- PTCA
- Laser angioplasty
- Vascular stents
- Thrombolytic therapy: streptokinase (Streptase)

● **Nursing interventions**
- Assess cardiovascular and neurovascular status
- Monitor and record vital signs, I/O, and laboratory studies

(Text continues on page 52.)

Common causes of PVD

- Atherosclerosis
- Inflammation

How PVD happens

- Arterial thickening and loss of elasticity
- Decreased perfusion and blood clot formation causes arterial blockage and ischemia

Key signs and symptoms of PVD

- Intermittent claudication
- Pain in extremities at rest
- Diminished or absent pulses in extremities
- Color changes in extremities: rubor, cyanosis, pallor

Diagnosing PVD

- Arteriography: location of obstruction
- Doppler studies: decreased blood flow and arterial pressure

Treating PVD

- Active ROM and isometric exercises, as tolerated
- Antiplatelet agent
- Vasodilator
- Anticoagulant
- Antilipemics

GO WITH THE FLOW

Managing diminished or absent pulse

A diminished or absent pulse can result from several life-threatening disorders. Your assessment and interventions will vary depending on whether the diminished or absent pulse is localized to one extremity or generalized. They will also depend on associated signs and symptoms. Use the decision tree here to help you establish priorities for managing this problem.

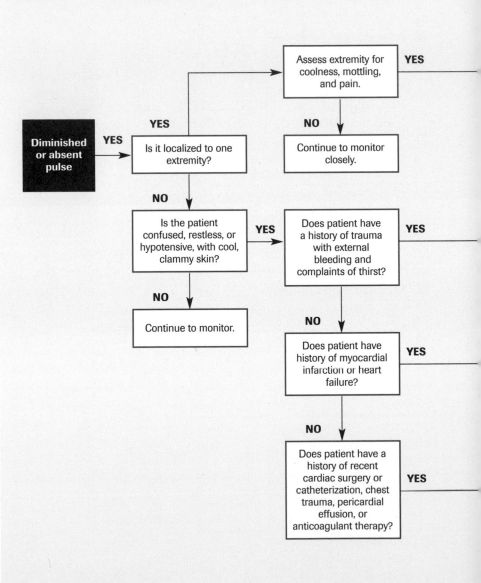

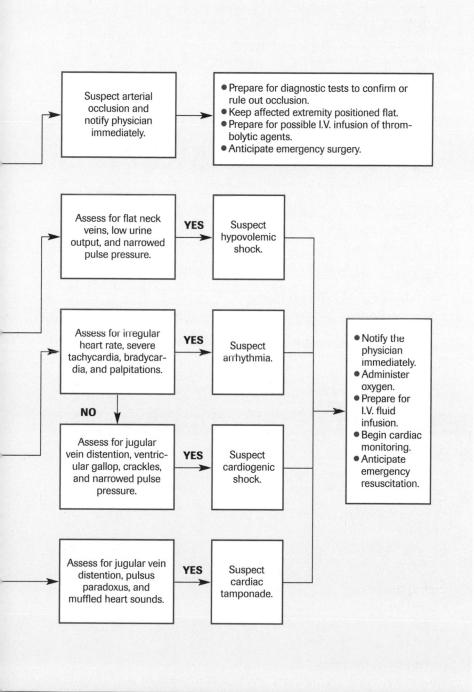

Suspect arterial occlusion and notify physician immediately.

- Prepare for diagnostic tests to confirm or rule out occlusion.
- Keep affected extremity positioned flat.
- Prepare for possible I.V. infusion of thrombolytic agents.
- Anticipate emergency surgery.

Assess for flat neck veins, low urine output, and narrowed pulse pressure.

YES → Suspect hypovolemic shock.

Assess for irregular heart rate, severe tachycardia, bradycardia, and palpitations.

YES → Suspect arrhythmia.

NO

Assess for jugular vein distention, ventricular gallop, crackles, and narrowed pulse pressure.

YES → Suspect cardiogenic shock.

Assess for jugular vein distention, pulsus paradoxus, and muffled heart sounds.

YES → Suspect cardiac tamponade.

- Notify the physician immediately.
- Administer oxygen.
- Prepare for I.V. fluid infusion.
- Begin cardiac monitoring.
- Anticipate emergency resuscitation.

Key nursing interventions for a patient with PVD

- Assess cardiovascular and neurovascular status.
- Check peripheral circulation.
- Encourage walking and leg exercises.
- Provide daily foot care.

Key complications of PVD

- Stasis ulcers
- Acute vascular occlusion

Key facts about thrombophlebitis

- Inflammation of the venous wall
- Clot formation occurs causing venous insufficiency

Common causes of thrombophlebitis

- Venous stasis
- Hypercoagulability

How thrombophlebitis happens

- Massing of RBCs in a fibrin network
- Obstruction of vein by enlarged thrombus

- Check peripheral circulation: pulses, color, temperature, and complaints of abnormal sensations, such as numbness or tingling
- Administer medications, as prescribed
- Encourage walking and other leg exercises
- Provide daily foot care
- Maintain the patient's prescribed diet
- Provide appropriate preoperative and postoperative care
- Individualize home care instructions
- Follow the disorder and treatment plan
  - Follow instructions for medication use
  - Comply with medical follow-up
  - Recognize the symptoms of decreased peripheral circulation
  - Monitor for skin breakdown
  - Care for the feet daily
  - Avoid activities or situations that will exacerbate the condition, such as temperature extremes, prolonged standing, constrictive clothing, or crossing the legs at the knee when seated

⬤ **Complications**
  - Gangrene
  - Septicemia
  - Stasis ulcers
  - Acute vascular occlusion

⬤ **Possible surgical interventions**
  - Bypass grafting
  - Endarterectomy
  - Sympathectomy
  - Amputation
  - Embolectomy

THROMBOPHLEBITIS

⬤ **Definition**
  - Inflammation of the venous wall, resulting in clot formation

⬤ **Causes**
  - Venous stasis (from varicose veins, pregnancy, heart failure, prolonged bed rest)
  - Hypercoagulability (from cancer, blood dyscrasias, oral contraceptives)
  - Injury to the venous wall (from I.V. injections, fractures, antibiotics)

⬤ **Pathophysiology**
  - Massing of RBCs in a fibrin network
  - Obstruction by enlarged thrombus, leading to venous insufficiency (common sites are deep veins and superficial veins)

⬤ **Assessment findings**
  - Superficial veins: red, warm skin that's tender to touch
  - Deep veins

- Major venous trunks: edema, positive Homans' sign, tender to touch, cramping pain, cyanosis, venous distention
- Small veins: tenderness, induration over muscle, minimal to no distention

● **Diagnostic test findings**
- Venography: venous-filling defects
- Ultrasound: decreased blood flow or occlusion
- Phlebography: venous-filling defects
- Hematology: increased WBC count

● **Medical management**
- Monitoring: vital signs and neurovascular checks
- Anticoagulants: heparin
- Position: elevation of the affected extremity
- Activity: bed rest; active and passive ROM and isometric exercises
- Laboratory studies: WBC, PT, and PTT
- Antiembolism stockings; warm, moist compresses
- Thrombolytic agent: streptokinase (Streptase)
- Anti-inflammatory agent: aspirin

● **Nursing interventions**
- Assess cardiovascular status
- Monitor and record vital signs, neurovascular checks, and laboratory studies
- Assess for Homans' sign
- Administer medications, as prescribed
- Monitor PTT and assess for bleeding
- Keep the patient in bed and elevate the affected extremity
- Apply warm, moist compresses
- Measure and record the circumference of thighs and calves
- Individualize home care instructions
- Follow the disorder and treatment plan
  - Follow instructions for medication use
  - Recognize the signs and symptoms of bleeding
  - Avoid prolonged sitting or standing, constrictive clothing, or crossing the legs when seated
  - Have blood drawn for prothrombin time if taking warfarin as directed

● **Complications**
- Pulmonary embolism
- Stroke
- MI
- Death

● **Possible surgical interventions**
- Vena cava filter
- Thrombectomy

ENDOCARDITIS

● **Definition**
  • Inflammation and infection of the endocardial lining

● **Causes**
  • Bacterial infection: beta-hemolytic streptococcus, *Staphylococcus aureus*
  • Rheumatic heart disease
  • Dental procedures or infection
  • Invasive monitoring
  • I.V. drug abuse

● **Pathophysiology**
  • Formation of bacterial colonies on the endocardial lining, destroying heart valve leaflets (see *Degenerative changes in endocarditis*)
  • Disrupted blood flow, resulting in murmurs
  • Vegetations that seed the bloodstream with bacteria

● **Assessment findings**
  • Elevated temperature
  • Heart murmur
  • Diaphoresis
  • Malaise
  • Anorexia
  • Chills
  • Dyspnea
  • Tachypnea
  • Crackles
  • Tachycardia
  • Arrhythmias
  • S_3, S_4
  • Peripheral edema
  • Clubbing of fingers and toes
  • Petechiae
  • Night sweats
  • Splinter hemorrhages in nail beds
  • Hematuria
  • Joint pain
  • Headache

● **Diagnostic test findings**
  • Blood cultures: positive for specific organism
  • Hematology: increased WBCs, ESR; decreased HCT
  • Echocardiography: valvular damage, vegetations

● **Medical management**
  • Oxygen therapy
  • Monitoring: vital signs, I/O, and neurovascular checks
  • Antibiotics: penicillin G potassium (Pentids), vancomycin (Vancocin), cefazolin (Ancef), depending on organism

---

Key facts about endocarditis

• Inflammation and infection of the endocardial lining
• Caused by formation of bacterial colonies on the endocardial lining, destroying heart valve leaflets

Common causes of endocarditis

• Bacterial infection
• Rheumatic heart disease

How endocarditis happens

• Bacterial colonies form on endocardial lining
• Heart valve leaflets are destroyed
• Blood flow is disrupted

Key signs and symptoms of endocarditis

• Elevated temperature
• Heart murmur
• Malaise

Diagnosing endocarditis

• Blood cultures: positive for specific organism
• Echocardiography: valvular damage, vegetations

Treating endocarditis

• Antibiotics
• Positive inotropic agents
• Antipyretics
• Anticoagulants

Degenerative changes in endocarditis

This illustration shows typical vegetations on the endocardium produced by fibrin and platelet deposits on infection sites.

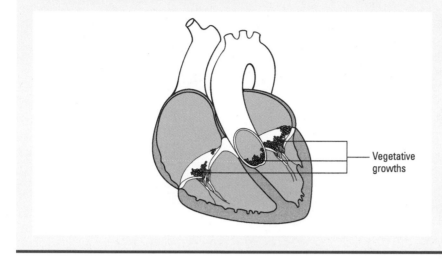

Vegetative growths

- Laboratory studies: blood cultures, WBC, and HCT
- I.V. therapy: hydration
- Activity: bed rest
- Positive inotropic agents: digoxin (Lanoxin), dobutamine (Dobutrex)
- Fluids: increased intake
- Antipyretic: aspirin
- Anticoagulant: warfarin (Coumadin)

● **Nursing interventions**
- Assess cardiovascular status
- Monitor and record vital signs, I/O, and laboratory studies
- Administer I.V. fluids, oxygen, and medications, as prescribed
- Encourage fluids
- Provide emotional support to allay the patient's anxiety
- Encourage rest periods
- Individualize home care instructions
- Follow the disorder and treatment plan
  - Follow instructions for medication use
  - Comply with medical follow-up
  - Follow activity limitations; alternate rest periods with activity, and adhere to the prescribed exercise regimen
  - Avoid exposure to people with infections; monitor self for infection, particularly after a dental or gynecologic examination; and seek treatment if infection develops
  - Wear medical identification

● **Complications**
- Embolism

Key complications of endocarditis

- Embolism
- Stroke
- Arrhythmias

Key facts about abdominal aortic aneurysm

- Dilation of or localized weakness in the medial layer of an abdominal artery
- Four types: saccular, fusiform, dissecting, and false

Common causes of abdominal aortic aneurysm

- Atherosclerosis
- Hypertension
- Smoking

How abdominal aortic aneurysm happens

- Degenerative changes weaken the medial layer of the artery
- Force of blood flow causes out-pouching

Key signs and symptoms of aortic aneurysm

- Lower abdominal pain, lower back pain
- Abdominal mass to the left of the midline
- Abdominal pulsations
- Bruits

- Heart failure
- Mycotic aneurysm
- Stroke
- Arrhythmias
- Brain abscess

● **Possible surgical intervention**
- Valve replacement

ABDOMINAL AORTIC ANEURYSM

● **Definition**
- Dilation of or localized weakness in the medial layer of an abdominal artery
- Four types: saccular, fusiform, dissecting, false (see *Types of aortic aneurysms*)

● **Causes**
- Most common
  - Atherosclerosis
  - Hypertension
  - Smoking
- Less common
  - Congenital defect
  - Trauma
  - Syphilis
  - Infection
  - Marfan syndrome

● **Pathophysiology**
- Degenerative changes from atherosclerosis, weakening the medial layer of artery
- Continued weakening from the force of blood flow, resulting in out-pouching of the artery

● **Assessment findings**
- Asymptomatic
- Lower abdominal pain, lower back pain
- Abdominal mass to the left of the midline
- Abdominal pulsations
- Bruits
- Diminished femoral pulses
- Systolic blood pressure in the legs lower than that in the arms
- Deep, diffuse chest pain
- Hoarse voice
- Coughing
- Dyspnea
- Dysphagia
- Jugular vein distention
- Edema

Types of aortic aneurysms

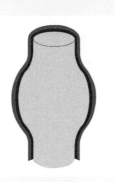
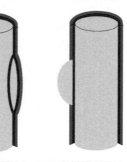
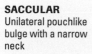
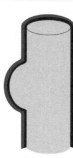

SACCULAR
Unilateral pouchlike bulge with a narrow neck

FUSIFORM
A spindle-shaped bulge encompassing the entire diameter of the vessel

DISSECTING
A hemorrhagic separation of the medial layer of the vessel wall, which creates a false lumen

FALSE ANEURYSM
A pulsating hematoma resulting from trauma and often mistaken for an abdominal aneurysm

Diagnostic test findings
- CT scan: reveals aneurysm size and location
- ECG: differentiation of aneurysm from MI
- Abdominal ultrasound: aneurysm
- Aortography: aneurysm

Medical management
- Monitoring: vital signs, I/O, and neurovascular checks
- Activity: bed rest
- Analgesic: oxycodone, morphine
- Beta-adrenergic blocker: propranolol (Inderal)
- Antihypertensives: methyldopa (Aldomet), hydralazine (Apresoline), prazosin (Minipress)

Nursing interventions
- Assess cardiovascular status
- Monitor and record vital signs, I/O, neurovascular checks, and laboratory studies
- Check peripheral circulation: pulses, temperature, color, and complaints of abnormal sensations
- Assess pain level
- Administer medications, as prescribed
- Provide emotional support to allay the patient's anxiety
- Observe the patient for signs of shock, such as anxiety; restlessness; decreased pulse pressure; increased thready pulse; and pale, cool, moist, clammy skin
- Provide preoperative and postoperative care, as indicated
- Individualize home care instructions

Types of abdominal aortic aneurysm
- Saccular: unilateral; pouchlike bulge
- Fusiform: spindle-shaped bulge; encompasses entire diameter of vessel
- Dissecting: hemorrhagic separation of medial layer of vessel wall; creates a false lumen
- False: pulsating hematoma; often mistaken for an abdominal aneurysm

Diagnosing abdominal aortic aneurysm
- Aneurysm apparent on chest X-ray, abdominal ultrasound, and aortography
- CT scan—reveals aneurysm size and location

Treating abdominal aortic aneurysm
- Analgesics
- Beta-adrenergic blockers
- Antihypertensives
- Resection with graft repair

Key nursing interventions for a patient with abdominal aortic aneurysm
- Check peripheral circulation: pulses, temperature, color, and complaints of abnormal sensations.
- Observe the patient for signs of shock, such as anxiety; restlessness; decreased pulse pressure; increased thready pulse; and pale, cool, moist, clammy skin.

- Follow the disorder and treatment plan
  - Follow instructions for medication use
  - Comply with medical follow-up
  - Recognize the signs and symptoms of decreased peripheral circulation, such as change in skin color or temperature, complaints of numbness or tingling, and absent pulses
  - Adhere to activity limitations, alternate rest periods with activity, and adhere to prescribed exercise regimen
  - Maintain a quiet environment

● **Complications**
- Rupture of aneurysm
- Hemorrhage
- Renal failure
- Death

● **Possible surgical interventions**
- Resection of aneurysm
- Endovascular graft repair

CARDIOMYOPATHY

● **Definition**
- Disease of the muscle of the heart impacting the structure and function of the ventricle
- Types
  - Congestive (dilated)
  - Hypertrophic—two types
    - More common form is caused by pressure overload-hypertension or aortic valve stenosis
    - Hypertrophic obstructive cardiomyopathy is due to a genetic abnormality
  - Restrictive (obliterative)

● **Causes**
- Viral infection
- Metabolic and immunologic disorders
- Pregnancy and postpartum disorders
- Congenital
- Ischemia
- Drug abuse
- Chronic alcoholism (congestive)
- Severe, chronic hypertension
- Idiopathic hypertrophic subaortic stenosis (hypertrophic)
- Amyloidosis (restrictive)
- Cancer and other infiltrative diseases (restrictive)

● **Pathophysiology**
- Weakened heart muscle occurs from primary disorder or infection

---

Key complications of abdominal aortic aneurysm

- Rupture
- Hemorrhage
- Renal failure

Key facts about cardiomyopathy

- Disease of the heart's muscle impacting the structure and function of the ventricle
- Types include:
- Congestive (dilated)
- Hypertrophic
- Hypertrophic obstructive
- Restrictive (obliterative)

Common causes of cardiomyopathy

- Viral infection
- Ischemia
- Metabolic and immunologic disorders

- Cardiac function is altered, resulting in decreased cardiac output
- Increased heart rate and increased muscle mass compensate in early stages
- Heart failure develops in later stages
- Myocardium becomes flabby

● **Assessment findings**
- Major manifestations
  - Dyspnea
  - Dry cough
  - Fatigue
  - Palpitations
  - Weakness
- Other manifestations
  - Signs and symptoms of heart failure
  - Paroxysmal nocturnal dyspnea
  - Jugular vein distention
  - Dependent pitting edema
  - Enlarged liver
  - Murmur
  - Crackles
  - S_3, S_4

● **Diagnostic test findings**
- ECG: left ventricular hypertrophy
- Echocardiogram: decreased myocardial function
- Cardiac catheterization: rule out CAD
- Chest X-ray: cardiomegaly

● **Medical management**
- Oxygen therapy
- Monitoring: vital signs, ECG, hemodynamic variables, and I/O
- Bed rest
- Position: semi-Fowler's
- Laboratory studies: ABGs, sodium, potassium, CK and LD with isoenzymes
- Diet: low-sodium, vitamin supplements
- I.V. therapy
- Left ventricular assist device
- IABP
- Arterial line for blood pressure monitoring
- Diuretics: furosemide (Lasix), bumetanide (Bumex), metolazone (Zaroxolyn)
- Beta-adrenergic blockers: propranolol (Inderal), nadolol (Corgard), metoprolol (Lopressor)
- Calcium channel blockers: verapamil (Calan), diltiazem (Cardizem), nifedipine (Procardia), nicardipine (Cardene)
- ACE inhibitors: captopril (Capoten), enalapril (Vasotec), lisinopril (Prinivil)

How cardiomyopathy happens
- Illness causes weakened heart muscle
- Cardiac function is altered
- Increased muscle mass develops with myocardium becoming flabby

Key signs and symptoms of cardiomyopathy
- Dyspnea
- Dry cough
- Fatigue
- Palpitations
- Weakness

Diagnosing cardiomyopathy
- ECG: left ventricular hypertrophy
- Echocardiogram: decreased myocardial function
- Chest X-ray: cardiomegaly

Treating cardiomyopathy
- Oxygen therapy
- Left ventricular assist device
- Diuretics
- Beta-adrenergic blockers
- Calcium channel blockers
- ACE inhibitors
- Anticoagulants

Key nursing interventions for a patient with cardiomyopathy

- Administer oxygen and medications as prescribed.
- Keep the patient in semi-Fowler's position.
- Monitor ECG results.

Key complications of cardiomyopathy

- Heart failure
- Death

Key facts about cardiac arrhythmias

- Abnormal electrical conduction or automaticity
- Alter heart rate and rhythm

Common causes of cardiac arrhythmias

- MI
- Electrolyte imbalance
- Acid-base imbalances

- Anticoagulant: warfarin (Coumadin)
- **Nursing interventions**
  - Assess cardiovascular and respiratory status
  - Monitor and record vital signs, I/O, hemodynamic variables, laboratory studies, and ECG results
  - Administer oxygen and medications, as prescribed
  - Maintain bed rest
  - Keep the patient in semi-Fowler's position
  - Provide emotional support to allay the patient's anxiety
  - Maintain the patient's prescribed diet
  - Provide information about the American Heart Association
  - Individualize home care instructions
  - Follow the disorder and treatment plan
    - Follow instructions for medication use
    - Comply with medical follow-up
    - Recognize signs and symptoms of heart failure
    - Avoid straining during bowel movements
    - Monitor pulses and blood pressure
    - Weigh daily and report increases over 3 lb (1.4 kg)
    - Demonstrate exercises to increase cardiac output (raising arms)
    - Refrain from smoking and drinking alcohol
- **Complications**
  - Heart failure
  - Arterial emboli
  - Arrhythmia
  - Death
- **Possible surgical interventions**
  - Ventricular myomectomy
  - Heart transplant

CARDIAC ARRHYTHMIAS

- **Definition**
  - Abnormal electrical conduction or automaticity causing changes in heart rate and rhythm
- **Causes**
  - Congenital
  - Myocardial ischemia
  - MI
  - Organic heart disease
  - Drug effects and toxicity
  - Conductive tissue degeneration
  - Electrolyte imbalance
  - Acid-base imbalances

- Cellular hypoxia
- **Pathophysiology**
  - Result from a disturbance in excitability, automaticity, or conductivity
  - Heart rate and rhythm are altered, reducing cardiac output
- **Assessment findings**
  - Asymptomatic
  - Palpitations
  - Chest pain
  - Dizziness
  - Weakness, fatigue
  - Feelings of impending doom
  - Irregular heart rhythm
  - Bradycardia or tachycardia
  - Hypotension
  - Syncope
  - Altered LOC
  - Diaphoresis
  - Pallor
  - Nausea, vomiting
  - Cold, clammy skin
  - Life-threatening arrhythmias may result in pulselessness, absence of respirations, and no palpable blood pressure
- **Possible diagnostic findings**
  - ECG: changes in heart rate, rhythm (see *Types of cardiac arrhythmias*, pages 62 to 69)
  - Blood chemistry: electrolyte imbalance, toxic drug levels
- **Medical management** (see *Types of cardiac arrhythmias*, pages 62 to 69)
- **Nursing interventions**
  - Assess cardiovascular, respiratory, and neurovascular status; observe for arrhythmias if the patient is receiving continuous cardiac monitoring
  - If the patient has an arrhythmia, promptly assess airway, breathing, and circulation
  - Perform cardiopulmonary resuscitation (CPR), if indicated, until other advanced cardiac life support (ACLS) measures are available and successful
  - Perform defibrillation for ventricular tachycardia and ventricular fibrillation
  - Administer medications, oxygen, and I.V. fluids, as needed
  - Prepare for procedures, such as cardioversion or pacemaker insertion, if indicated
  - Assess for predisposing factors (such as fluid and electrolyte imbalance) and signs of drug toxicity, especially digoxin; correct the underlying cause—for example, if the patient has a toxic reaction to a drug, withhold the next dose

(Text continues on page 69.)

How cardiac arrhythmias happen

- Disturbance in excitability, automaticity, or conductivity occurs
- Heart rate and rhythm are altered

Key signs and symptoms of cardiac arrhythmia

- Chest pain
- Irregular heart rhythm
- Bradycardia or tachycardia
- Hypotension
- Syncope
- Diaphoresis

Diagnosing cardiac arrhythmias

- ECG: changes in heart rate and rhythm
- Blood chemistry: electrolyte imbalance

Key nursing interventions for a patient with a cardiac arrhythmia

- Observe for arrhythmias.
- If the patient has an arrhythmia, promptly assess airway, breathing, and circulation.
- Perform CPR, if indicated, until other ACLS measures are available and successful.
- Perform defibrillation for ventricular tachycardia and ventricular fibrillation.
- Prepare for procedures, such as cardioversion or pacemaker insertion, if indicated.

ECG characteristics: Sinus arrhythmia

- Irregular atrial and ventricular rhythms
- Normal P wave preceding each QRS complex

ECG characteristics: Sinus tachycardia

- Atrial and ventricular rhythms regular
- Rate > 100 beats/minute; rarely > 160 beats/minute
- Normal P wave preceding each QRS complex

ECG characteristics: Sinus bradycardia

- Atrial and ventricular rhythms regular
- Rate < 60 beats/minute
- Normal P waves preceding each QRS complex

Types of cardiac arrrhythmias

This chart reviews many common cardiac arrhythmias and outlines their features, causes, and treatments. Use a normal electrocardiogram strip, if available, to compare normal cardiac rhythm configurations with the rhythm strips below. Characteristics of normal sinus rhythm include:

- ventricular and atrial rates of 60 to 100 beats/minute
- regular and uniform QRS complexes and P waves
- PR interval of 0.12 to 0.20 second
- QRS duration < 0.12 second
- identical atrial and ventricular rates, with consistent PR interval.

ARRHYTHMIA AND FEATURES	CAUSES	TREATMENT
Sinus arrhythmia 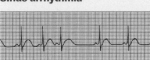 • Irregular atrial and ventricular rhythms • Normal P wave preceding each QRS complex	• A normal variation of normal sinus rhythm in athletes, children, and elderly people • Also seen with digoxin toxicity and inferior wall myocardial infarction (MI)	• Atropine if rate decreases below 40 beats/minute and the patient is symptomatic
Sinus tachycardia • Atrial and ventricular rhythms regular • Rate > 100 beats/minute; rarely, > 160 beats/minute • Normal P wave preceding each QRS complex	• Normal physiologic response to fever, exercise, anxiety, pain, dehydration; may also accompany shock, left ventricular failure, cardiac tamponade, hyperthyroidism, anemia, hypovolemia, pulmonary embolism, and anterior wall MI • May also occur with atropine, epinephrine, isoproterenol, quinidine, caffeine, alcohol, and nicotine use	• Correction of underlying cause • Beta-adrenergic blockers or calcium channel blockers for symptomatic patients
Sinus bradycardia • Atrial and ventricular rhythms regular • Rate < 60 beats/minute • Normal P waves preceding each QRS complex	• Normal, in well-conditioned heart, as in an athlete • Increased intracranial pressure; increased vagal tone due to straining during defecation, vomiting, intubation, mechanical ventilation; sick sinus syndrome, hypothyroidism; inferior wall MI • May also occur with anticholinesterase, beta-adrenergic blocker, digoxin, and morphine use	• Correction of underlying cause • For low cardiac output, dizziness, weakness, altered level of consciousness, or low blood pressure; advanced cardiac life support (ACLS) protocol for administration of atropine • Temporary pacemaker or permanent pacemaker • Dopamine or epinephrine infusion

Types of cardiac arrhythmias *(continued)*

ARRHYTHMIA AND FEATURES	CAUSES	TREATMENT
Sinoatrial arrest or block (sinus arrest) ![ECG strip] • Atrial and ventricular rhythms regular except for missing complex • Normal P waves preceding each QRS complex, missing during pause • Pause not equal to a multiple of the previous sinus rhythm	• Acute infection • Coronary artery disease, degenerative heart disease, acute inferior wall MI • Vagal stimulation, Valsalva's maneuver, carotid sinus massage • Digoxin, quinidine, or salicylate toxicity • Pesticide poisoning • Pharyngeal irritation caused by endotracheal (ET) intubation • Sick sinus syndrome	• Correction of underlying cause • Treat symptoms with atropine I.V. • Temporary or permanent pacemaker for repeated symptomatic episodes
Wandering atrial pacemaker ![ECG strip] • Atrial and ventricular rhythms slightly irregular • PR interval varies • P waves irregular with changing configuration, indicating that they're not all from sinoatrial (SA) node or single atrial focus; may appear after the QRS complex • QRS complexes uniform in shape but irregular in rhythm	• Rheumatic carditis due to inflammation involving the SA node • Digoxin toxicity • Sick sinus syndrome	• No treatment if patient is asymptomatic • Treatment of underlying cause if patient is symptomatic
Premature atrial contraction (PAC) 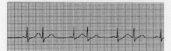 • Premature, abnormal-looking P waves that differ in configuration from normal P waves • QRS complexes after P waves, except in very early or blocked PACs • P wave often buried in the preceding T wave or identified in the preceding T wave	• Coronary or valvular heart disease, atrial ischemia, coronary atherosclerosis, heart failure, acute respiratory failure, chronic obstructive pulmonary disease (COPD), electrolyte imbalance, and hypoxia • Digoxin toxicity; use of aminophylline, adrenergics, or caffeine • Anxiety	• Usually no treatment needed • Treatment of underlying cause

(continued)

ECG characteristics: Sinoatrial arrest or block

• Atrial and ventricular rhythms regular except for missing complex
• Normal P waves preceding each QRS complex, missing during pause
• Pause not equal to a multiple of the previous sinus rhythm

ECG characteristics: Wandering atrial pacemaker

• Atrial and ventricular rhythms slightly irregular
• PR interval varies
• P waves irregular with changing configuration, indicating that they aren't all from SA node or single atrial focus; may appear after the QRS complex
• QRS complexes uniform in shape but irregular in rhythm

ECG characteristics: Premature atrial contraction

• Premature, abnormal-looking P waves that differ in configuration from normal P waves
• QRS complexes after P waves, except in very early or blocked PACs
• P wave often buried in the preceding T wave or identified in the preceding T wave

ECG characteristics: Paroxysmal supraventricular tachycardia

- Atrial and ventricular rhythms regular
- Heart rate > 160 beats/minute; rarely exceeds 250 beats/minute
- P waves regular but aberrant; difficult to differentiate from preceding T wave
- P wave preceding each QRS complex
- Sudden onset and termination of arrhythmia

ECG characteristics: Atrial flutter

- Atrial rhythm regular, rate 250 to 400 beats/minute
- Ventricular rate variable, depending on degree of AV block (usually 60 to 100 beats/minute)
- Sawtooth P-wave configuration possible (F waves)
- QRS complexes uniform in shape but often irregular in rate

ECG characteristics: Atrial fibrillation

- Atrial rhythm grossly irregular; rate > 400 beats/minute
- Ventricular rate grossly irregular
- QRS complexes of uniform configuration and duration
- PR interval indiscernible
- No P waves, or P waves that appear as erratic, irregular, baseline fibrillatory waves

---

Types of cardiac arrhythmias *(continued)*

ARRHYTHMIA AND FEATURES	CAUSES	TREATMENT
Paroxysmal supraventricular tachycardia 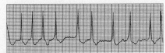 ● Atrial and ventricular rhythms regular ● Heart rate > 160 beats/minute; rarely exceeds 250 beats/minute ● P waves regular but aberrant; difficult to differentiate from preceding T wave ● P wave preceding each QRS complex ● Sudden onset and termination of arrhythmia	● Intrinsic abnormality of atrioventricular (AV) conduction system ● Physical or psychological stress, hypoxia, hypokalemia, cardiomyopathy, congenital heart disease, MI, valvular disease, Wolff-Parkinson-White syndrome, cor pulmonale, hyperthyroidism, and systemic hypertension ● Digoxin toxicity; use of caffeine, marijuana, or central nervous system stimulants	● If patient is unstable: immediate cardioversion ● If patient is stable: vagal stimulation, Valsalva's manuever, and carotid sinus massage ● If cardiac function is preserved, treatment priority: adenosine, calcium channel blocker, beta-adrenergic blocker, digoxin, and cardioversion; then consider amiodarone, procainamide, or sotalol if each preceding treatment is ineffective in rhythm conversion ● If the ejection fraction is less than 40% or if the patient is in heart failure, treatment order: digoxin, amiodarone, then diltiazem.
Atrial flutter ● Atrial rhythm regular, rate 250 to 400 beats/minute ● Ventricular rate variable, depending on degree of AV block (usually 60 to 100 beats/minute) ● Sawtooth P-wave configuration possible (F waves) ● QRS complexes uniform in shape but often irregular in rate	● Heart failure, tricuspid or mitral valve disease, pulmonary embolism, cor pulmonale, inferior wall MI, and carditis ● Digoxin toxicity	● If patient is unstable with a ventricular rate > 150 beats/minute, immediate cardioversion. ● If patient is stable, drug therapy may include calcium channel blockers, diltiazem, beta-adrenergic blockers, or antiarrhythmics. ● Anticoagulation therapy (heparin, enoxparin [Lovenox], or warfarin) may also be necessary ● Radiofrequency ablation to control rhythm
Atrial fibrillation ● Atrial rhythm grossly irregular; rate > 400 beats/minute ● Ventricular rate grossly irregular ● QRS complexes of uniform configuration and duration ● PR interval indiscernible ● No P waves, or P waves that appear as erratic, irregular, baseline fibrillatory waves	● Heart failure, COPD, thyrotoxicosis, constrictive pericarditis, ischemic heart disease, sepsis, pulmonary embolus, rheumatic heart disease, hypertension, mitral stenosis, atrial irritation, complication of coronary bypass or valve replacement surgery ● Nifedipine and digoxin use	● If patient is unstable with a ventricular rate > 150 beats/minute, immediate cardioversion. ● If patient is stable, follow ACLS protocol for cardioversion and drug therapy which may include calcium channel blockers, beta-adrenergic blockers, or antiarrhythmics ● Anticoagulants, such as heparin, enoxaparin, or warfarin

Types of cardiac arrhythmias *(continued)*

ARRHYTHMIA AND FEATURES	CAUSES	TREATMENT
Atrial fibrillation *(continued)*		• Class III antiarrhythmic, dofetilide (Tikosyn) for conversion of atrial fibrillation and atrial flutter to normal sinus rhythm • Radiofrequency catheter ablation to the His bundle to interrupt all conduction between atria and the ventricles (in resistant patients with recurring symptomatic atrial fibrillation) • Maze procedure in which sutures are placed in stragetic places in the atrial myocardium to prevent electrical circuits from developing perpetuating atrial fibrillation
Premature junctional contractions (junctional premature beats) • Atrial and ventricular rhythms irregular • P waves inverted; may precede, be hidden within, or follow QRS complex • PR interval < 0.12 second if P wave precedes QRS complex • QRS complex configuration and duration normal	• MI or ischemia • Digoxin toxicity and excessive caffeine or amphetamine use	• Correction of underlying cause • Discontinuation of digoxin if appropriate
Junctional rhythm • Atrial and ventricular rhythms regular; atrial rate 40 to 60 beats/minute; ventricular rate usually 40 to 60 beats/minute (60 to 100 beats/minute is accelerated junctional rhythm) • P waves preceding, hidden within (absent), or after QRS complex; inverted if visible • PR interval (when present) < 0.12 second • QRS complex configuration and duration normal, except in aberrant conduction	• Inferior wall MI or ischemia, hypoxia, vagal stimulation, sick sinus syndrome • Acute rheumatic fever • Valve surgery • Digoxin toxicity	• Correction of underlying cause • Atropine for symptomatic slow rate • Pacemaker insertion if patient doesn't respond to drugs • Discontinuation of digoxin if appropriate

(continued)

ECG characteristics: Premature junctional contractions

- Atrial and ventricular rhythms irregular
- P waves inverted; may precede, be hidden within, or follow QRS complex
- PR Interval < 0.12 second if P wave precedes QRS complex
- QRS complex configuration and duration normal

ECG characteristics: Junctional rhythm

- Atrial and ventricular rhythms regular; atrial rate 40 to 60 beats/minute; ventricular rate usually 40 to 60 beats/minute (60 to 100 beats/minute is accelerated junctional rhythm)
- P waves preceding, hidden within (absent), or after QRS complex; inverted if visible
- PR interval (when present) < 0.12 second
- QRS complex configuration and duration normal, except in aberrant conduction

ECG characteristics: Junctional tachycardia

- Atrial and ventricular rhythms regular
- Atrial rate > 100 beats/minute
- Ventricular rate > 100 beats/ minute
- P wave inverted; may occur before or after QRS complex, may be hidden in QRS complex, or may be absent
- QRS complex configuration and duration normal

ECG characteristics: First-degree AV block

- Atrial and ventricular rhythms regular
- PR interval > 0.20 second
- P wave precedes QRS complex
- QRS complex normal

ECG characteristics: Second-degree AV block (Mobitz I)

- Atrial rhythm regular
- Ventricular rhythm irregular
- Atrial rate exceeds ventricular rate
- PR interval progressively longer with each cycle until QRS complex disappears; PR interval shorter after dropped beat

ECG characteristics: Second-degree AV block (Mobitz II)

- Atrial rhythm regular
- Ventricular rhythm regular or ir- regular; varying degree of block
- PR interval constant except with dropped beat
- QRS complexes periodically absent

Types of cardiac arrhythmias *(continued)*

ARRHYTHMIA AND FEATURES	CAUSES	TREATMENT
Junctional tachycardia • Atrial and ventricular rhythms regular • Atrial rate > 100 beats/minute; however, P waves may be absent, hidden in QRS complex, or preceding T wave • Ventricular rate > 100 beats/minute • P wave inverted; may occur before or after QRS complex, may be hidden in QRS complex, or may be absent • QRS complex configuration and duration normal	• Myocarditis, cardio-myopathy, inferior wall MI or ischemia, acute rheumatic fever, complication of valve replacement surgery • Digoxin toxicity	• Correction of underlying cause • Beta-adrenergic blockers, calcium channel blockers, or amiodarone • Discontinuation of digoxin if appropriate
First-degree AV block • Atrial and ventricular rhythms regular • PR interval > 0.20 second • P wave precedes QRS complex • QRS complex normal	• May be seen in a healthy person • Inferior wall MI or ischemia, hypothyroidism, hypokalemia, hyperkalemia • Digoxin toxicity; use of quinidine, procainamide, or beta-adrenergic or calcium channel blockers, or amiodarone	• Correction of underlying cause • Possibly atropine if severe bradycardia develops, and the patient is symptomatic • Cautious use of digoxin, calcium channel blockers, and beta-adrenergic blockers
Second-degree AV block Mobitz I (Wenckebach) • Atrial rhythm regular • Ventricular rhythm irregular • Atrial rate exceeds ventricular rate • PR interval progressively longer, but only slightly, with each cycle until QRS complex disappears (dropped beat); PR interval shorter after dropped beat	• Inferior wall MI, cardiac surgery, acute rheumatic fever, and vagal stimulation • Digoxin toxicity; use of propranolol, quinidine, or procainamide	• Treatment of underlying cause • Atropine or temporary pacemaker for symptom-producing bradycardia • Discontinuation of digoxin if appropriate
Second-degree AV block Mobitz II • Atrial rhythm regular • Ventricular rhythm regular or irregular, with varying degree of block • PR interval constant, except with dropped beat • QRS complexes periodically absent	• Severe coronary artery disease, anterior wall MI, acute myocarditis • Digoxin toxicity	• Temporary or permanent pacemaker • Atropine, dopamine, or epinephrine for symptom-producing bradycardia • Discontinuation of digoxin if appropriate

Types of cardiac arrhythmias *(continued)*

ARRHYTHMIA AND FEATURES	CAUSES	TREATMENT
Third-degree AV block (complete heart block) • Atrial rhythm regular • Ventricular rate slow and rhythm regular • No relation between P waves and QRS complexes • No constant PR interval • QRS interval normal (nodal pacemaker) or wide and bizarre (ventricular pacemaker) rates regular • PR interval varies • P wave may be buried in QRS complexes or T wave • QRS complex normal	• Inferior or anterior wall MI, congenital abnormality, rheumatic fever, hypoxia, postoperative complication of mitral valve replacement, Lev's disease (fibrosis and calcification that spreads from cardiac structures to the conductive tissue), Lenegre's disease (conductive tissue fibrosis) • Digoxin toxicity	• Temporary or permanent pacemaker • Atropine may be used cautiously; likely ineffective in a wide-complex QRS rhythm • Dopamine or epinephrine for symptom-producing bradycardia
Premature ventricular contraction (PVC) • Atrial rhythm regular • Ventricular rhythm irregular • QRS complex premature, usually followed by a complete compensatory pause • QRS complex wide and distorted, usually > 0.14 second • Premature QRS complexes occurring singly, in pairs, or in threes, alternating with normal beats; focus from one or more sites • Ominous when clustered, multifocal, with R wave on T pattern	• Heart failure; old or acute MI, ischemia, or contusion; myocardial irritation by ventricular catheter or a pacemaker; hypercapnia; hypokalemia; hypocalcemia • Drug toxicity (cardiac glycosides, aminophylline, tricyclic antidepressants, beta-adrenergic blockers [isoproterenol or dopamine]) • Caffeine, tobacco, or alcohol use • Psychological stress, anxiety, pain, exercise	• If warranted, amiodarone, procainamide, or lidocaine I.V. • Treatment of underlying cause • Discontinuation of drug causing toxicity • Potassium chloride rider I.V. if PVC induced by hypokalemia • Magnesium sulfate I.V. if PVC induced by hypomagnesemia

ECG characteristics: Third-degree AV block

- Atrial rhythm regular
- Ventricular rate slow and rhythm regular
- No relation between P waves and QRS complexes
- No constant PR interval
- QRS interval normal (nodal pacemaker) or wide and bizarre (ventricular pacemaker) rates regular
- PR interval varies
- P wave may be buried in QRS complexes or T wave
- QRS complex normal

ECG characteristics: PVC

- Atrial rhythm regular
- Ventricular rhythm irregular
- QRS complex premature, usually followed by a complete compensatory pause
- QRS complex wide and distorted, usually > 0.14 second
- Premature QRS complexes occurring singly, in pairs, or in threes, alternating with normal beats; focus from one or more sites
- Ominous when clustered, multifocal, with R wave on T pattern

(continued)

ECG characteristics: Ventricular tachycardia

- Ventricular rate 140 to 220 beats/minute, rhythm regular or irregular
- QRS complexes wide, bizarre, and independent of P waves
- P waves not discernible
- May start and stop suddenly

ECG characteristics: Ventricular fibrillation

- Ventricular rhythm chaotic; rate rapid
- QRS complexes wide and irregular; no visible P waves

Types of cardiac arrhythmias *(continued)*

ARRHYTHMIA AND FEATURES	CAUSES	TREATMENT
Ventricular tachycardia 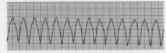 • Ventricular rate 140 to 220 beats/minute, rhythm regular or irregular • QRS complexes wide, bizarre, and independent of P waves • P waves not discernible • May start and stop suddenly	• Myocardial ischemia, infarction, or aneurysm; coronary artery disease; rheumatic heart disease; mitral valve prolapse; heart failure; cardiomyopathy; ventricular catheters; hypokalemia; hypercalcemia; pulmonary embolism • Digoxin, procainamide, epinephrine, or quinidine toxicity • Anxiety	• Pulseless: Initiate cardiopulmonary resuscitation (CPR); follow ACLS protocol for defibrillation, ET intubation, and administration of epinephrine or vasopressin, followed by amiodarone or lidocaine; if ineffective, magnesium sulfate or procainamide. • With pulse: If hemodynamically stable monomorphic VT follow ACLS protocol for administration of amiodarone, procainamide, sotalol, or lidocaine; if drugs are ineffective, initiate synchronized cardioversion. • If polymorphic VT, follow ACLS protocol for administration of amiodarone, beta-adrenergic blockers, lidocaine, procainamide, or sotalol. If drugs are ineffective, initiate synchronized cardioversion. • If torsades: administer magnesium, then overdose pacing if rythm perisists; isoproterenol, phenytoin, or lidocaine may also be given. • Implanted cardioverter defibrillator if recurrent VT
Ventricular fibrillation 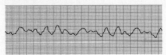 • Ventricular rhythm chaotic; rate rapid • QRS complexes wide and irregular; no visible P waves	• Myocardial ischemia or infarction, untreated ventricular tachycardia, R-on-T phenomenon, hypokalemia, hyperkalemia, hypercalcemia, alkalosis, electric shock, hypothermia • Digoxin, epinephrine, or quinidine toxicity	• Initiate CPR; follow ACLS protocol for defibrillation, ET intubation, and administration of epinephrine or vasopressin, followed by amiodarone, lidocaine or, if ineffective, magnesium sulfate or procainamide. • Implantable cardioverter defibrillator if risk for recurrent ventricular fibrillation

Types of cardiac arrhythmias *(continued)*

ARRHYTHMIA AND FEATURES	CAUSES	TREATMENT
Asystole • No atrial or ventricular rate or rhythm • No discernible P waves, QRS complexes, or T waves	• Myocardial ischemia or infarction, aortic valve disease, heart failure, hypoxia, hypokalemia, severe acidosis, electric shock, ventricular arrhythmia, AV block, pulmonary embolism, heart rupture, cardiac tamponade, hyperkalemia, electromechanical dissociation • Cocaine overdose	• Initiate CPR, follow ACLS protocol for ET intubation, transcutaneous pacing, administration of epinephrine and atropine

- Monitor and record vital signs, I/O, hemodynamic variables, laboratory studies, medication levels, and ECG readings
- Maintain prescribed diet
- Maintain bed rest, until patient is stable
- Provide support to the patient and family
- Individualize home care instructions
- Follow the disorder (specific arrhythmia) and treatment plan
  - Know the signs and symptoms of an arrhythmia to report
  - Take pulse regularly and report abnormal values
  - Understand all procedures, such as pacemaker insertion
  - Comply with medical follow-up

● **Complications**
  - Stroke
  - MI
  - Hypotension
  - Heart failure
  - Shock
  - Death

● **Possible surgical interventions**
  - Pacemaker insertion
  - Catheter ablation therapy
  - Endocardial resection

PERICARDITIS

● **Definition**
  - Inflammation of the pericardium, the fibrous sac that envelops, supports, and protects the heart

Common causes of pericarditis

- Bacterial, fungal, or viral infection
- Neoplasms (primary or metastases from lungs, breasts, or other organs)
- Postcardiac injury such as MI

How pericarditis happens

- Irritation to the pericardium causes inflammatory response
- Chest pain results
- Exudate may develop

Key signs and symptoms of acute pericarditis

- Sharp, sudden pain over the sternum that increases with deep inspiration
- Pericardial friction rub
- Pain decreases when sitting up and leaning forward

Diagnosing pericarditis

- Echocardiography
- Detects pericarditis and pericardial effusion
- ECG
- Elevated ST segments
- QRS segments may be diminished with pericardial effusion
- Rhythm changes may occur, including atrial ectopic rhythms, such as atrial fibrillation and sinus arrhythmia

● **Causes**
  - Bacterial, fungal, or viral infection
  - Neoplasms (primary or metastases from lungs, breasts, or other organs)
  - High dose radiation to the chest
  - Hypersensitivity or autoimmune disease, such as acute rheumatic fever (most common cause of pericarditis in children)
  - Medications, such as hydralazine or procainamide
  - Postcardiac injury, such as MI (which later causes an autoimmune reaction in the pericardium), trauma, and surgery that leaves the pericardium intact but allows blood to leak into the pericardial cavity
  - Aortic aneurysm with pericardial leakage (less common)
  - Myxedema with cholesterol deposits in the pericardium (less common)

● **Pathophysiology**
  - A pathogen or other substance attacks the pericardium starting the inflammatory response and causing chest pain
  - Acute pericarditis may be fibrinous or effusive, with serous, purulent, or hemorrhagic exudate
  - Chronic pericarditis (also called constrictive pericarditis) is characterized by dense, fibrous pericardial thickening

● **Assessment findings**
  - Acute pericarditis
    - Sharp, sudden pain over the sternum, radiating to the neck, shoulders, back, and arms
    - Pain increases with deep inspiration or when lying down and decreases when sitting up and leaning forward
    - Pericardial friction rub
    - Distant heart sounds
    - Increased cardiac dullness
    - Diminished or absent apical impulse
  - Chronic pericarditis
    - Increased systemic venous pressure
    - Signs similar to chronic right-sided heart failure, including fluid retention, ascites, and hepatomegaly

● **Diagnostic test findings**
  - Echocardiography: detects pericarditis and pericardial effusion
  - Hematologic studies: WBC may normal or elevated, especially in infectious pericarditis; ESR is elevated
  - Blood chemistries: Serum CK-MB levels are slightly elevated with associated myocarditis; BUN levels detect uremia
  - Serologic testing: antistreptolysin-O titers detect rheumatic fever
  - Skin testing: purified protein derivative skin test detects tuberculosis
  - Cultures: pericardial fluid culture may identify causative organism in bacterial or fungal pericarditis

- ECG: elevated ST segments; QRS segments may be diminished with pericardial effusion; rhythm changes may occur, including atrial ectopic rhythms, such as atrial fibrillation and sinus arrhythmia

- **Medical management**
  - Oxygen therapy
  - Bed rest as long as fever and pain persist
  - Nonsteroidal anti-inflammatory drugs: aspirin, indomethacin (Indocin)
  - Corticosteroids, if the cause isn't tuberculosis
  - Antibiotics: depending on causative organism
  - Pericardiocentesis

- **Nursing interventions**
  - Assess cardiovascular and respiratory status
  - Monitor and record vital signs, I/O, and hemodynamic variables
  - Administer I.V. fluids, oxygen, and medications, as prescribed
  - Assess pain, provide analgesics as prescribed, and evaluate effect
  - Maintain complete bed rest
  - Monitor for signs of cardiac compression and cardiac tamponade, such as decreased blood pressure, increased CVP, and pulsus paradoxus
  - Provide reassurance and explain all test, procedures, and treatments
  - Place the patient in an upright position
  - Individualize home care instructions
  - Follow the disorder and treatment plan
    - Follow instructions for medication use
    - Comply with medical follow-up
    - Follow activity restrictions
    - Report signs and symptoms of pericarditis, pericardial effusion, and cardiac tamponade to physician immediately

- **Complications**
  - Pericardial effusion
  - Heart failure
  - Chronic right-sided heart failure
  - Cardiac tamponade
  - Arrhythmias
  - Stroke
  - Death

- **Possible surgical intervention**
  - Pericardectomy

ARTERIAL OCCLUSIVE DISEASE

- **Definition**
  - Obstruction or narrowing of the aorta's lumen and its major branches, causing an interruption of blood flow, usually to the legs and feet

---

Treating pericarditis

- Oxygen therapy
- Bed rest as long as fever and pain persist
- Nonsteroidal anti-inflammatory drugs
- Corticosteroids
- Antibiotics
- Pericardectomy

Key nursing interventions for a patient with pericarditis

- Maintain complete bed rest.
- Place the patient in an upright position.
- Monitor and record vital signs, I/O, and hemodynamic variables.
- Assess pain and provide analgesics, as prescribed

Key complications of pericarditis

- Pericardial effusion
- Cardiac tamponade
- Arrhythmias

Key facts about arterial occlusive disease

- Obstruction or narrowing of the aorta's lumen and it's major branches that causes an interruption of blood flow
- Usually affects legs and feet

Common causes of arterial occlusive disease

- Atherosclerosis
- Emboli
- Thrombosis
- Trauma or fracture

How arterial occlusive disease happens

- Endogenous or exogenous mechanism causes arterial occlusion
- Reduced perfusion causes tissue ischemia, skin ulceration and gangrene

Key signs and symptoms of arterial occlusive disease

- Femoral, popliteal, or innominate arteries
- Decreased pulses distal to the occlusion
- Mottling and pallor of the extremity
- Paralysis and paresthesia in the affected extremity
- Sudden and localized pain in the affected extremity (most common symptom)
- Internal and external carotid arteries
- Stroke
- TIA

● **Causes and risk factors**
- Causes
  - Atherosclerosis
  - Emboli
  - Thrombosis
  - Trauma or fracture
- Risk factors
  - Age
  - Diabetes mellitus
  - Family history of vascular disorders, MI, or stroke
  - Hyperlipidemia
  - Hypertension
  - Smoking

● **Pathophysiology**
- Occlusive mechanism may be endogenous, due to emboli formation or thrombosis, or exogenous, due to trauma or fracture
- Arteries unable to respond to increased needs related to physical activity or sympathetic nervous system responses
- Reduced perfusion results in tissue ischemia, skin ulceration, and gangrene
- May affect carotid, vertebral, innominate, subclavian, mesenteric, celiac, femoral, and popliteal arteries

● **Assessment findings**
- Femoral, popliteal, or innominate arteries
  - Decreased pulses distal to the occlusion
  - Mottling of the extremity
  - Pallor
  - Paralysis and paresthesia in the affected arm or leg
  - Sudden and localized pain in the affected arm or leg (most common symptom)
  - Temperature change that occurs distal to the occlusion
- Internal and external carotid arteries
  - Absent or decreased pulsation with an auscultatory bruit over affected arteries
  - Stroke
  - TIAs
- Subclavian artery
  - Subclavian steal syndrome (characterized by the backflow of blood from the brain through the vertebral artery on the same side as the occlusion, into the subclavian artery distal to the occlusion; clinical effects of vertebrobasilar occlusion and exercise-induced arm claudication)
- Vertebral and basilar arteries
  - TIAs

● **Diagnostic test findings**
- Arteriography: demonstrates the type (thrombus or embolus), location, and degree of obstruction, and the collateral circulation
- Doppler ultrasonography and plethysmography: show decreased blood flow distal to the occlusion in acute disease
- EEG and computed tomography scan: to rule out brain lesions
- Ophthalmodynamometry: Determines the degree of obstruction in the internal carotid artery by comparing ophthalmic artery pressure to brachial artery pressure on the affected side

● **Medical management**
- Anticoagulants: heparin, warfarin (Coumadin)
- Diet: low-cholesterol
- Antilipemics: atorvastatin (Lipitor), simvastatin (Zocor), ezetimibe (Zetia)
- Antiplatelets: aspirin, ticlopidine (Ticlid), clopidogrel (Plavix)
- Pentoxifylline (Trental)
- Thrombolytics: alteplase (Activase), streptokinase (Streptase), urokinase (Abbokinase)
- Smoking cessation
- Activity: walking

● **Nursing interventions**
- Assess distal pulses, skin color, and temperature
- Assess pain level and provide pain relief as needed
- Assist the patient to gradually increase activity as tolerated
- Maintain prescribed diet
- Administer I.V. fluids, oxygen, and medications, as prescribed
- Monitor and record vital signs, I/O, laboratory values, and hemodynamic variables
- Monitor the patient with carotid, innominate, vertebral, or subclavian artery occlusion for signs of stroke

● **Complications**
- Amputation
- Stroke
- Gangrene
- Kidney failure

● **Possible surgical interventions**
- Surgery: atherectomy, balloon angioplasty, bypass grafting, embolectomy, laser angioplasty, patch grafting, stent placement, thromboendarterectomy, or amputation

NCLEX CHECKS

It's never too soon to begin your NCLEX preparation. Now that you've reviewed this chapter, carefully read each of the following questions and choose the best answer. Then compare your responses to the correct answers.

Diagnosing arterial occlusive disease

- Arteriography: type (thrombus or embolus), location, and degree of obstruction, collateral circulation
- Doppler ultrasonography: decreased blood flow distal to the occlusion

Treating arterial occlusive disease

- Anticoagulants
- Antiplatelets
- Thrombolytics
- Embolectomy

Key nursing interventions for a patient with arterial occlusive disease

- Assess distal pulses, skin color, and temperature.
- Assess pain level and provide pain relief as needed.
- Administer I.V. fluids, oxygen, and medications, as prescribed.
- Monitor the patient with carotid, innominate, vertebral, or subclavian artery occlusion for signs of stroke.

Key complications of arterial occlusive disease

- Amputation
- Stroke

TOP 10

Items to study for your next test on the cardiovascular system

1. Myocardial blood supply
2. Cardiac conduction system
3. Significance of assessment findings, such as chest pain, edema, and blood pressure changes
4. Patient preparation and post-operative care for diagnostic procedures such as cardiac catheterization
5. Modifiable and nonmodifiable risk factors for developing cardiovascular disorders
6. Patient preparation and post-operative care for surgical procedures, such as coronary artery bypass grafting, aneurysm repair, and pacemaker insertion
7. Assessment of ABCs and rapid response to cardiac arrhythmias
8. Medication use for such disorders as hypertension, MI, CAD, and heart failure
9. Nursing interventions for key disorders, such as CAD, hypertension, heart failure, and MI
10. Patient teaching points

1. While auscultating the heart sounds of a client with mitral insufficiency, the nurse hears an extra heart sound immediately after the S_2. The nurse should document this extra heart sound as a:
- ☐ **1.** S_1.
- ☒ **2.** S_3.
- ☐ **3.** S_4.
- ☐ **4.** mitral murmur.

2. A nurse administers heparin to a client with deep vein thrombophlebitis. Which laboratory value should the nurse monitor to determine the effectiveness of heparin?
- ☒ **1.** PTT
- ☐ **2.** HCT
- ☐ **3.** CBC
- ☐ **4.** PT

3. A client has just returned from cardiac catheterization. Which nursing intervention would be most appropriate?
- ☐ **1.** Help the client ambulate to the bathroom.
- ☐ **2.** Restrict fluids.
- ☒ **3.** Monitor peripheral pulses.
- ☐ **4.** Insert an indwelling urinary catheter.

4. A client is in the first postoperative day after left femoropopliteal revascularization. Which position would be most appropriate for this client?
- ☐ **1.** On his left side
- ☐ **2.** In high Fowler's position
- ☒ **3.** On his right side
- ☐ **4.** In a left lateral decubitus position

5. A nurse is evaluating a client with left-sided heart failure. Which finding should the nurse expect to assess?
- ☐ **1.** Ascites
- ☒ **2.** Dyspnea
- ☐ **3.** Hepatomegaly
- ☐ **4.** Jugular vein distention

6. A client has developed acute pulmonary edema. Which test result should the nurse expect?
- ☒ **1.** Interstitial edema by chest X-ray
- ☐ **2.** Metabolic alkalosis by ABG analysis
- ☐ **3.** Bradycardia by ECG
- ☐ **4.** Decreased PAWP by hemodynamic monitoring

7. A nurse is performing discharge teaching for a client with PVD. The nurse should teach the client to:
- ☐ **1.** inspect his feet weekly.
- ☒ **2.** begin a daily walking program.
- ☐ **3.** wear constrictive clothing.
- ☐ **4.** stand rather than sit when possible.

8. If a nurse knows a client's heart rate, what other value and formula does she need to know to calculate CO? _____ $CO = JV \times HR$ _____
 → Amount of blood ejected w̅ each Heart beat

9. A client comes to the clinic and states he has a history of hypertension. Which type of medication might the nurse expect the client to be taking to control his blood pressure?

☐ **1.** Antilipemics
☐ **2.** Antibiotics
☒ **3.** ACE inhibitors
☐ **4.** Antidiabetics

10. A nurse is caring for a client with junctional tachycardia. Identify the area where this arrhythmia originates.

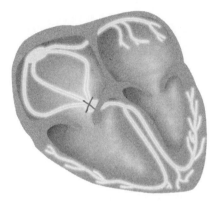

ANSWERS AND RATIONALES

1. CORRECT ANSWER: 2
An S_3 is heard following an S_2. This indicates that the client is experiencing heart failure and results from increased filling pressures. An S_1 is a normal heart sound made by the closing of the mitral and tricuspid valves. An S_4 is heard before S_1 and is caused by resistance to ventricular filling. A murmur of mitral insufficiency occurs during systole and is heard when there's turbulent blood flow across the valve.

2. CORRECT ANSWER: 1
The therapeutic effectiveness of heparin is determined by monitoring the patient's PTT. PT, HCT, and CBC don't monitor the therapeutic effectiveness of heparin. Monitoring the PT determines warfarin's effectiveness.

3. CORRECT ANSWER: 3
After cardiac catheterization, monitor peripheral pulses to assess peripheral perfusion. Helping the client ambulate to the bathroom is incorrect because the client should be on bed rest for 4 to 8 hours after the procedure to reduce the

risk of bleeding at the insertion site. Restricting fluids is incorrect because the client should be encouraged to drink fluids after the procedure, unless contraindicated. Adequate hydration reduces the risk of nephrotoxicity that can occur with the use of contrast dye. Although urine output is monitored following cardiac catheterization, the insertion of a urinary catheter isn't necessary.

4. CORRECT ANSWER: 3

Following revascularization, avoid positioning the client on the surgical side. Because this client had left femoropopliteal revascularization, he may be positioned on the right side. Placing the client on the left side is incorrect because this would position the client on the operative side. Positioning the client in high Fowler's position is incorrect because the client should avoid flexion at the surgical site. Placing the client in a left lateral decubitus position is incorrect because this would place the client on the surgical side and cause flexion at the site.

5. CORRECT ANSWER: 2

Dyspnea may occur in a client with left-sided heart failure. Ascites, hepatomegaly, and jugular vein distention are assessment findings in right-sided heart failure.

6. CORRECT ANSWER: 1

The chest X-ray of a client with acute pulmonary edema shows interstitial edema as a result of the heart's failure to pump adequately. Metabolic alkalosis is incorrect because the ABG analysis of a client in acute pulmonary edema shows respiratory alkalosis or acidosis. Bradycardia is incorrect because the ECG would most likely indicate tachycardia. Decreased PAWP is incorrect because PAWP rises in the client with acute pulmonary edema.

7. CORRECT ANSWER: 2

The nurse should encourage the client with PVD to follow a program of walking and other leg exercises. Inspecting the feet weekly is incorrect because the nurse should teach the client to inspect his feet daily. Wearing constrictive clothing is incorrect because the client should wear loose clothing that doesn't restrict circulation. Standing when possible—rather than sitting—is incorrect because the client should avoid standing for long periods.

8. CORRECT ANSWER: STROKE VOLUME

Cardiac output equals stroke volume (the amount of blood ejected with each beat) times heart rate. [CO = SV × HR]

9. CORRECT ANSWER: 3

ACE inhibitors may be prescribed to help control high blood pressure. Other types of medications that may be prescribed include diuretics, calcium channel blockers, angiotensin II receptor blockers, and beta-adrenergic blockers. Antilipemics help lower serum cholesterol levels, antibiotics are used to fight infection, and antidiabetics help control serum glucose levels.

10. CORRECT ANSWER:

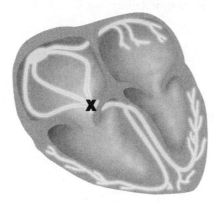

In junctional tachycardia, the AV node fires rapidly. The atria are depolarized by retrograde conduction; however, conduction through the ventricle remains normal.

2

Respiratory system

PRETEST

1. Modifiable risk factors for a client to prevent the development of a respiratory disorder include:

- ☒ 1. tobacco use.
- ☐ 2. family history.
- ☐ 3. aging.
- ☐ 4. allergies.

CORRECT ANSWER: 1

2. Which nursing diagnosis would most apply to a client with respiratory disease?

- ☒ 1. Activity intolerance
- ☐ 2. Imbalanced nutrition: More than body requirements
- ☐ 3. Disturbed body image
- ☐ 4. Deficient fluid volume

CORRECT ANSWER: 1

3. An important nursing intervention to help prevent respiratory complications is:

- ☐ 1. recommending support services.
- ☒ 2. teaching the correct use of incentive spirometry.
- ☐ 3. documenting vital signs and intake and output.
- ☐ 4. establishing effective communication techniques.

CORRECT ANSWER: 2

4. A complication of pulmonary emboli may be:

☐ 1. status asthmaticus.

☐ 2. aspiration pneumonia.

☐ 3. cor pulmonale.

☒ 4. death.

CORRECT ANSWER: 4

5. A client is admitted to the hospital with an acute exacerbation of asthma. Auscultation reveals almost absent breath sounds. Thirty minutes after administering albuterol (Proventil) by nebulizer, the nurse auscultates diffuse inspiratory and expiratory wheezes throughout all lung fields. This finding most likely represents:

☒ 1. increased airflow.

☐ 2. no change in airflow.

☐ 3. decreased airflow.

☐ 4. no correlation with airflow.

CORRECT ANSWER: 1

LEARNING OBJECTIVES

After studying this chapter, you should be able to:

● Describe the psychosocial impact of respiratory disorders.

● Differentiate between modifiable and nonmodifiable risk factors in the development of a respiratory disorder.

● List three probable and three possible nursing diagnoses for a patient with a respiratory disorder.

● Identify the nursing interventions for a patient with a respiratory disorder.

● Write three goals for teaching a patient with a respiratory disorder.

CHAPTER OVERVIEW

Caring for the patient with a respiratory disorder requires a sound understanding of respiratory anatomy and physiology as well as the diffusion of oxygen. A thorough assessment is essential to planning and implementing appropriate care. The assessment should include a complete history, a physical examination, diagnostic testing, identification of modifiable and nonmodifiable risk factors, and information related to the psychosocial impact of respiratory dysfunction on the patient.

Nursing interventions are geared toward improving gas exchange and breathing abilities. Nursing diagnoses focus primarily on ineffective breathing patterns and impaired gas exchange. Patient teaching—a crucial nursing activity—involves giving the patient information about medication regimens, signs and symptoms of possible complications, reducing modifiable risk factors (avoiding people with infections, activity and diet restrictions, stress management, and smoking cessation), and medical follow-up.

ANATOMY AND PHYSIOLOGY REVIEW

Key facts about nares
- Filter out particles
- Humidify inspired air
- Contain olfactory receptor sites

- **Nares**
  - Filter out particles
  - Humidify inspired air
  - Contain olfactory receptor sites
- **Paranasal sinuses**
  - Air-filled, cilia-lined cavities
  - Function: to trap particles
- **Pharynx**
  - Serves as a passageway to digestive and respiratory tracts
  - Maintains air pressure in the middle ear
  - Contains a mucosal lining that humidifies and warms inspired air and traps particles
- **Larynx**
  - Known as the "voice box"
  - Connects the upper and lower airways
  - Contains vocal cords that produce sounds and initiate the cough reflex
- **Trachea**
  - Consists of smooth muscle
  - Contains C-shaped cartilaginous rings
  - Connects the larynx to the bronchi

Key facts about bronchi
- Formed by trachea branching
- Right main bronchus is slightly larger and more vertical than the left
- Bronchioles branch into terminal bronchioles

- **Bronchi and bronchioles**
  - Formed by branching of the trachea
  - Right main bronchus is slightly larger and more vertical than the left
  - Bronchioles branch into terminal bronchioles, which end in alveoli

- **Alveoli**
  - Clustered microscopic sacs enveloped by capillaries
  - Site of gas exchange
  - Coating of surfactant reduces surface tension to keep alveoli from collapsing
  - Diffusion of gases occurs across the alveolar-capillary membrane
- **Lungs**
  - Composed of three lobes on the right side and two lobes on the left side
  - Covered by pleura
  - Regulate air exchange by concentration gradient
- **Pleura**
  - Visceral pleura covers the lungs
  - Parietal pleura lines the thoracic cavity
  - Pleural fluid lubricates the pleura to reduce friction during respiration

ASSESSMENT FINDINGS

- **History**
  - Difficulty breathing, shortness of breath, dyspnea
  - Chest pain
  - Cough
  - Hoarseness
  - Dysphagia
  - Fatigue
  - Weight change
- **Physical examination**
  - Respiratory system changes
    - Nasal flaring
    - Decreased respiratory excursion
    - Decreased diaphragmatic excursion
    - Accessory muscle use
    - Retractions
    - Heaving
  - Sputum characteristics, including color and amount of sputum
  - Clubbing of fingers
  - Adventitious breath sounds: crackles, rhonchi, wheezing, and pleural friction rub (see *Abnormal breath sounds,* page 82)
  - Fremitus
  - Crepitus
  - Abnormal pattern and character of respirations
  - Shape of thoracic anatomy (such as barrel chest)
  - Change in mentation
  - Cyanosis
  - Diaphoresis or cold, clammy skin

Key facts about alveoli
- Site of gas exchange
- Occurs across the alveolar-capilillary exchange

Key facts about lungs
- Three lobes on the right side
- Two lobes on the left side
- Covered by pleura
- Regulate air exchange

Key signs and symptoms of a respiratory disorder
- Dyspnea
- Fatigue
- Cough
- Accessory muscle use
- Retractions
- Adventitious sounds: crackles, rhonchi, wheezing, and pleural friction rub
- Abnormal pattern and character of respirations
- Change in mentation
- Cyanosis

Abnormal breath sounds

Characteristics of abnormal breath sounds are described here.

- *Crackles*—intermittent, nonmusical, crackling sounds heard during inspiration; classified as fine or coarse
- *Wheezes*—high-pitched sounds heard on exhalation that are caused by blocked airflow
- *Rhonchi*—low-pitched snoring or rattling sound heard primarily on exhalation
- *Stridor*—loud, high-pitched sound heard during inspiration
- *Pleural friction rub*—low-pitched, grating sound heard during inspiration and expiration; accompanied by pain

Abnormal breath sounds found in respiratory disorders

- Crackles
- Wheezes
- Rhonchi
- Stridor
- Pleural friction rub

Key facts about bronchoscopy

- Allows for visualization of the trachea and bronchial tree
- Used to obtain biopsies and allows for deep tracheal suctioning
- Intervention: check cough and gag reflexes after procedure

Key facts about chest X-ray

- Provides radiographic picture of lung tissue
- Intervention: determine pregnancy status for the female patient

Key facts about pulmonary angiography

- Allows for radiographic examination of pulmonary circulation
- Interventions:
- note allergies to iodine, seafood, and radiopaque dyes before test
- assess insertion site for bleeding after test

DIAGNOSTIC TESTS AND PROCEDURES

- **Bronchoscopy**
  - Definition and purpose
    - Procedure using a bronchoscope for direct visualization of the trachea and bronchial tree
    - Used to obtain biopsies and perform deep tracheal suctioning
  - Nursing interventions before the procedure
    - Explain the procedure and what to expect following the procedure
    - Withhold food and fluids
    - Allay the patient's anxiety
    - Place obtained written informed consent in the patient's chart
  - Nursing interventions after the procedure
    - Check cough and gag reflexes—this minimizes the risk of aspiration
    - Assess sputum
    - Assess respiratory status
    - Withhold food and fluids until gag reflex returns
    - Check vasovagal response
    - Monitor pulse oximetry

- **Chest X-ray**
  - Definition and purpose
    - Noninvasive examination
    - Radiographic picture of lung tissue
  - Nursing interventions
    - Explain the procedure to the patient
    - Determine the patient's ability to inhale and hold breath
    - Ensure that the patient removes jewelry
    - Determine pregnancy status, for the female patient

- **Pulmonary angiography**
  - Definition and purpose
    - Procedure using an injection of a radiopaque dye through a catheter
    - Radiographic examination of the pulmonary circulation

- Nursing interventions before the procedure
  - Explain the procedure to the patient
  - Note the patient's allergies to iodine, seafood, and radiopaque dyes
  - Instruct the patient about possible flushing of the face or burning in the throat after the dye is injected
  - Place obtained written informed consent in the patient's chart
- Nursing interventions after the procedure
  - Assess neurovascular status
  - Check the insertion site for bleeding
  - Monitor for delayed allergic response

● **Sputum studies**
- Definition and purpose
  - Laboratory test
  - Microscopic evaluation of sputum that includes culture and sensitivity, Gram stain, and acid-fast bacillus
- Nursing interventions
  - Explain the procedure to the patient
  - Obtain early-morning sterile specimen from suctioning or expectoration

● **Thoracentesis**
- Definition and purpose
  - Procedure using needle aspiration of intrapleural fluid under local anesthesia
  - Specimen examination or removal of pleural fluid
- Nursing interventions before the procedure
  - Explain the procedure to the patient
  - Place obtained signed informed consent in the patient's chart
  - Place the patient in the proper position (either sitting on the edge of the bed or lying partially on the side, partially on the back)
- Nursing interventions after the procedure
  - Assess the patient's respiratory status
  - Monitor vital signs frequently
  - Position the patient on the affected side, as ordered, for at least 1 hour to seal the puncture site
  - Check the puncture site for fluid leakage
  - Auscultate lungs and assist with postprocedure chest X-ray to assess for pneumothorax
  - Monitor oxygen saturation (SaO_2) levels

● **Pulmonary function tests (PFTs)**
- Definition and purpose
  - Noninvasive test
  - Measurement of lung volume, ventilation, and diffusing capacity
- Nursing interventions
  - Explain the procedure to the patient
  - Document bronchodilators or narcotics used before testing

Key facts about sputum culture

- Microscopic evaluation of sputum: culture and sensitivity, Gram stain, and acid-fast bacillus
- Intervention: obtain early-morning sterile specimen

Key facts about thoracentesis

- Allows for removal of pleural fluid and specimen examination
- Interventions:
- before the procedure: place the patient in the proper position
- after the procedure: place the patient on affected side for 1 hour and assess for pneumothorax

Key facts about PFTs

- Measure lung volume, ventilation, and diffusing capacity
- Intervention: document bronchodilators or narcotics used before testing

Key facts about ABG analysis

- Arterial blood measurements of tissue oxygenation, and acid-base status
- Intervention: apply pressure to puncture site for 5 minutes after procedure

Key facts about lung scan

- Provides imaging of distribution and blood flow in lungs
- Interventions:
- Assess for allergies to isotopes
- Check catheter insertion site for bleeding after lung scan

Key facts about Mantoux test

- Skin test to detect TB antibodies
- Intervention: circle and record the test site
- Reading should be obtained 48 to 72 hours after injection

Key facts about laryngoscopy

- Direct visualization of larynx through use of a laryngoscope
- Interventions:
- Withhold food and fluids for 6 to 8 hours before test
- Withhold flood and fluids after test until gag reflex returns

– Allay the patient's anxiety during testing

● **Arterial blood gas (ABG) analysis**
- Definition and purpose
  - Laboratory test
  - Assessment of arterial blood for tissue oxygenation, ventilation, and acid-base status
- Nursing interventions before the procedure
  - Explain the procedure to the patient
  - Note temperature
  - Document oxygen and assisted mechanical ventilation used
- Nursing interventions after the procedure
  - Apply pressure to the site for 5 minutes
  - Apply a pressure dressing

● **Lung scan**
- Definition and purpose
  - Procedure using inhalation or I.V. injection of radioisotopes
  - Imaging of distribution and blood flow in the lungs
- Nursing interventions before the procedure
  - Explain the procedure to the patient
  - Allay the patient's anxiety
  - Determine the patient's ability to lie still during the procedure
  - Assess for allergies to injected radioisotopes
- Nursing interventions after the procedure
  - Check the catheter insertion site for bleeding
  - Increase fluid intake, unless contraindicated

● **Mantoux intradermal skin test**
- Definition and purpose
  - Procedure involving the administration of tuberculin
  - Detection of tuberculosis (TB) antibodies
- Nursing interventions
  - Explain the procedure to the patient
  - Document current dermatitis or rashes
  - Cancel test if history of positive results in past skin testing
  - Note history of receiving the bacille Calmette-Guèrin vaccine as a child (may be contraindication for Mantoux skin test)
  - Circle and record the test site
  - Note date for follow-up reading (48 to 72 hours after injection)

● **Laryngoscopy**
- Definition and purpose
  - Procedure using a laryngoscope
  - Direct visualization of the larynx
- Nursing interventions before the procedure
  - Explain the procedure to the patient
  - Withhold food and fluids for 6 to 8 hours before the test

– Explain to the patient that he'll receive a sedative to promote relaxation
– Provide emotional support to allay the patient's anxiety
– Place obtained written informed consent in the patient's chart
• Nursing interventions after the procedure
– Assess the patient's respiratory status
– Withhold food and fluids until gag reflex returns
– Assess for trauma to oropharynx
– Assess for hemoptysis

Lung biopsy

• Definition and purpose
– Procedure involving the percutaneous removal of a small amount of lung tissue
– Histologic evaluation
• Nursing interventions before the procedure
– Explain the procedure to the patient
– Withhold food and fluids
– Place obtained written informed consent in the patient's chart
• Nursing interventions after the procedure
– Observe the patient for signs of pneumothorax and air embolism
– Check the patient for hemoptysis and hemorrhage
– Monitor and record vital signs
– Check the insertion site for bleeding
– Monitor for signs of respiratory distress

Hematologic studies

• Definition and purpose
– Laboratory test of a blood sample
– Analysis for red blood cells (RBCs), white blood cells (WBCs), prothrombin time (PT), partial thromboplastin time (PTT), erythrocyte sedimentation rate (ESR), platelets, hemoglobin (Hb), and hematocrit (HCT)
• Nursing interventions
– Explain the procedure to the patient
– Note current drug therapy before the procedure
– Check the site for bleeding after the procedure

Blood chemistry

• Definition and purpose
– Laboratory test of a blood sample
– Analysis for potassium, sodium, calcium, phosphorus, glucose, bicarbonate, blood urea nitrogen (BUN), creatinine, protein, albumin, osmolality, and alpha$_1$-antitrypsin levels
• Nursing interventions
– Explain the procedure to the patient
– Check the site for bleeding after the procedure

Key facts about lung biopsy

• Removal of a small amount of lung tissue for histologic evaluation
• Intervention: observe the patient for signs of pneumothorax and air embolism after procedure

Key facts about hematologic studies

• Blood test
• Analysis of:
– RBCs
– WBCs
– PT and PTT
– ESR
– Platelets
– Hb and HCT
• Intervention: check the site for bleeding after the procedure

Key facts about blood chemistry

• Blood test
• Analysis of:
– Potassium, sodium, calcium, phosphorus
– Glucose
– Bicarbonate
– BUN and creatinine
– Protein and albumin
– Osmolality
– Alpha$_1$-antitrypsin
• Intervention: check the site for bleeding after the procedure

TOP 4

Ways a respiratory disease impacts a patient's life

1. Fear of dying
2. Restrictions in work activity
3. Changes in leisure activities, sexual function, and role performance
4. Social isolation

Key risk factors for a respiratory disorder

- Modifiable: cigarette or pipe smoking, obesity, alcohol use
- Nonmodifiable: aging, history of allergies, previous respiratory illness, family history

Key probable nursing diagnoses for a respiratory disorder

- Ineffective breathing pattern
- Impaired gas exchange
- Ineffective airway clearance
- Impaired physical mobility

PSYCHOSOCIAL IMPACT OF RESPIRATORY DISORDERS

- **Developmental impact**
  - Decreased self-esteem
  - Fear of dying
- **Economic impact**
  - Disruption or loss of employment
  - Cost of hospitalizations and home health care
- **Occupational and recreational impact**
  - Restrictions in or loss of work activity
  - Changes in leisure activities
- **Social impact**
  - Social isolation
  - Changes in role performance
  - Changes in sexual function

RISK FACTORS

- **Modifiable risk factors**
  - Inadequate knowledge of risk factors
  - Cigarette or pipe smoking
  - Use of chewing tobacco
  - Alcohol abuse
  - Obesity
  - Crowded living conditions
  - Exposure to chemical and environmental pollutants
- **Nonmodifiable risk factors**
  - Aging
  - History of allergies
  - Previous respiratory illness
  - Family history of respiratory illness
  - Family history of allergies

NURSING DIAGNOSES

- **Probable nursing diagnoses**
  - Ineffective breathing pattern
  - Impaired gas exchange
  - Ineffective airway clearance
  - Impaired physical mobility
  - Insomnia
  - Activity intolerance
  - Ineffective tissue perfusion (cardiopulmonary)
  - Deficient knowledge (discuss process treatment)

● **Possible nursing diagnoses**
- Impaired spontaneous ventilation
- Dysfunctional ventilatory weaning response
- Anxiety
- Fear
- Imbalanced nutrition: Less than body requirements
- Impaired verbal communication
- Noncompliance (treatment plan)
- Risk for aspiration
- Ineffective health maintenance

LARYNGECTOMY

● **Description**
- Partial laryngectomy: surgical excision of a lesion on one vocal cord
- Total laryngectomy: surgical removal of the larynx, hyoid bone, and tracheal rings, with closure of the pharynx and formation of a permanent tracheostomy

● **Preoperative nursing interventions**
- Complete patient and family preoperative teaching
  - Explain the procedure to the patient
  - Describe the operating room, postanesthesia care unit (PACU), and preoperative and postoperative routines
  - Demonstrate postoperative turning, coughing, deep breathing, use of incentive spirometry, and range-of-motion (ROM) exercises
  - Explain the postoperative need for monitoring devices, drainage tubes, surgical dressings, oxygen therapy, I.V. therapy, and pain control
- Complete a preoperative checklist; check that a signed informed consent is in the patient's chart
- Administer preoperative medications as prescribed
- Allay the patient's and his family's anxiety about surgery
- Document the patient's history and physical assessment database
- Establish methods of communication: writing, call bell, "magic slate," picture board
- Encourage the patient to express his feelings about changes in his body image and loss of his voice

● **Postoperative nursing interventions**
- Assess respiratory status
- Monitor and record vital signs, intake and output (I/O), laboratory studies, and pulse oximetry
- Assess pain level, administer postoperative analgesics as prescribed, and evaluate effect
- Assess gag and cough reflexes and ability to swallow
- Observe for hemorrhage and edema in the neck

Key nursing interventions after laryngectomy

- Assess respiratory status.
- Keep the patient in semi-Fowler's position.
- Provide tracheal suction.
- Administer high-humidity oxygen.
- Observe for hemorrhage and edema in the neck.
- Monitor and maintain position and patency of drainage tubes.
- Assess the color, amount, and consistency of sputum.
- Encourage the patient to express feelings about changes in body image and loss of voice.
- Provide oral hygiene.
- Reinforce method of communication established preoperatively.
- Reinforce speech therapy.
- Assess gag and cough reflex and ability to swallow.

Key facts about radical neck dissection

- Excision of:
- Sternocleidomastoid and omohyoid muscles
- Muscles of the floor of the mouth
- Submaxillary gland
- Internal jugular vein
- External carotid artery
- Cervical chain of lymph nodes
- Laryngectomy

- Assess for return of peristalsis; provide solid foods and liquids, as tolerated; increase calories and protein and provide supplements, as needed
- Administer I.V. fluids and enteric feedings
- Provide emotional support to allay the patient's anxiety
- Provide wound care
- Encourage coughing, deep breathing, and use of incentive spirometry
- Keep the patient in semi-Fowler's position
- Provide tracheal suction as needed
- Increase activity as tolerated
- Administer oxygen via high-humidity tracheostomy mask
- Monitor and maintain position and patency of drainage tubes: wound drainage
- Assess the color, amount, and consistency of sputum
- Encourage the patient to express his feelings about changes in his body image and loss of his voice
- Provide oral hygiene
- Reinforce method of communication established preoperatively
- Reinforce speech therapy
- Provide stoma and laryngectomy care
- Reinforce increased intake of fluids
- Arrange referrals to community agencies
- Individualize home care instructions
    - Know about the disorder and its implications
    - Follow instructions for medication use and be aware of possible adverse effects
    - Communicate using esophageal speech or artificial larynx
    - Avoid swimming, showering, and using aerosol sprays
    - Complete stoma and laryngectomy care daily
    - Suction laryngectomy using clean technique
    - Protect the neck from injury
    - Demonstrate ways to prevent debris from entering the stoma

● **Possible complications**
- Hemorrhage
- Atelectasis
- Pneumonia
- Aspiration
- Depession
- Infection

RADICAL NECK DISSECTION

● **Description**
- Surgical excision of the sternocleidomastoid and omohyoid muscles, muscles of the floor of the mouth, submaxillary gland, internal jugular vein, external carotid artery, and cervical chain of lymph nodes, in addition to laryngectomy

● Preoperative nursing interventions

- Complete patient and family preoperative teaching
  - Explain the procedure to the patient
  - Describe the operating room, PACU, and preoperative and postoperative routines
  - Demonstrate postoperative turning, coughing, deep breathing, incentive spirometry, and ROM exercises
  - Explain the postoperative need for monitoring devices, drainage tubes, surgical dressings, incentive spirometer, oxygen therapy, I.V. therapy, and pain control
- Complete a preoperative checklist; check that a signed informed consent is in the patient's chart
- Administer preoperative medications as prescribed
- Allay the patient's and his family's anxiety about surgery
- Document the patient's history and physical assessment database
- Establish methods of communication: writing, call bell, "magic slate," picture board
- Discuss alteration in body image and function

● Postoperative nursing interventions

- Assess cardiac, respiratory, and neurologic status
- Assess pain and administer postoperative analgesics, as prescribed
- Administer oxygen via high-humidity tracheostomy mask
- Monitor and record vital signs, I/O, laboratory studies, and pulse oximetry
- Assess gag and cough reflexes and ability to swallow
- Observe the patient for hemorrhage and edema in the neck
- Assess for the return of peristalsis; provide nutrition and liquids, as indicated
- Administer I.V. fluids, nasogastric (NG) tube feedings, and transfusion therapy, as prescribed
- Provide emotional support to allay the patient's anxiety
- Provide wound care, as directed
- Reinforce turning, coughing, and deep breathing
- Keep the patient in high Fowler's position
- Provide tracheal suction as needed
- Maintain activity: active and passive ROM and isometric exercises, as tolerated
- Monitor and maintain position and patency of drainage tubes: NG, indwelling urinary catheter, and wound drainage
- Encourage the patient to express his feelings about changes in his body image and loss of his voice
- Provide stoma and laryngectomy care; arrange for referrals to community agencies for follow-up care
- Reinforce increased intake of fluids
- Reinforce method of communication established preoperatively
- Reinforce speech therapy

Key nursing interventions before radical neck dissection

- Demonstrate turning, coughing, deep breathing, incentive spirometry, and ROM exercises.
- Establish methods of communication.

Key nursing interventions after radical neck dissection

- Assess cardiac, respiratory, and neurologic status.
- Reinforce turning, coughing, and deep breathing.
- Keep the patient in high Fowler's position.
- Provide tracheal suction.
- Observe the patient for hemorrhage and edema in the neck.
- Administer high-humidity oxygen.
- Monitor and maintain position and patency of drainage tubes.
- Assess gag and cough reflexes and ability to swallow.
- Encourage the patient to express his feelings about changes in his body image and loss of his voice.
- Provide stoma and laryngectomy care.

- Individualize home care instructions
  - Know about the disorder and its implications
  - Communicate using esophageal speech or artificial larynx
  - Recognize the signs and symptoms of tracheostomy stenosis
  - Avoid swimming, showers, and using aerosol sprays
  - Protect the neck from injury
  - Suction laryngectomy using clean technique
  - Complete incision, stoma, and laryngectomy care daily
  - Demonstrate ways to prevent debris from entering the stoma
  - Complete ROM exercises for arms, shoulders, and neck daily

● **Possible complications**
- Tracheostomy stenosis
- Aspiration
- Pneumonia
- Hemorrhage
- Infection
- Depression

LUNG RESECTION

● **Description**
- Lobectomy: surgical removal of one lobe of the lung
- Wedge resection: surgical removal of a wedge-shaped section of a lobe
- Pneumonectomy: surgical removal of a lung

● **Preoperative nursing interventions**
- Complete patient and family preoperative teaching
  - Explain the procedure to the patient
  - Describe the operating room, PACU, and preoperative and postoperative routines
  - Demonstrate postoperative turning, coughing, deep breathing, , and ROM exercises, and the use of incentive spirometry
  - Explain the postoperative need for monitoring devices, drainage tubes, chest tubes, surgical dressings, oxygen therapy, I.V. therapy, and pain control (see *Checking in on chest tubes*)
- Complete a preoperative checklist; check that a signed informed consent is in the patient's chart
- Administer preoperative medications as prescribed
- Allay the patient's and his family's anxiety about surgery
- Document the patient's history and physical assessment database

● **Postoperative nursing interventions**
- Assess cardiac and respiratory status
- Maintain the patient's position: for pneumonectomy patient, keep him on his back or on the side of the surgery; for lobectomy or wedge resection patient, keep him on his back or on the side opposite the surgery

---

Key facts about lung resection

- Lobectomy: removal of lobe of lung
- Wedge resection: removal of section of lung
- Pneumonectomy: removal of entire lung

Key nursing interventions before pulmonary resection

- Demonstrate postoperative turning, coughing, deep breathing, ROM exercises, and the use of incentive spirometry.
- Explain the postoperative need for monitoring devices, drainage tubes, chest tubes, surgical dressings, oxygen therapy, I.V. therapy, and pain control.

Checking in on chest tubes

Caring for a patient with a chest tube requires taking actions to ensure the patient's health. Here are typical nursing steps regarding chest tubes, beginning when the chest tube is first placed:

- First, have the patient take several deep breaths to fully inflate the lungs and help push pleural air out through the tube.
- Next, palpate his chest around the tube for subcutaneous emphysema and notify the physician if any is present.
- Routinely assess the function of the chest tube. Describe and record the amount of drainage on the intake and output sheet every shift.

If there's a leak:
- Bubbling in the water-seal chamber or air leak meter indicates that there's an air leak. If there's no air leak, the water level in this chamber will rise and fall with the patient's respirations, reflecting normal pressure changes in the pleural cavity.

- If the water fluctuates with respirations (for example, fluctuation occurs on exhalation in the patient breathing spontaneously), the lung is most likely the source of the air leak.
- If the lung isn't the source of the air leak, check and tighten the connections. If the leak is in the tubing, replace the unit.

If the tube becomes dislodged:
- Cover the opening immediately with petroleum gauze and apply pressure to prevent negative inspiratory pressure from sucking air into the patient's chest. Call the physician and continue to keep the opening closed. Then get ready to start the chest tube process over.
- If the chest tube becomes cracked, place the distal end of the tube in sterile water and call the physician.

Key facts about chest tube care

- If there's an air leak:
- Lung may be the source.
- Check and tighten connections.
- Replace the unit if the leak is in the tubing.
- If the tube becomes dislodged:
- Cover chest opening with petroleum gauze and apply pressure.
- Notify the physician.
- If the chest tube is cracked:
- Place distal end of tube in sterile water.
- Notify the physician.

- Administer oxygen and maintain endotracheal tube to ventilator, if indicated
- Monitor and record vital signs, I/O, laboratory studies, electrocardiogram (ECG), hemodynamic variables, and pulse oximetry
- Assess chest tube insertion site for subcutaneous air and drainage (except pneumonectomy)
- Reinforce turning, coughing, and deep breathing; use of incentive spirometry; and splinting of incision
- Assess pain level, administer postoperative analgesics as prescribed, and evaluate effect
- Assess for return of peristalsis; provide solid foods and liquids, as tolerated
- Administer I.V. fluids
- Provide emotional support to allay the patient's anxiety
- Provide wound care
- Provide suction, chest physiotherapy, and postural drainage
- Maintain activity: active and passive ROM and isometric exercises, as tolerated
- Monitor and maintain position and patency of drainage tubes: NG tube, indwelling urinary catheter, and chest tube

Key nursing interventions after lung resection

- Assess cardiac and respiratory status.
- Reinforce turning, coughing, and deep breathing; use of incentive spirometry; and splinting of incision.
- Maintain the patient's position: for pneumonectomy patient, keep him on his back or on the side of the surgery; for lobectomy or wedge resection patient, keep him on his back or on the side opposite the surgery.
- Monitor and maintain position and patency of drainage tubes: NG tube, indwelling urinary catheter, and chest tube.
- Assess chest tube insertion site for subcutaneous air and drainage (except pneumonectomy).

- Encourage the patient to express his feelings about his surgery
- Administer antibiotics as prescribed
- Individualize home care instructions
    - Recognize the signs and symptoms of respiratory distress
    - Complete incision care daily and recognize signs and symptoms of infection
    - Maintain active ROM exercises to operative shoulder

● **Possible complications**
- Hemorrhage
- Pneumonia
- Respiratory failure

PULMONARY EMBOLECTOMY

● **Description**
- Removal of pulmonary emboli from the pulmonary artery using a balloon-tipped catheter with a cup device and syringe suction

● **Preoperative nursing interventions**
- Complete patient and family preoperative teaching
    - Explain the procedure to the patient
    - Describe the operating room, PACU, and preoperative and postoperative routines
    - Demonstrate postoperative turning, coughing, deep breathing, incentive spirometry, and ROM exercises
    - Explain the postoperative need for surgical dressings, oxygen therapy, I.V. therapy, and pain control
- Complete a preoperative checklist; check that a signed informed consent is in the patient's chart
- Administer preoperative medications as prescribed
- Allay the patient's and his family's anxiety about surgery
- Document the patient's history and physical assessment database
- Administer anticoagulants as prescribed
- Administer thrombolytics as prescribed

● **Postoperative nursing interventions**
- Assess cardiac, respiratory, and neurologic status
- Administer oxygen
- Monitor and record vital signs, I/O, laboratory studies, neurovascular checks, and pulse oximetry
- Check site for bleeding
- Maintain pressure dressing
- Assess pain level, administer postoperative analgesics as prescribed, and evaluate effect
- Assess for return of peristalsis; provide solid foods and liquids, as tolerated
- Administer I.V. fluids
- Provide emotional support to allay the patient's anxiety

Key facts about embolectomy

- Removal of an embolus from an artery
- Involves use of a balloon-tipped catheter

Key nursing interventions before embolectomy

- Administer thrombolytics as prescribed.
- Demonstrate postoperative turning, coughing, deep breathing, incentive spirometry, and ROM exercises.

Key nursing interventions after embolectomy

- Assess cardiac, respiratory, and neurologic status.
- Provide wound care.
- Monitor and record vital signs, I/O, laboratory studies, neurovascular checks, and pulse oximetry.
- Reinforce turning, coughing, deep breathing, and use of incentive spirometry.
- Keep the patient in semi-Fowler's position.
- Administer anticoagulants as prescribed.

- Provide wound care
- Reinforce turning, coughing, deep breathing, and use of incentive spirometry
- Keep the patient in semi-Fowler's position
- Maintain activity: active and passive ROM and isometric exercises, as tolerated
- Administer anticoagulants as prescribed
- Individualize home care instructions
  - Recognize the signs and symptoms of bleeding
  - Avoid prolonged sitting
  - State precautions of long-term anticoagulant therapy
  - Complete incision care daily and recognize signs and symptoms of infection

● **Possible complications**
- Hemorrhage
- Recurrent embolism
- Thrombosis
- Respiratory distress
- Infection
- Respiratory failure

VENA CAVAL FILTER INSERTION AND PLICATION OF INFERIOR VENA CAVA

● **Description**
- Vena caval filter (for example, Greenfield filter) insertion: surgical placement of an intracaval filter (umbrella) to partially occlude the inferior vena cava and prevent pulmonary emboli
- Plication: surgical suturing and placement of Teflon clips to partially occlude the inferior vena cava and prevent pulmonary emboli

● **Preoperative nursing interventions**
- Complete patient and family preoperative teaching
  - Explain the procedure to the patient
  - Describe the operating room, PACU, and preoperative and postoperative routines
  - Demonstrate postoperative turning, coughing, deep breathing, incentive spirometry, and ROM exercises
  - Explain the postoperative need for surgical dressings, oxygen therapy, I.V. therapy, and pain control
- Complete a preoperative checklist; check that a signed informed consent is in the patient's chart
- Administer preoperative medications as prescribed
- Allay the patient's and his family's anxiety about surgery
- Document the patient's history and physical assessment database

Key facts about vena caval filter insertion and plication of inferior vena cava

- Vena caval filter insertion: surgical placement of an intracaval filter (umbrella) to partially occlude inferior vena cava
- Plication: surgical suturing and placement of Teflon clips to partially occlude inferior vena cava

Key nursing interventions before vena caval filter insertion and plication of inferior vena cava

- Demonstrate turning, coughing, deep breathing, incentive spirometry, and ROM exercises.
- Provide emotional support to the patient and his family.

Key nursing interventions after vena caval filter insertion and plication of inferior vena cava

- Check the insertion site for bleeding and hematoma.
- Assess peripheral edema.
- Apply antiembolism stockings.

● **Postoperative nursing interventions**
  - Assess cardiac and respiratory status
  - Check the insertion site for bleeding and hematoma
  - Monitor and record vital signs, I/O, laboratory studies, neurovascular checks, and pulse oximetry
  - Assess pain level, administer postoperative analgesics, as prescribed, and evaluate effect
  - Assess for return of peristalsis; provide solid foods and liquids, as tolerated
  - Administer I.V. fluids
  - Provide emotional support to allay the patient's anxiety
  - Inspect the surgical dressing and change it, as directed
  - Reinforce turning, coughing, deep breathing, and use of incentive spirometry
  - Keep the patient in semi-Fowler's position, with the foot of the bed elevated
  - Maintain activity: active and passive ROM and isometric exercises, as tolerated
  - Administer oxygen therapy
  - Assess peripheral edema
  - Apply antiembolism stockings
  - Avoid hip flexion
  - Individualize home care instructions
    - Recognize the signs and symptoms of respiratory distress
    - Avoid prolonged sitting or crossing legs when sitting
    - Complete incision care daily and recognize the signs and symptoms of infection
    - Perform daily exercise per physician's instructions
    - Elevate legs when sitting
    - Wear antiembolism stockings
    - Adhere to long-term anticoagulant therapy

● **Possible complications**
  - Recurrent embolism
  - Infection

PNEUMONIA

Key facts about pneumonia

- Inflammation of alveolar spaces
- Alveolar fluid increases
- Ventilation decreases

Common causes of pneumonia

- Organisms
- Aspiration
- Chemical irritants

● **Definition**
  - Bacterial, viral, parasitic, or fungal infection that causes inflammation of the alveolar spaces

● **Causes**
  - Organisms: *Streptococcus pneumoniae, Escherichia coli, Haemophilus influenzae, Staphylococcus aureus, Pneumocystis carinii, Pneumococcus,* and *Pseudomonas* (see Pneumocystis carinii *pneumonia*)
  - Aspiration of food or gastric contents
  - Chemical irritants

Pneumocystis carinii pneumonia

Pneumocystis carinii pneumonia (PCP) is a communicable, opportunistic infection frequently associated with human immunodeficiency virus (HIV) infection as well as other immunocompromising conditions, such as organ transplantation, leukemia, lymphoma, and steroid use.

It has an insidious onset, with increasing shortness of breath and a nonproductive cough. Other signs and symptoms include low-grade, intermittent fever; tachypnea and dyspnea; cyanosis (with acute illness); dullness on percussion (with consolidation); crackles; and decreased breath sounds.

Diagnostic tests may include chest X-ray, arterial blood gas analysis to check for hypoxemia, and fiber-optic bronchoscopy to obtain lung tissue specimens for culture. PCP may respond to drug therapy with co-trimoxazole or pentamidine (which may be administered I.V. or in aerosol form). Prophylactic therapy with co-trimoxazole in the patient with HIV with low immune function has prevented PCP from high mortality rates.

Care for a patient with PCP resembles that of a patient with other types of pneumonia. Key nursing interventions include administering oxygen and an analgesic, as needed; assessing the patient's respiratory status frequently; practicing good hand-washing techniques throughout care; limiting activity and encouraging rest periods; and teaching techniques to reduce the spread of infection and reduce stress.

Key facts about PCP
- Communicable, opportunistic infection associated with immunocompromised conditions
- Causes shortness of breath and nonproductive cough
- Treatment: drug therapy, oxygen, and analgesics

● **Pathophysiology**
- Microorganisms enter the alveolar spaces by droplet inhalation
- Inflammation occurs and alveolar fluid increases
- Ventilation decreases as secretions thicken

● **Assessment findings**
- Cough
- Malaise
- Chills
- Shortness of breath
- Dyspnea
- Elevated temperature
- Crackles
- Rhonchi
- Pleural friction rub
- Pleuritic pain
- Sputum production
  - Rusty, green, or bloody (pneumococcal pneumonia)
  - Yellow-green (bronchopneumonia)

● **Diagnostic test findings**
- Sputum culture: identification of organism
- Chest X-ray: pulmonary infiltrates
- Hematology: increased WBCs, ESR

Key signs and symptoms of pneumonia
- Cough
- Chills
- Dyspnea
- Elevated temperature
- Crackles
- Rhonchi
- Pleural friction rub
- Sputum production

Diagnosing pneumonia
- Sputum culture: positive for specific organism
- Chest X-ray: pulmonary infiltrates
- ABG analysis: respiratory alkalosis

Patient teaching for respiratory disorders

- Smoking cessation
- Self-monitoring for infection
- Medication therapy
- Dietary and exercise recommendations
- Follow-up care

Treating pneumonia

- Oxygen therapy
- Antibiotics
- Antipyretics
- Bronchodilators

Key nursing interventions for a patient with pneumonia

- Administer oxygen.
- Assess respiratory status.
- Monitor and record vital signs, I/O, laboratory studies, and pulse oximetry.
- Monitor and record color, consistency, and amount of sputum.
- Encourage fluids to 3 to 4 L/day.

TIME-OUT FOR TEACHING

Patients with respiratory disorders

Be sure to include these topics in your teaching plan for the patient with a respiratory disorder.

- Smoking cessation; avoidance of irritants
- Self-monitoring for infection, including avoiding exposure to people with infections
- Signs of infection and respiratory distress
- Optimal weight maintenance

- Medication therapy, including action, adverse effects, and scheduling
- Dietary recommendations and restrictions
- Rest and activity patterns
- Community agencies and resources
- Follow-up appointments

- ABG analysis: hypoxemia, respiratory alkalosis

Medical management

- Oxygen therapy with intubation and mechanical ventilation, if needed
- Monitoring: vital signs, ABG values, and I/O
- Treatments: indwelling urinary catheter, chest physiotherapy, postural drainage, incentive spirometry, and high-flow nebulizer treatments
- Antibiotics: penicillin G (Pentids), ampicillin (Omnipen), pentamidine (NebuPent), amoxicillin and clavulanate (Augmentin)
- Diet: high-calorie, high-protein
- Dietary recommendation: encourage fluids
- I.V. therapy: hydration, saline lock
- Position: semi-Fowler's
- Activity: bed rest, active and passive ROM and isometric exercises
- Laboratory studies: WBCs, sputum culture, blood culture, and throat culture
- Antipyretics: aspirin, acetaminophen (Tylenol)
- Bronchodilators: metaproterenol (Alupent), albuterol (Proventil)
- Specialized bed: rotation (Rotorest)
- Pulse oximetry

Nursing interventions

- Administer oxygen
- Assess respiratory status
- Monitor and record vital signs, I/O, laboratory studies, and pulse oximetry
- Administer medications as prescribed
- Monitor and record color, consistency, and amount of sputum
- Keep the patient in semi-Fowler's position
- Reposition the patient every 2 hours; encourage coughing, deep breathing, and use of incentive spirometry
- Maintain the patient's diet
- Encourage fluids to 3 to 4 qt (3 to 4 L)/day
- Administer I.V. fluids

- Encourage the patient to express his feelings about difficulty breathing
- Provide emotional support to allay the patient's anxiety
- Prevent spread of infection
- Provide oral hygiene
- Provide information about the American Lung Association
- Individualize home care instructions (for more information about teaching, see *Patients with respiratory disorders*)
  - Know about the disorder and its implications
  - Follow instructions for medication use and be aware of possible adverse effects
  - Recognize the signs and symptoms of respiratory infection
  - Avoid exposure to people with infections
  - Increase fluid intake to 3 qt (3 L)/day

● **Complications**
- Heart failure
- Pulmonary edema
- Respiratory failure
- Death

● **Possible surgical interventions**
- None

CHRONIC OBSTRUCTIVE PULMONARY DISEASE (COPD)

● **Definition**
- COPD is group of diseases that results in persistent obstruction of bronchial airflow
- Diseases include emphysema, asthma, bronchiectasis, and chronic bronchitis
- In emphysema, the stimulus to breathe is low partial pressure of arterial oxygen (PaO_2) instead of increased partial pressure of arterial carbon dioxide ($PaCO_2$)

● **Causes**
- Cigarette smoke (primary and secondary)
- Polluted air, chemical irritants
- Respiratory tract infections
- Genetic predisposition

● **Pathophysiology**
- Bronchiectasis: infection destroys the bronchial mucosa, which is replaced by fibrous scar tissue; loss of resilience and dilation of airways causes pooling of secretions, obstruction of air flow, and decreased perfusion
- Asthma: irritants to bronchial tree cause bronchoconstriction, resulting in narrowed inflamed airways, dyspnea, and mucus production—all of which are reversible

Key complications of pneumonia
- Respiratory failure
- Heart failure
- Death

Key facts about COPD
- Persistent obstruction of bronchial airflow
- In emphysema, the stimulus to breathe is low PaO_2 instead of increased $PaCO_2$
- Four types
- Bronchiectasis
- Asthma
- Bronchitis
- Emphysema

Common causes of COPD
- Cigarette smoke
- Irritants
- Infection
- Genetic

Key signs and symptoms of COPD

- Cough
- Dyspnea
- Sputum production
- Clubbing of fingers
- Use of accessory muscles

Diagnosing COPD

- Chest X-ray: congestion, hyperinflation
- ABG analysis: respiratory acidosis
- PFTs: increased residual volume and functional residual capacity; decreased vital capacity

Treating COPD

- Oxygen therapy
- High-calorie diet with fluids to 3 qt (3 L)/day
- Antibiotics
- Bronchodilators
- Corticosteroids
- Beta-adrenergic medication
- Mast cell stabilizers

- Bronchitis: excessive bronchial mucus production causes chronic or recurrent productive cough
- Emphysema: destruction of elastin alters alveolar walls and narrows airways, resulting in enlargement of air spaces distal to terminal bronchioles, trapped air, and coalesced alveoli

● Assessment findings

- Cough
- Dyspnea
- Sputum production
- Weight loss
- Barrel chest (emphysema)
- Hemoptysis
- Exertional dyspnea
- Clubbing of fingers
- Malaise
- Wheezes
- Crackles
- Anemia
- Anxiety
- Diaphoresis
- Use of accessory muscles
- Orthopnea

● Diagnostic test findings

- Chest X-ray: congestion, hyperinflation
- ABG analysis: respiratory acidosis, hypoxemia
- Sputum studies: positive identification of organism
- PFTs: increased residual volume, increased functional residual capacity, decreased vital capacity

● Medical management

- Oxygen therapy: 2 to 3 L/minute
- Intubation and mechanical ventilation if necessary
- Monitoring: vital signs, I/O, pulse oximetry, and respiratory status
- Position: high Fowler's
- Treatments: chest physiotherapy, postural drainage, intermittent positive pressure breathing, high-flow nebulizer treatments, and incentive spirometry
- Diet: high-calorie diet
- Dietary recommendations: fluids to 3 qt (3 L)/day if not contraindicated
- I.V. therapy: saline lock
- Activity: as tolerated
- Laboratory studies: ABG values, WBCs, and sputum studies
- Bronchodilators: terbutaline (Brethine), aminophylline (Truphylline), isoproterenol (Isuprel), theophylline (Theo-Dur); via nebulizer: albuterol (Proventil), ipratropium (Atrovent), metaproterenol (Alupent)

- Corticosteroids: hydrocortisone (Solu-Cortef), methylprednisolone (Solu-Medrol)
- Expectorant: guaifenesin (Robitussin)
- Antibiotics: ampicillin (Omnipen), tetracycline (Achromycin), cefixime (Suprax)
- Antacid: aluminum hydroxide gel (AlternaGEL)
- Beta-adrenergic medication: epinephrine (Adrenalin)
- Mast cell stabilizer: cromolyn (Intal)

● **Nursing interventions**
  - Assess respiratory status
  - Administer low-flow oxygen
  - Monitor and record vital signs, I/O, pulse oximetry, and laboratory studies
  - Provide chest physiotherapy, intermittent positive pressure breathing, turning, postural drainage, and suction; encourage coughing, deep breathing, and use of incentive spirometer
  - Keep the patient in high Fowler's position
  - Administer medications as prescribed
  - **Reinforce pursed-lip breathing to prolong exhalation and to increase airway pressure**
  - Maintain the patient's diet
  - Administer small, frequent feedings
  - Encourage fluids
  - Encourage the patient to express his feelings about difficulty breathing
  - Allow activity as tolerated
  - Monitor and record the color, amount, and consistency of sputum
  - Provide emotional support to allay the patient's anxiety
  - Weigh the patient daily
  - Provide information about the American Lung Association
  - Individualize home care instructions
    - Know about the disorder and its implications
    - Follow instructions for medication use and be aware of possible adverse effects
    - Stop smoking and avoid second-hand smoke
    - Control weight and follow dietary recommendations
    - Identify ways to reduce stress
    - Recognize the signs and symptoms of respiratory infection and respiratory distress
    - Adhere to activity limitations
    - Know proper use of home oxygen
    - Demonstrate pursed-lip and diaphragmatic breathing
    - Avoid exposure to chemical irritants and pollutants
    - Demonstrate deep-breathing and coughing exercises

● **Complications**
  - Carbon dioxide narcosis
  - Acute respiratory failure

Key nursing interventions for a patient with COPD

- Assess respiratory status.
- Administer low-flow oxygen.
- Provide chest physiotherapy, intermittent positive pressure breathing, turning, postural drainage, and suction; encourage coughing, deep breathing, and use of incentive spirometer.
- Keep the patient in high Fowler's position.
- Reinforce pursed-lip breathing to prolong exhalation and to increase airway pressure.
- Administer small, frequent feedings.
- Encourage fluids.

Key complications of COPD

- Acute respiratory failure
- Pneumonia
- Right-sided heart failure (emphysema)

- Pneumonia
- From emphysema
  - Pulmonary hypertension
  - Right-sided heart failure
  - Spontaneous pneumothorax

● **Possible surgical intervention**
- None

ACUTE RESPIRATORY DISTRESS SYNDROME (ARDS, SHOCK LUNG)

● **Definition**
- Respiratory failure that occurs in critically ill patients with underlying illnesses (such as pneumonia, septic shock, or trauma)

● **Causes**
- Viral pneumonia
- Fat emboli
- Aspiration of gastric contents
- Drug overdose
- Pulmonary contusions
- Idiosyncratic drug reaction
- Inhalation of noxious gases
- Near drowning
- Burn injury
- Sepsis
- Trauma
- Oxygen toxicity
- Multiple blood transfusions

● **Pathophysiology**
- Damaged capillary membranes cause interstitial edema and intra-alveolar hemorrhage (see *What happens in ARDS*)
- Decreased gas exchange results
- Cellular damage causes decreased surfactant production, resulting in hypoxemia

● **Assessment findings**
- Dyspnea
- Tachypnea
- Tachycardia
- Cyanosis
- Intercostal and substernal retractions
- Cough
- Crackles
- Rhonchi
- Anxiety

Key facts about ARDS

- Clinical syndrome of respiratory insufficiency
- Damaged capillary membranes cause interstitial edema and intra-alveolar hemorrhage
- Hypoxemia results

Common causes of ARDS

- Viral pneumonia
- Fat emboli
- Sepsis
- Decreased surfactant production

Key signs and symptoms of ARDS

- Dyspnea
- Tachypnea
- Crackles
- Rhonchi
- Anxiety
- Decreased breath sounds

GO WITH THE FLOW

What happens in ARDS

This flowchart shows the process and progress of acute respiratory distress syndrome (ARDS).

Injury reduces blood flow to the lungs, allowing platelets to aggregate.

These platelets release substances, such as serotonin, bradykinin and, especially, histamine. These substances inflame and damage the alveolar membrane and later increase capillary permeability. At this early stage, signs and symptoms of ARDS are undetectable.

Histamines and other inflammatory substances increase capillary permeability, allowing fluid to shift into the interstitial space. As a result, the patient may experience tachypnea, dyspnea, and tachycardia.

As capillary permeability increases, proteins and more fluid leak out, increasing interstitial osmotic pressure and causing pulmonary edema. At this stage, the patient may experience increased tachypnea, dyspnea, and cyanosis. Hypoxia (usually unresponsive to increased fraction of inspired oxygen), decreased pulmonary compliance, and crackles and rhonchi may also develop.

Fluid in the alveoli and decreased blood flow damage surfactant in the alveoli, reducing the cells' ability to produce more. Without surfactant, alveoli collapse, impairing gas exchange. Look for thick, frothy sputum and marked hypoxemia with increased respiratory distress.

The patient breathes faster, but sufficient oxygen can't cross the alveolocapillary membrane. Carbon dioxide, however, crosses more easily and is lost with every exhalation. Oxygen and carbon dioxide levels in the blood decrease. Look for increased tachypnea, hypoxemia, and hypocapnia.

Pulmonary edema worsens. Meanwhile, inflammation leads to fibrosis, which further impedes gas exchange. The resulting hypoxemia leads to metabolic acidosis. At this stage, look for increased partial pressure of arterial carbon dioxide; decreased pH, partial pressure of arterial oxygen, and bicarbonate levels; and mental confusion.

Pathophysiology of ARDS

- Lung injury causes platelets to aggregate.
- Platelets release substances that inflame and damage the alveolar membrane, increasing capillary permeability.
- Fluids shift into the interstitial space.
- As capillary permeability increases, pulmonary edema results.
- Alveoli collapse, impairing gas exchange.
- Oxygen and carbon dioxide levels in the blood decrease.
- Pulmonary edema worsens, inflammation leads to fibrosis, and gas exchange is further impeded.
- Metabolic acidosis results.

Diagnosing ARDS

- ABG analysis: respiratory acidosis, hypoxemia that doesn't respond to increased percentage of oxygen
- Chest X-ray: interstitial edema

Treating ARDS

- Oxygen therapy
- Intubation and mechanical ventilation using PEEP
- Antibiotics
- Steroids
- Sedatives
- Neuromuscular blocking agents

Key nursing interventions for a patient with ARDS

- Assess respiratory status.
- Monitor mechanical ventilation.
- Monitor and record vital signs, hemodynamic variables, I/O, laboratory studies, and pulse oximetry.
- Administer medications.

- Restlessness
- Hypotension
- Altered level of consciousness
- Motor dysfunction
- Decreased breath sounds

● **Diagnostic test findings**
- ABG analysis: respiratory acidosis, hypoxemia that doesn't respond to increased percentage of oxygen
- Chest X-ray: interstitial edema
- Sputum culture: may identify offending organism
- Blood cultures: may identify offending organism

● **Medical management**
- Oxygen therapy
- Intubation and mechanical ventilation using positive end expiratory pressure (PEEP)
- Monitoring: vital signs, I/O, pulse oximetry, central venous pressure (CVP), ECG, and hemodynamic variables
- Treatments: chest physiotherapy, postural drainage, and suction
- Diet: restrict fluid intake
- I.V. therapy: saline lock
- Position: high-Fowler's
- Activity: bed rest; active ROM and isometric exercises
- Laboratory studies: ABG values, sputum studies, blood cultures, Hb, and HCT
- Transfusion therapy: platelets, packed RBCs
- Deep vein thrombosis prophylaxis
- Antibiotics: amoxicillin (Amoxil), ampicillin (Omnipen)
- Analgesic: morphine
- Diuretics: furosemide (Lasix), ethacrynic acid (Edecrin)
- Anticoagulant: heparin
- Steroids: hydrocortisone (Solu-Cortef), methylprednisolone (Solu-Medrol)
- Antacid: aluminum hydroxide gel (AlternaGEL)
- Sedative: lorazepam (Ativan)
- Neuromuscular blocking agents: pancuronium (Pavulon), vecuronium (Norcuron)
- Mucosal barrier fortifier: sucralfate (Carafate)

● **Nursing interventions**
- Assess respiratory status
- Monitor mechanical ventilation
- Monitor and record vital signs, hemodynamic variables, I/O, laboratory studies, and pulse oximetry
- Provide suction, turning, and postural drainage; encourage coughing and deep breathing
- Keep the patient in high Fowler's position

- Maintain fluid restrictions
- Administer I.V. fluids
- Administer total parenteral nutrition (TPN)
- Administer medications as prescribed
- Encourage the patient to express his feelings about difficulty breathing
- Provide rest periods between activities
- Weigh the patient daily
- Provide emotional support to allay the patient's anxiety
- Maintain bed rest
- Individualize home care instructions
    - Know about the disorder and its implications
    - Follow instructions for medication use and be aware of possible adverse effects
    - Recognize the signs and symptoms of respiratory distress
    - Demonstrate deep breathing and coughing exercises
    - Avoid exposure to chemical irritants and pollutants

● **Complications**
- Multiple organ failure
- Ventilator-associated pneumonia
- Death

● **Possible surgical intervention**
- Tracheostomy for prolonged respiratory failure

TUBERCULOSIS, PULMONARY

● **Definition**
- Airborne, infectious, communicable disease that can occur acutely or chronically

● **Causes**
- *Mycobacterium tuberculosis*
- Risk factors: immunocompromised, exposure to active TB

● **Pathophysiology**
- Alveoli become the focus of infection from inhaled droplets containing bacteria
- Tubercle bacilli multiply, spread through the lymphatics, and drain into the systemic circulation
- In the lung tissue, macrophages surround the bacilli and form tubercles
- Tubercles go through the process of caseation, liquefaction, and cavitation

● **Assessment findings**
- Fatigue
- Malaise
- Irritability
- Night sweats
- Tachycardia

Key complications of ARDS
- Ventilator-associated pneumonia
- Death

Key facts about TB
- Airborne, infectious, communicable disease
- Can occur acutely or chronically

Common causes of TB
- *M. tuberculosis*
- Risk increases in immunocompromised patient

Key signs and symptoms of TB
- Night sweats
- Elevated temperature
- Yellow and mucoid sputum
- Cough
- Dyspnea

Diagnosing TB

- Chest X-ray: active or calcified lesions
- Sputum cultures: positive acid-fast bacillus; positive *M. tuberculosis*
- Mantoux skin test: positive

Treating TB

- Standard and airborne precautions
- Antituberculosis medications: isoniazed, ethambutol, rifampin

Key nursing interventions for a patient with TB

- Assess respiratory status.
- Monitor and record vital signs, pulse oximetry, I/O, and laboratory studies.
- Maintain airborne precautions.
- Place patient in a negative pressure room.
- Maintain the patient's diet.
- Provide suctioning, turning, chest physiotherapy, and postural drainage; encourage coughing, deep breathing, and use of incentive spirometry.
- Encourage fluids.
- Provide frequent oral hygiene.

- Weight loss
- Anorexia
- Cough
- Yellow and mucoid sputum
- Dyspnea
- Hemoptysis
- Crackles
- Elevated temperature

● Diagnostic test findings

- Chest X-ray: active or calcified lesions
- Sputum cultures: positive acid-fast bacillus; positive *M. tuberculosis*
- Hematology: increased WBCs, ESR
- Mantoux skin test: positive

● Medical management

- Monitoring: vital signs and I/O
- Treatments: chest physiotherapy, postural drainage, and incentive spirometry
- Precautions: standard and airborne
- Antituberculosis: isoniazid (INH), ethambutol (Myambutol), rifampin (Rifadin), pyrazinamide (pms-Pyrazinamide)
- Diet: high-carbohydrate, high-protein, high-vitamin B_6 and C, high-calorie
- I.V. therapy: saline lock
- Activity: bed rest, active ROM and isometric exercises
- Laboratory studies: ABG values, hepatic studies (due to medications), and sputum studies
- Antibiotic: streptomycin (Streptomycin)

● Nursing interventions

- Assess respiratory status
- Monitor and record vital signs, pulse oximetry, I/O, and laboratory studies
- Place patient in a negative pressure room and maintain airborne precautions
- Administer medications as prescribed
- Provide suctioning, turning, chest physiotherapy, and postural drainage; encourage coughing, deep breathing, and use of incentive spirometry
- Maintain the patient's diet
- Provide small, frequent meals
- Provide emotional support to allay the patient's anxiety
- Encourage fluids
- Instruct the patient to cover nose and mouth when sneezing or coughing
- Provide frequent oral hygiene
- Provide information about the American Lung Association
- Individualize home care instructions
  - Know about the disorder and its implications

– Follow instructions for medication use and be aware of possible adverse effects

– Demonstrate methods to prevent spread of sputum droplets

– Reinforce need to finish entire course of medication (6 to 18 months)

● **Complications**
- Atelectasis
- Spontaneous pneumothorax
- Pleural effusion
- Respiratory failure
- Death

● **Possible surgical intervention**
- Lobectomy

PNEUMOTHORAX

● **Definition**
- Collapse of the lung due to loss of negative intrapleural pressure
- Types include spontaneous, open, tension

● **Causes**
- Chest trauma
- Rupture of a bleb
- Invasive procedure
- Mechanical ventilation

● **Pathophysiology**
- The loss of negative intrapleural pressure causes lung collapse
- Surface area for gas exchange is reduced, resulting in hypoxia and hypercarbia
- Spontaneous pneumothorax occurs with bleb rupture
- Open pneumothorax occurs when an opening through the chest wall allows positive atmospheric pressure to enter the pleural space
- Tension pneumothorax occurs when positive pressure builds up in the pleural space

● **Assessment findings**
- Sharp chest pain that increases with exertion
- Diminished or absent breath sounds on affected side
- Dyspnea
- Tracheal shift
- Restlessness
- Anxiety
- Diaphoresis
- Tachycardia
- Tachypnea
- Unequal chest expansion

Key complications of TB
- Pleural effusion
- Pneumothorax
- Death

Key facts about pneumothorax
- Loss of negative intrapleural pressure
- Results in collapse of the lung
- Three types: spontaneous, open, and tension

Common causes of pneumothorax
- Chest trauma
- Rupture of a bleb
- Invasive procedure

Key signs and symptoms of pneumothorax
- Sharp pain that increases with exertion
- Diminished or absent breath sounds unilaterally
- Dyspnea
- Tachypnea

- Subcutaneous emphysema
- Pallor, cyanosis
- Cough

● Diagnostic test findings
- Chest X-ray: pneumothorax
- ABG analysis: respiratory acidosis, hypoxemia
- Ventilation-perfusion ($\dot{V}/\dot{Q}$) scintigraphy: decreased
- $\dot{V}/\dot{Q}$ defects: $\dot{V}/\dot{Q}$ mismatches

● Medical management
- Oxygen therapy
- Needle decompression (tension pneumothorax)
- Insertion: chest tube to water-seal drainage
- Monitoring: vital signs, pulse oximetry, and I/O
- Laboratory studies: ABG values
- Position: high Fowler's
- Activity: out of bed to chair, active ROM exercises to affected arm
- Treatments: incentive spirometry
- Analgesic: oxycodone (Tylox)

● Nursing interventions
- Assess respiratory status
- Administer oxygen
- Keep the patient in high Fowler's position
- Monitor and record vital signs, chest tube drainage, air leak or subcutaneous emphysema, and laboratory studies
- Administer medications as prescribed
- Turn the patient and encourage coughing, deep breathing, and the use of incentive spirometry
- Maintain chest tube to water-seal drainage
- Allay the patient's anxiety
- Assess the patient's pain
- Individualize home care instructions
    - Know about the disorder and its implications
    - Follow instructions for medication use and be aware of possible adverse effects
    - Recognize the signs and symptoms of pneumothorax and respiratory infection
    - Avoid heavy lifting

● Complications
- Cardiac arrhythmia
- Respiratory failure
- Infection
- Death

● Possible surgical interventions
- Pleurodesis with talc
- Video-assisted thorascopic surgery

Treating pneumothorax

- Oxygen therapy
- Needle decompression (tension pneumothorax)
- Insertion: chest tube to water-seal drainage

Key nursing interventions for a patient with pneumothorax

- Assess respiratory status.
- Monitor vital signs and chest tube drainage.
- Administer medications as prescribed.

Key complications of pneumothorax

- Respiratory failure
- Death

PULMONARY EMBOLISM

- **Definition**
  - Undissolved substance in the pulmonary vasculature that obstructs blood flow
  - Three types
    - Fat
    - Air
    - Thrombus

- **Causes**
  - Flat or long bone fractures
  - Thrombophlebitis
  - Venous stasis
  - Hypercoagulable state
  - Risk factors
    - Pregnancy
    - Immobility
    - Cancer
    - Joint replacement surgery
    - Trauma
    - Central line insertion
    - Smoking; hormonal contraceptive use (see *Who's at risk for pulmonary embolism?* page 108)

- **Pathophysiology**
  - Air, fat, or the tail of a thrombus that breaks off travels from the venous circulation to the right side of the heart and pulmonary artery
  - The embolism obstructs blood flow, resulting in pulmonary hypertension and possible infarction

- **Assessment findings**
  - Chest pain
  - Dyspnea
  - Tachycardia
  - Elevated temperature
  - Cough
  - Frothy, pink-tinged sputum
  - Hemoptysis
  - Tachypnea
  - Anxiety
  - Crackles
  - Hypotension
  - Arrhythmias

- **Diagnostic test findings**
  - Spiral computed tomography (CT) scan: identifies pulmonary embolism
  - Lung scan: decreased pulmonary circulation, blood flow obstruction
  - Angiography: location of embolism, filling defect of pulmonary artery

Key facts about pulmonary embolism

- Undissolved substance in pulmonary vasculature obstructs blood flow
- Three types: fat, air, and thrombus

Common causes of pulmonary embolism

- Flat or long bone fractures
- Thrombophlebitis
- Venous stasis

Key signs and symptoms of pulmonary embolism

- Chest pain
- Dyspnea
- Frothy, pink-tinged sputum
- Tachypnea
- Crackles

TOP 5

Conditions that increase risk for pulmonary embolism

1. Surgery
2. Prolonged bed rest
3. Atrial fibrillation
4. Cancer
5. Central lines

Diagnosing pulmonary embolism

- ABG analysis: respiratory alkalosis, hypoxemia
- Lung scan: decreased pulmonary circulation, blood flow obstruction
- Angiography: location of embolism, filling defect of pulmonary artery

Treating pulmonary embolism

- Oxygen therapy
- Intubation and mechanical ventilation
- Anticoagulants
- Thrombolytics

Who's at risk for pulmonary embolism?

Many disorders and treatments heighten the risk of pulmonary embolism. At particular risk are surgical patients. The anesthetic used during surgery can injure lung vessels, and surgery or prolonged bed rest can promote venous stasis, which compounds the risk.

PREDISPOSING DISORDERS
- Cardiac arrhythmia (especially atrial fibrillation)
- Lung disorders, especially chronic types
- Cardiac disorders
- Infection
- Diabetes mellitus
- History of thromboembolism, thrombophlebitis, or vascular insufficiency
- Sickle cell disease
- Autoimmune hemolytic anemia
- Polycythemia
- Osteomyelitis
- Long-bone fracture
- Presence of central lines

VENOUS STASIS
- Prolonged bed rest or immobilization
- Obesity

- Older than age 40
- Burns
- Recent childbirth
- Orthopedic casts

VENOUS INJURY
- Surgery, particularly of the legs, pelvis, abdomen, or thorax
- Leg or pelvic fractures or injuries
- I.V. drug abuse
- I.V. therapy

INCREASED BLOOD COAGULABILITY
- Cancer
- Use of high-estrogen hormonal contraceptives
- Hypercoagulable condition

- Chest X-ray: dilated pulmonary arteries
- ABG analysis: respiratory alkalosis, hypoxemia
- Blood chemistry: increased lactate dehydrogenase
- ECG: tachycardia, nonspecific ST changes

● **Medical management**
- Oxygen therapy with intubation and mechanical ventilation, if needed
- Monitoring: vital signs, pulse oximetry, CVP, ECG, I/O, and neurovascular checks
- Thrombolytics: streptokinase, urokinase, tissue plasminogen activator
- Anticoagulants: heparin, warfarin (Coumadin)
- I.V. therapy: hydration, saline lock
- Position: high Fowler's
- Activity: bed rest; active and passive ROM and isometric exercises
- Laboratory studies: ABG analysis, PT, and PTT
- Treatments: indwelling urinary catheter, incentive spirometry
- Analgesics: meperidine (Demerol), oxycodone and acetaminophen (Percocet, Tylox)
- Diuretics: furosemide (Lasix), ethacrynic acid (Edecrin)

Nursing interventions
- Assess respiratory status
- Administer oxygen
- Monitor vital signs, CVP, I/O, signs and symptoms of bleeding, laboratory studies, and pulse oximetry
- Administer medications as prescribed
- Encourage coughing, deep breathing, and use of incentive spirometry
- Keep the patient in high Fowler's position
- Administer I.V. fluids
- Provide emotional support to allay the patient's anxiety
- Monitor and record color, consistency, and amount of sputum
- Assess for positive Homans' sign
- Monitor PT and PTT to maintain therapeutic anticoagulation levels
- Individualize home care instructions
  - Know about the disorder and its implications
  - Follow instructions for medication use and be aware of possible adverse effects
  - Recognize the signs and symptoms of respiratory distress
  - Avoid activities that promote venous stasis
    · Prolonged sitting and standing
    · Wearing constrictive clothing
    · Crossing legs when seated
    · Using hormonal contraceptives; smoking
  - Recognize signs and symptoms of bleeding

Complications
- Pulmonary infarction
- Respiratory failure
- Bleeding
- Death

Possible surgical interventions
- Pulmonary embolectomy
- Vena cava filter insertion
- Percutaneous thrombectomy

LUNG CANCER

Definition
- Malignant tumor of the lung that may be primary or metastatic

Causes
- Cigarette smoke (primary or secondary)
- Exposure to environmental pollutants
- Exposure to occupational pollutants

Pathophysiology
- Unregulated cell growth and uncontrolled cell division result in the development of a neoplasm

Types of lung cancer

- Epidermoid
- Adenocarcinoma
- Large cell anaplastic
- Small cell anaplastic

Key signs and symptoms of lung cancer

- Cough
- Hemoptysis
- Weight loss
- Anorexia

Diagnosing lung cancer

- Bronchoscopy: positive biopsy
- Chest X-ray, CT scan, MRI, and lung scan: mass
- Pulmonary angiography: involvement of pulmonary artery or veins
- Sputum studies: positive cytology for cancer cells

Treating lung cancer

- Radiation therapy
- Antineoplastics
- Surgery

- Four histologic types include epidermoid (squamous), adenocarcinoma, large cell anaplastic, and small cell anaplastic
- The lungs are a common target site for metastasis from other organs

● **Assessment findings**
- Cough
- Dyspnea
- Hoarseness
- Hemoptysis
- Chest pain
- Chills
- Fever
- Weight loss
- Weakness
- Anorexia
- Wheezing
- Fatigue

● **Diagnostic test findings**
- Chest X-ray, CT scan, or magnetic resonance imaging (MRI): lesion or mass
- Positron emission tomography scan: cancerous tumors
- Bronchoscopy: malignant cells
- Pulmonary angiography: involvement of pulmonary artery or pulmonary veins
- Sputum culture: positive cytology for cancer cells

● **Medical management**
- Radiation therapy
- Antineoplastics: cisplatin (Platinol), cyclophosphamide (Cytoxan), doxorubicin (Adriamycin), vinblastine (Velban)
- Oxygen therapy with intubation and mechanical ventilation, if needed
- Monitoring: vital signs, pulse oximetry, and I/O
- Analgesics: morphine (Roxanol), hydromorphone (Dilaudid)
- Diet: high-protein, high-calorie
- I.V. therapy: hydration, saline lock
- Position: semi-Fowler's
- Activity: active and passive ROM exercises, as tolerated
- Laboratory studies: ABG analysis
- Nutritional support: TPN
- Treatment: incentive spirometry
- Isotope implant
- Laser photocoagulation
- Diuretics: furosemide (Lasix), ethacrynic acid (Edecrin)
- Antiemetic: prochlorperazine (Compazine), ondansetron (Zofran)

● **Nursing interventions**
- Assess respiratory status
- Administer oxygen

- Monitor and record vital signs, pulse oximetry, I/O, and laboratory studies
- Administer medications as prescribed
- Assess the patient's pain level, administer analgesics, as prescribed, and evaluate effect
- Maintain the patient's diet
- Encourage fluids
- Administer I.V. fluids
- Provide suction and turning; encourage coughing and deep breathing
- Keep the patient in semi-Fowler's position
- Administer TPN
- Encourage the patient to express his feelings about his diagnosis
- Provide emotional support to allay the patient's anxiety
- Provide postchemotherapeutic and postradiation nursing care
    - Provide skin and mouth care
    - Monitor dietary intake
    - Administer antiemetics and antidiarrheals, as prescribed
    - **Monitor for bleeding, infection, and electrolyte imbalance**
    - Provide rest periods
- Provide information about the American Cancer Society
- Individualize home care instructions
    - Know about the disorder and its implication
    - Follow instructions for medication use and be aware of possible adverse effects
    - Demonstrate deep breathing and coughing exercises
    - Alternate rest periods with activity
    - Follow dietary recommendations and restrictions
    - Know the location of local support services

● **Complications**
- Respiratory failure
- Pneumonia
- Depression
- Metastasis
- Death

● **Possible surgical interventions**
- Lung resection
- Lobectomy
- Wedge resection
- Pneumonectomy

LARYNGEAL CANCER

● **Definition**
- Malignant tumor or lesion of the larynx
- Intrinsic tumor located on the vocal cords
- Extrinsic tumor located on another part of the larynx

Common causes of laryngeal cancer

- Cigarette smoking
- Alcohol abuse
- Environmental pollutants
- Radiation

Key signs and symptoms of laryngeal cancer

- Throat pain
- Palpable mass in neck
- Dysphagia
- Persistent hoarseness

Diagnosing laryngeal cancer

- Laryngoscopy: lesions, ulcerations, positive biopsy
- Biopsy: cytology positive for cancer cells

Treating laryngeal cancer

- Radiation therapy
- Antineoplastics
- Surgery
- Speech therapy

● **Causes**
  - Cigarette smoking
  - Alcohol abuse
  - Exposure to environmental pollutants
  - Exposure to radiation

● **Pathophysiology**
  - Unregulated cell growth and uncontrolled cell division result in the development of a neoplasm through the growth of abnormal cells
  - Most laryngeal cancers are squamous cell carcinomas

● **Assessment findings**
  - Persistent hoarseness
  - Throat pain
  - Burning sensation
  - Palpable mass in neck
  - Dysphagia
  - Dyspnea
  - Cough
  - Hemoptysis
  - Weakness
  - Weight loss
  - Foul breath

● **Diagnostic test findings**
  - Laryngoscopy: lesions, ulcerations, positive biopsy
  - Biopsy: cytology positive for cancer cells
  - CT scan: laryngeal tumor
  - MRI: laryngeal tumor

● **Medical management**
  - Radiation therapy
  - Antineoplastics: methotrexate (Amethopterin), vincristine (Oncovin), bleomycin (Blenoxane), cisplatin (Platinol)
  - Oxygen therapy
  - Monitoring: vital signs and I/O
  - Diet: high-calorie, high-vitamin, high-protein
  - I.V. therapy: hydration, saline lock
  - Position: semi-Fowler's
  - Activity: as tolerated
  - Laboratory studies: Hb, HCT, and ABG analysis
  - Nutritional support: TPN, NG tube feedings, or gastrostomy feedings
  - Speech therapy
  - Treatment: incentive spirometry
  - Analgesic: oxycodone and acetaminophen (Percocet, Tylox), hydromorphone (Dilaudid)
  - Antiemetic: prochlorperazine (Compazine), ondansetron (Zofran)

● **Nursing interventions**
- Assess respiratory status
- Administer oxygen
- Monitor and record vital signs, pulse oximetry, I/O, and laboratory studies
- Administer medications as prescribed
- Monitor and record the color, amount, and consistency of sputum
- Maintain high-calorie, high-vitamin, high-protein diet
- Administer I.V. fluids
- Turn the patient and encourage coughing, deep breathing, and use of incentive spirometer
- Maintain activity as tolerated
- Keep the patient in semi-Fowler's position
- Administer TPN, NG tube feedings, or gastrostomy feedings
- Encourage the patient to express his feelings about his diagnosis
- Provide emotional support to allay the patient's anxiety
- Provide postchemotherapeutic and postradiation nursing care
  - Provide prophylactic skin and mouth care
  - Monitor dietary intake
  - Administer antiemetics and antidiarrheals, as prescribed
  - Monitor for bleeding, infection, and electrolyte imbalance
  - Provide rest periods
- Provide information about the Lost Chord Club, New Voice Club, and International Association of Laryngectomies
- Individualize home care instructions
  - Know about the disorder and its implications
  - Follow instructions for medication use and be aware of possible adverse effects
  - Recognize the signs and symptoms of respiratory distress
  - Limit using voice
  - Demonstrate tracheostomy care, suctioning, alternative communication
  - Know the location of local support services

● **Complications**
- Laryngeal obstruction
- Respiratory distress
- Depression
- Metastasis
- Dysphagia

● **Possible surgical interventions**
- Partial laryngectomy
- Total laryngectomy
- Radical neck dissection

Key nursing interventions in caring for a patient with laryngeal cancer
- Assess respiratory status.
- Administer oxygen.
- Provide emotional support.
- Provide postchemotherapeutic and postradiation nursing care.

Key complications of laryngeal cancer
- Depression
- Laryngeal obstruction
- Respiratory distress

Key facts about occupational lung disease

- Obstructive or restrictive respiratory disorders
- Occurs with exposure to occupational fumes, dust, vapors, or gases
- Four main categories:
- Occupational asthma
- Pneumoconiosis
- Diffuse interstitial fibrosis
- Extrinsic allergic alveolitis

Common causes of occupational lung disease

- Fumes, dust, vapors, or gases
- Cigarette smoke

Key signs and symptoms of occupational lung disease

- Exertional dyspnea
- Blood-streaked sputum
- Cough
- Tachypnea

OCCUPATIONAL LUNG DISEASE

● **Definition**
- Obstructive or restrictive respiratory disorders that result from exposure to occupational fumes, dust, vapors, or gases
- Four main categories of occupational lung disease: occupational asthma, pneumoconiosis, diffuse interstitial fibrosis, and extrinsic allergic alveolitis

● **Causes**
- Exposure to occupational fumes, dust, vapors, or gases
- Cigarette smoke

● **Pathophysiology**
- Occupational asthma is associated with variable airway narrowing related to an exposure in the workplace
- Pneumoconiosis is due to lodging of inhaled dust in the lungs
    - Silicosis is caused by long-term inhalation of free crystalline silica dust
    - Coal miner's pneumoconiosis (black lung disease) is due to deposits of coal dust in the lungs
- Diffuse interstitial fibrosis is caused by occupational exposure to irritants
    - Asbestosis: common among asbestos miners, millers, and those employed in building trades and shipping yards (see *A close look at asbestosis*)
    - Talcosis occurs after years of exposure to high concentrations of talc dust
    - Berylliosis, a chronic granulomatous disorder, caused by inhalation of beryllium
- Extrinsic allergic alveolitis is a hypersensitivity pneumonitis caused by an immunologic response to inhaled organic dust or chemicals containing bacteria or fungal antigens
    - Includes farmer's lung, bird fancier's lung, and machine operator's lung

● **Assessment findings**
- Exertional dyspnea
- Anxiety
- Frequent respiratory infections
- Blood-streaked sputum
- Cough
- Tachypnea

● **Diagnostic test findings**
- Chest X-ray: nodular lesions, enlarged hilar nodes
- Lung biopsy: to establish diagnosis
- PFTs: reveal decreased volume and forced vital capacity
- ABG analysis: may reveal decreased PaO_2 and SaO_2 levels; increased $PaCO_2$

A close look at asbestosis

After years of exposure to asbestos, healthy lung tissue progresses to massive pulmonary fibrosis, as shown here.

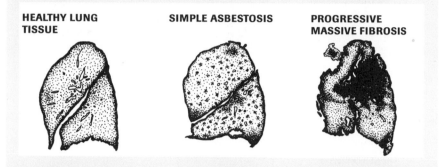

HEALTHY LUNG TISSUE   **SIMPLE ASBESTOSIS**   **PROGRESSIVE MASSIVE FIBROSIS**

● **Medical management**
- Oxygen therapy: 1 to 2 L/minute; mechanical ventilation in advanced cases
- Treatments: chest physiotherapy, turning, coughing, deep breathing, postural drainage, and intermittent positive pressure breathing
- Dietary recommendations: increase fluids, unless contraindicated
- Aerosol therapy
- Bronchodilators: aminophylline (Phyllocontin), theophylline (Theo-Dur), metaproterenol (Alupent), cromolyn (Intal)
- Corticosteroids: oral prednisone or aerosol corticosteroid
- Inhaled mucolytic therapy: acetylcysteine (Mucomyst)
- Antibiotics: according to susceptibility of infecting organism
- Diuretic: furosemide (Lasix)
- Cardiac glycoside: digoxin (Lanoxin)
- Fluid restriction for cor pulmonale
- Activity: as tolerated
- Monitoring: vital signs, pulse oximetry, and I/O
- Laboratory studies: ABG analysis, WBCs, and sputum studies
- I.V. therapy: hydration, saline lock

● **Nursing interventions**
- Assess cardiovascular and respiratory status
- Administer oxygen
- Provide chest physiotherapy, intermittent positive pressure breathing, turning, and postural drainage; encourage coughing, deep breathing, and use of incentive spirometry
- Monitor and record vital signs, I/O, and laboratory studies
- Administer medications as prescribed
- Monitor sputum for amount, color, and consistency
- Maintain patient's diet
- Administer small, frequent feedings

Key complications of occupational lung disease

- Right-sided heart failure
- Respiratory infection
- Respiratory failure

Key facts about acute respiratory failure

- Acute deterioration in ABG values with corresponding clinical deterioration
- With normal lung tissue, acute respiratory failure usually means $PaCO_2$ above 50 mm Hg and PaO_2 below 50 mm Hg
- COPD patient usually has consistently high $PaCO_2$ and low PaO_2

Common causes of acute respiratory failure

- Respiratory infection
- Bronchospasm
- CNS depression
- Cardiovascular disorders

- Encourage fluids, unless the patient has cor pulmonale
- Encourage activity as tolerated
- Individualize home care instructions
  - Know about the disorder and its implications
  - Follow instructions for medication use and be aware of possible adverse effects
  - Prevent infection by avoiding crowds and persons with respiratory infections
  - Receive influenza and pneumococcal vaccines
  - Pace activities and provide rest periods
  - Know proper use of home oxygen
  - Stop smoking
  - Know the location of local support services

● **Complications**
- Cor pulmonale
- Right-sided heart failure
- Respiratory infection
- TB
- Respiratory failure

● **Possible surgical interventions**
- Tracheostomy for chronic respiratory failure

ACUTE RESPIRATORY FAILURE

● **Definition**
- Impaired arterial oxygenation or inadequate carbon dioxide elimination that leads to tissue hypoxia

● **Causes**
- Respiratory infection, such as bronchitis or pneumonia (most common)
- Bronchospasm
- Accumulating secretions secondary to cough suppression
- Head or chest trauma
- Injudicious use of sedatives, opioids, tranquilizers, or oxygen
- Central nervous system (CNS) depression
- Myocardial infarction
- Heart failure, pulmonary edema, or pulmonary emboli
- Airway irritants
- Myxedema
- Metabolic alkalosis
- Pneumothorax
- Thoracic or abdominal surgery

● **Pathophysiology**
- In the patient with normal lung tissue, acute respiratory failure usually means $PaCO_2$ above 50 mm Hg and PaO_2 below 50 mm Hg

Identifying respiratory failure

Use these measurements to identify respiratory failure:
- vital capacity less than 15 cc/kg
- tidal volume less than 3 cc/kg
- negative inspiratory force less than -25 cm H_2O
- respiratory rate more than twice the normal rate
- diminished partial pressure of arterial oxygen despite increased fraction of inspired oxygen
- elevated partial pressure of arterial carbon dioxide, with pH lower than 7.25.

- These limits don't apply to the patient with COPD, who commonly has a consistently high $PaCO_2$ and low PaO_2
- Acute respiratory failure may develop in the patient with COPD as a result of any condition that increases the work of breathing and decreases the respiratory drive
- Increased $\dot{V}/\dot{Q}$ mismatch and reduced alveolar ventilation decrease PaO_2 (hypoxemia) and increase $PaCO_2$ (hypercapnia)
- The resulting hypoxemia and acidemia affect all body organs, especially the CNS and respiratory and cardiovascular systems

Assessment findings
- Increased or normal respiratory rate, depending on cause
- Shallow or deep respirations, or alternating between the two
- Air hunger
- Cyanosis
- Crackles, rhonchi, wheezes, or diminished breath sounds
- Restlessness
- Confusion
- Loss of concentration
- Irritability
- Coma
- Tachycardia
- Arrhythmias
- Jugular vein distention
- Hepatomegaly
- Peripheral edema

Diagnostic test findings
- ABG analysis: progressive deterioration in ABG levels and pH
- Blood chemistry: increased bicarbonate, indicating metabolic alkalosis or metabolic compensation for chronic respiratory acidosis; hypokalemia and hypochloremia from diuretic and corticosteroid therapies that treat acute respiratory failure (see *Identifying respiratory failure*)
- Hematology: elevated WBCs due to bacterial infection
- Chest X-ray: identifies pathologic conditions, such as emphysema, atelectasis, lesions, pneumothorax, infiltrates, or effusions

Key signs and symptoms of acute respiratory failure
- Tachypnea
- Abnormal breath sounds
- Restlessness
- Confusion
- Tachycardia
- Arrhythmias

Diagnosing acute respiratory failure
- ABG analysis: progressive deterioration
- Chest X-ray: identifies pathologic conditions
- ECG: arrhythmias

- ECG: arrhythmias suggest cor pulmonale or myocardial hypoxia

● **Medical management**
- Oxygen therapy: use minimum fraction of inspired air (FIO_2) required, by nasal prongs or Venturi mask, to maintain ventilation or oxygen saturation greater than 85%
- Intubation and mechanical ventilation
- Bronchodilators: terbutaline (Brethine), aminophylline (Phyllocontin), isoproterenol (Isuprel), theophylline (Theo-Dur); via nebulizer: albuterol (Proventil), ipratropium (Atrovent), metaproterenol (Alupent)
- Corticosteroids: hydrocortisone (Solu-Cortef), methylprednisolone (Solu-Medrol)
- Treatments: chest physiotherapy, postural drainage, intermittent positive pressure breathing, and incentive spirometry
- Position: high Fowler's
- Activity: as tolerated
- Monitoring: vital signs, pulse oximetry, and I/O
- Laboratory studies: ABG analysis, WBCs, and sputum studies
- Fluid restriction
- Antibiotics: ampicillin (Omnipen), tetracycline (Achromycin), cefixime (Suprax)
- Diuretic: furosemide (Lasix)
- Vasopressor: dopamine
- Antacid: aluminum hydroxide gel (AlternaGEL)
- I.V. therapy: saline lock

● **Nursing interventions**
- Assess cardiovascular and respiratory status
- Administer oxygen therapy
- Monitor and record vital signs, pulse oximetry, I/O, and laboratory studies
- Provide chest physiotherapy, intermittent positive pressure breathing, turning, postural drainage, and suctioning; encourage coughing, deep breathing, and use of incentive spirometer
- Administer medications as prescribed
- Monitor and record the color, amount, and consistency of sputum
- Maintain the patient's diet
- Administer small, frequent feedings
- Encourage fluids, unless contraindicated
- Reinforce pursed-lip breathing
- Keep the patient in high Fowler's position
- Encourage the patient to express concerns, and allay his anxieties
- Allow activity as tolerated
- Weigh the patient daily
- Individualize home care instructions
  - Know about the disorder and its implications
  - Follow instructions for medication use and be aware of possible adverse effects

- Recognize the signs and symptoms of respiratory infection and hypoxia
- Adhere to activity limitations
- Know proper use of home oxygen
- Demonstrate pursed-lip breathing and coughing exercises
- Receive influenza and pneumococcal vaccines

● **Complications**
  - Chronic respiratory failure
  - Ventilator-associated pneumonia
  - Death

● **Surgical interventions**
  - Tracheostomy for chronic respiratory failure

ASTHMA

● **Definition**
  - A chronic inflammatory airway disorder characterized by airflow obstruction and airway hyperresponsiveness to various stimuli
  - Two forms
    - Extrinsic (atopic) asthma is caused by sensitivity to specific external allergens
    - Intrinsic (nonatopic) asthma is caused by a reaction to internal, nonallergic factors

● **Causes**
  - Extrinsic asthma
    - Allergens (pollen, dust, dander, sulfite food additives)
  - Intrinsic asthma
    - Endocrine changes
    - Noxious fumes
    - Respiratory infection
    - Stress
    - Temperature and humidity

● **Pathophysiology**
  - Bronchial linings overreact to various stimuli, causing episodic spasms and inflammation that severely restrict the airways
  - Narrowed airways trap the air; as the airways becomes occluded by thick secretions, the lungs hyperinflate

● **Assessment findings**
  - Absent or diminished breath sounds during severe obstruction
  - Chest tightness
  - Dyspnea
  - Productive cough with thick mucus
  - Prolonged expiration
  - Tachypnea

Key complications of acute respiratory failure
- Ventilator-associated pneumonia
- Death

Key facts about asthma
- Form of COPD
- Heightened response to various stimuli causes widespread airway constriction

Common causes of asthma
- Extrinsic asthma is caused by sensitivity to specific external allergens
- Intrinsic asthma is caused by a reaction to internal, nonallergic factors

Key signs and symptoms of asthma
- Absent or diminished breath sounds during severe obstruction
- Usually asymptomatic between attacks
- Wheezing, primarily on expiration, but also sometimes on inspiration

Diagnosing asthma

- Decreased forced expiratory volumes that improve with bronchodilator therapy
- Increased residual volume and total lung capacity

Treating asthma

- Oxygen therapy
- Bronchodilators
- Corticosteroids
- Recognition and avoidance of precipitating factors
- Desensitization of allergens

Key nursing interventions for a patient with asthma

- Administer low-flow oxygen.
- Encourage fluids.
- Keep the patient in high Fowler's position.
- Monitor color, amount, and consistency of sputum.

- Tachycardia
- Use of accessory muscles
- Usually asymptomatic between attacks
- Wheezing, primarily on expiration, but also sometimes on inspiration

● **Diagnostic test findings**
- ABG analysis: in severe acute asthma, decreased PaO_2 and decreased, normal, or increased $PaCO_2$
- Laboratory values: serum immunoglobulin E may increase from an allergic reaction; WBC count may reveal increased eosinophil count
- Chest X-ray: hyperinflated lungs with air trapping during an attack
- PFTs: during attacks show decreased forced expiratory volumes that improve with bronchodilation therapy, and increased residual volume and total lung capacity
- Skin tests: may identify allergens

● **Medical management**
- Oxygen therapy with intubation and mechanical ventilation, if respiratory status worsens
- Bronchodilators: terbutaline (Brethine), aminophylline (Phyllocontin), theophylline (Theo-Dur); via nebulizer: albuterol (Proventil), ipratropium (Atrovent), metaproterenol (Alupent)
- Corticosteroids: hydrocortisone (Solu-Cortef), methylprednisolone (Solu-Medrol); via nebulizer: beclomethasone (Vanceril), triamcinolone (Azmacort)
- Position: high Fowler's
- Monitoring: vital signs, I/O, pulse oximetry, and laboratory values
- Treatments: turning, coughing, deep breathing, and breathing retraining
- Dietary recommendations: encourage fluids to 3 L/day as tolerated
- Activity: as tolerated
- Recognition and avoidance of precipitating factors
- Desensitization to allergens
- Antacid: aluminum hydroxide gel (AlternaGEL)
- Antibiotics: according to sensitivity of infective organism
- Mast cell stabilizer: cromolyn (Intal)
- Leukotriene antagonists: zileuton (Zyflo), zafirlukast (Accolate)
- Beta-adrenergics: epinephrine (Adrenalin), salmeterol (Serevent)
- I.V. therapy: saline lock

● **Nursing interventions**
- Administer low-flow oxygen
- Assess respiratory status
- Keep the patient in high Fowler's position
- Maintain the patient's diet as tolerated
- Administer small, frequent feedings
- Encourage fluids
- Provide turning; teach pursed-lip and diaphragmatic breathing; and encourage coughing and deep breathing

- Monitor and record vital signs, I/O, and laboratory studies
- Administer medications as prescribed
- Encourage patient to express his feelings about his fear of suffocation
- Allow activity as tolerated
- Monitor and record the color, amount, and consistency of sputum
- Individualize home care instructions
    - Know about the disorder and its implications
    - Follow instructions for medication use and be aware of possible adverse effects
    - Identify triggers to asthma attacks
    - Demonstrate use of a metered-dose inhaler and peak flow meter
    - Demonstrate pursed-lip and diaphragmatic breathing
    - Recognize early signs and symptoms of respiratory infection and hypoxia

● **Complications**
- Asphyxia
- Status asthmaticus
- Death

● **Possible surgical interventions**
- None

BLUNT CHEST TRAUMA INJURY

● **Definition**
- Trauma to the chest caused by sudden compression or positive pressure to the chest wall

● **Causes**
- Motor vehicle accidents
- Trauma
- Falls
- Sports injuries

● **Pathophysiology**
- Blunt trauma may result in rib fracture, flail chest, pneumothorax, tension pneumothorax, and cardiac tamponade
- Rib fracture causes pain with resultant hypoventilation, leading to atelectasis (see *A close look at atelectatic alveoli,* page 122)
- Flail chest results in paradoxical breathing and inadequate ventilation
- Pneumothorax impairs lung expansion, compromising gas exchange
- With cardiac tamponade, intrapericardial pressure increases, compressing the heart; cardiac output decreases; and cardiogenic shock occurs

● **Assessment findings**
- Cardiac tamponade
    - Chest pain

Key complications of asthma
- Status asthmaticus
- Death

Key facts about blunt chest trauma injury
- Trauma to the chest
- Caused by sudden compression or positive pressure to chest wall
- With cardiac tamponade, intrapericardial pressure increases, compressing the heart; cardiac output decreases; and cardiogenic shock occurs

Key signs and symptoms of cardiac tamponade

- Muffled heart sounds
- Restlessness
- Jugular vein distention
- Narrowed pulse pressure and paradoxical pulse

Key signs and symptoms of flail chest pain

- Pain on inspiration and on palpation of the injured area
- Paradoxical movement of the flail segment

Key signs and symptoms of pneumothorax

- Asymmetrical lung expansion
- Dyspnea
- Decreased or absent breath sounds on the affected side
- Restlessness
- Signs of mediastinal shift and tension pneumothorax

Key signs and symptoms of rib fractures

- Pain on inspiration
- Pain and tenderness of injured area upon palpation

A close look at atelectatic alveoli

Normally, air-filled alveoli exchange oxygen and carbon dioxide with capillary blood. However, in atelectasis, airless, shrunken alveoli can't accomplish gas exchange.

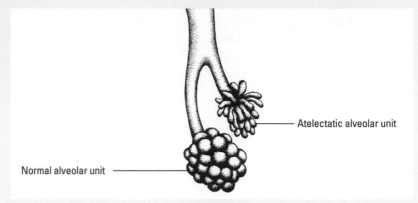

Atelectatic alveolar unit

Normal alveolar unit

- Hypotension
- Muffled heart sounds
- Tachycardia
- Cyanosis
- Diaphoresis
- Restlessness
- Jugular vein distention
- Narrowed pulse pressure and paradoxical pulse
- Flail chest
  - Paradoxical movement of the flail segment
  - Increased respiratory effort
  - Pain on inspiration and on palpation of the injured area
  - Cyanosis
  - Dyspnea
- Pneumothorax
  - Asymmetrical chest movement
  - Chest pain
  - Crepitus
  - Dyspnea
  - Decreased or absent breath sounds on the affected side
  - Restlessness
  - Signs of mediastinal shift and tension pneumothorax
- Rib fractures
  - Pain on inspiration
  - Pain and tenderness of injured area upon palpation
  - Hypoventilation

- Tension pneumothorax
  - Asymmetrical lung expansion and tracheal deviation to the affected side
  - Cyanosis
  - Hypotension
  - Decreased or absent breath sounds on the affected side
  - Jugular vein distention
  - Severe chest pain and respiratory distress
  - Subcutaneous emphysema

● Diagnostic test findings

- Chest X-rays: may confirm rib and sternal fractures, pneumothorax, flail chest, pulmonary contusions, lacerated or ruptured aorta, diaphragmatic rupture, lung compression, or atelectasis with hemothorax
- ECG: with cardiac damage, may show abnormalities, including tachycardia, atrial fibrillation, bundle-branch block, ST-segment changes, and ventricular arrhythmias
- Laboratory tests: serial aspartate aminotransferase, alanine aminotransferase, lactate dehydrogenase, creatine kinase, CK-MB, troponin I, and troponin T levels are elevated
- Retrograde aortography and transesophageal echocardiography: reveal aortic laceration or rupture
- Contrast studies and liver and spleen scans: detect diaphragmatic rupture
- Echocardiography, CT scans, and MRI: show the injury's extent

● Medical management

- Oxygen therapy
- Intubation and mechanical ventilation using positive pressure
- Position: semi-Fowler's (unless patient requires shock position)
- Monitoring: vital signs, I/O, hemodynamic parameters, ECG, and pulse oximetry
- Analgesic: morphine
- Supportive medications to control heart failure and arrhythmias
- Treatments: indwelling urinary catheter, chest tube, turning, coughing, deep breathing, incentive spirometry, and suction
- Diet: food and oral fluids restriction
- I.V. therapy: rapid I.V. fluids with lactated Ringer's or normal saline solution, if hypovolemic
- Activity: bed rest
- Laboratory studies: ABG analysis, complete blood count, cardiac enzymes, type, and crossmatch
- Transfusion therapy: RBCs, whole blood, plasma, autotransfusion
- Corticosteroids
- Pericardiocentesis

● Nursing interventions

- Assess cardiovascular and respiratory status
- Administer oxygen therapy

Key signs and symptoms of tension pneumothorax

- Asymmetrical lung expansion and tracheal deviation to the affected side
- Hypotension
- Decreased or absent breath sounds on the affected side
- Jugular vein distention
- Severe chest pain and respiratory distress
- Subcutaneous emphysema

Diagnosing blunt chest trauma injury

- Chest X-ray
- Echocardiography, CT scan, MRI

Treating blunt chest trauma injury

- Food and oral fluids restriction
- I.V. therapy: rapid I.V. fluids with lactated Ringer's or normal saline solution, if hypovolemic
- Oxygen therapy: high flow rates
- Intubation and mechanical ventilation using positive pressure
- Position: semi-Fowler's (unless patient requires shock position)
- Monitoring: vital signs, I/O, hemodynamic parameters, ECG, and pulse oximetry
- Transfusion therapy: RBCs, whole blood, plasma, autotransfusion
- Supportive medications to control heart failure and arrhythmias
- Pericardiocentesis

Key nursing interventions for a patient with blunt chest trauma injury

- Assess cardiovascular and respiratory status.
- Monitor and record vital signs, hemodynamic variables, I/O, laboratory studies, ABG values, and pulse oximetry.
- Monitor mechanical ventilation.
- Assess for pain and provide analgesics, as indicated.
- Maintain and monitor chest tubes and chest tube drainage
- Administer oxygen therapy.
- Provide suctioning and turning; encourage coughing, deep breathing, and use of incentive spirometer.
- Teach the patient to splint the chest to minimize pain and maximize lung expansion in flail chest.

Key complications of blunt chest trauma injury

- Hemothorax
- Pneumothorax
- Cardiac arrhythmia
- Death

- Monitor and record vital signs, hemodynamic variables, I/O, laboratory studies, ABG values, and pulse oximetry
- Monitor mechanical ventilation
- Assess for pain level, provide analgesics as prescribed, and evaluate effect
- Administer medications as ordered
- Maintain food and oral fluid restrictions
- Administer I.V. fluids
- Maintain bed rest or shock position
- Maintain and monitor chest tubes; monitor chest tube drainage
- Provide suctioning and turning; encourage coughing, deep breathing, and the use of incentive spirometer
- Support the patient during this potentially life-threatening event
- Teach the patient to splint the chest to minimize pain and maximize lung expansion in flail chest
- Monitor for complications, such as tension pneumothorax, hemorrhagic shock, and cardiac tamponade
- Individualize home care instructions
  - Know about the disorder and its implications
  - Follow instructions for medication use and be aware of possible adverse effects
  - Demonstrate coughing and deep-breathing exercises
  - Recognize signs and symptoms of respiratory distress
  - Take analgesics for pain as needed
  - Splint chest to relieve pain

● Complications
- Hemothorax
- Pneumothorax
- Hemorrhagic shock
- Diaphragmatic rupture
- Tension pneumothorax
- Cardiac arrhythmia
- Death

● Possible surgical interventions
- Surgical repair of injured area, such as flail rib segments, myocardial rupture, septal perforation, and aortic rupture
- Thorocotomy

NCLEX CHECKS

It's never too soon to begin your NCLEX preparation. Now that you've reviewed this chapter, carefully read each of the following questions and choose the best answer. Then compare your responses to the correct answers.

1. In a client with emphysema, the initiative to breathe is triggered by:
- ☐ **1.** high $PaCO_2$ levels.
- ☐ **2.** low $PaCO_2$ levels.
- ☐ **3.** high PaO_2 levels.
- ☒ **4.** low PaO_2 levels.

2. Extrinsic asthma is caused by:
- ☐ **1.** temperature changes.
- ☒ **2.** sensitivity to specific allergens.
- ☐ **3.** respiratory tract infection.
- ☐ **4.** emotional stress.

3. A nurse is assessing a client with suspected pneumothorax. Which key signs and symptoms should she expect? Select all that apply.
- ☐ **1.** Barrel chest
- ☐ **2.** Night sweats
- ☒ **3.** Diminished or absent breath sounds unilaterally
- ☐ **4.** Dysphagia
- ☒ **5.** Dyspnea

4. A nurse is teaching a client about the respiratory system. She explains that which of the following is the basic unit of gas exchange?
- ☒ **1.** Alveoli
- ☐ **2.** Larynx
- ☐ **3.** Bronchioles
- ☐ **4.** Surfactant

5. A nurse is assessing a client with fractured ribs from a motor vehicle accident. Which finding indicates the client has flail chest?
- ☐ **1.** Mediastinal shift
- ☒ **2.** Paradoxical chest movement
- ☐ **3.** Muffled heart sounds
- ☐ **4.** Subcutaneous emphysema

6. In which position should a nurse place a client who has just had a pneumonectomy?
- ☒ **1.** On his back or on the side of surgery
- ☐ **2.** On his abdomen or on the side opposite the surgery
- ☐ **3.** Prone
- ☐ **4.** Any position is acceptable

7. When planning the care of a client suspected of having TB, a nurse understands that which mechanism transmits TB?
- ☒ **1.** Airborne
- ☐ **2.** Fomites
- ☐ **3.** Hand to mouth
- ☐ **4.** Blood

TOP 10

Items to study for your next test on the respiratory system

1. Role of alveoli in gas exchange
2. Signs of respiratory changes
3. Abnormal breath sounds
4. Care of the patient with a chest tube
5. Preoperative and postoperative care of the patient with lung surgery
6. Types of pulmonary infection, such as pneumonia and TB
7. Care of the patient with COPD
8. Pathophysiologic changes with ARDs
9. Recognition of life-threatening respiratory disorders, such as pulmonary embolism, pneumothorax, and acute respiratory failure
10. Management and nursing interventions for the patient with lung or laryngeal cancer

8. A nurse is teaching a client with chronic bronchitis how to do pursed-lip breathing. What's the rationale for this type of exercise?
- [ ] **1.** Provides more time for gas exchange
- [x] **2.** Increases airway pressure
- [ ] **3.** Increases the oxygen concentration
- [ ] **4.** Stimulates coughing

9. A client with right-middle-lobe pneumonia is being cared for in the intensive care unit. While assessing the client, the nurse auscultates crackles in the right lower to mid lung fields and decreased airflow in the upper fields. What would be an appropriate treatment for this client?
- [ ] **1.** Administration of a diuretic
- [x] **2.** Administration of a bronchodilator
- [ ] **3.** Fluid restriction
- [ ] **4.** Endotracheal intubation

10. A client with ARDS is intubated and placed on mechanical ventilation. Which studies should be monitored to help regulate ventilator settings?
- [ ] **1.** PFTs
- [ ] **2.** Sputum and blood cultures
- [ ] **3.** Hb levels
- [x] **4.** ABG values

ANSWERS AND RATIONALES

1. CORRECT ANSWER: 4
Because of long-standing hypercapnia, low PaO_2 levels trigger breathing in a client with emphysema. In a client with a normal respiratory drive, increased $PaCO_2$ levels trigger the initiative to breathe.

2. CORRECT ANSWER: 2
Extrinsic, or atopic, asthma is caused by sensitivity to specific external allergens, such as pollen, dust, and dander. Temperature changes, respiratory tract infection, and emotional stress cause intrinsic (nonatopic) asthma.

3. CORRECT ANSWER: 3, 5
Diminished or absent breath sounds unilaterally and dyspnea are key signs and symptoms of a pneumothorax. A barrel chest typically develops with emphysema. Night sweats may occur with TB, and dysphagia may occur with laryngeal cancer.

4. CORRECT ANSWER: 1
The alveoli are the basic unit of gas exchange in the lungs. The larynx contains the vocal cords that produce sounds and initiate the cough reflex. The bronchioles are formed by the branching of the trachea, and aren't involved in gas exchange. Surfactant reduces surface tension to keep alveoli from collapsing.

5. CORRECT ANSWER: 2

Multiple rib fractures may cause flail chest, in which a portion of the chest wall moves in during inspiration, creating a paradoxical chest movement. Mediastinal shift may occur with pneumothorax. Muffled heart sounds may occur in cardiac tamponade. Subcutaneous emphysema is found in the client with tension pneumothorax.

6. CORRECT ANSWER: 1

Immediately following a pneumonectomy, place the client on his back or on the side of surgery. Positioning the client on the unaffected side or in another position may increase the stress on the bronchial stump and risk disruption of the suture line.

7. CORRECT ANSWER: 1

TB is transmitted by droplet nuclei produced when the infected person coughs or sneezes. It isn't spread by fomites, hand to mouth, or through blood.

8. CORRECT ANSWER: 2

Pursed-lip breathing is a technique that uses the mild resistance of partially opposed lips to prolong exhalation and to increase airway pressure, causing a delay of the airway's dynamic compression and minimizing the effects of airway trapping. Pursed-lip breathing doesn't provide more time for air exchange, increase the oxygen concentration, or stimulate coughing.

9. CORRECT ANSWER: 2

With pneumonia, inflammation occurs and alveolar fluid increases, causing crackles, rhonchi, and narrowed airways. A bronchodilator helps expand the airway, which allows the client increased airflow and may improve expectoration of secretions.

10. CORRECT ANSWER: 4

ABG values identify the oxygen, carbon dioxide, and bicarbonate levels in the client's system as well as the blood pH. Analysis of these values allows for adjustment in ventilator settings to maximize the client's gas exchange and achieve or maintain a normal pH.

3

Nervous system

1. The Glasgow Coma Scale, a tool used to help assess neurologic status, grades which responses?

☐ 1. Eye opening, motor and verbal responses
☐ 2. Pupil reaction, motor and verbal responses
☐ 3. Eye opening, cough and gag relfexes
☐ 4. Cough and gag reflexes, corneal and oculovestibular reflexes

CORRECT ANSWER: 1

2. Which nursing diagnosis would most apply to a client with seizure disorder?

☐ 1. Activity intolerance
☐ 2. Imbalanced nutrition: More than body requirements
☐ 3. Disturbed body image
☐ 4. Risk for injury

CORRECT ANSWER: 4

3. Conditions that increase a client's risk for experiencing a stroke include:

☐ 1. hypertension.
☐ 2. asthma.
☐ 3. Bell's palsy.
☐ 4. pneumonia.

CORRECT ANSWER: 1

4. A complication of amyotrophic lateral sclerosis may be:
- ☐ 1. urinary tract infection.
- ☐ 2. respiratory failure.
- ☐ 3. cor pulmonale.
- ☐ 4. increased intracerebral pressure.

CORRECT ANSWER: 2

5. A client is admitted to the hospital with a suspected spinal cord injury. An important nursing intervention until an exact diagnosis is made would be:
- ☐ 1. turning the patient every 1 to 2 hours.
- ☐ 2. performing range-of-motion exercises.
- ☐ 3. applying and maintaining a cervical collar.
- ☐ 4. administering blood products.

CORRECT ANSWER: 3

LEARNING OBJECTIVES

After studying this chapter, you should be able to:

- Describe the psychosocial impact of nervous system disorders.
- Differentiate between modifiable and nonmodifiable risk factors in the development of a nervous system disorder.
- List three probable and three possible nursing diagnoses for a patient with a nervous system disorder.
- Identify nursing interventions for a patient with a nervous system disorder.
- Write three goals for teaching a patient with a nervous system disorder.

CHAPTER OVERVIEW

Caring for the patient with a neurologic disorder requires a sound understanding of the anatomy and physiology of the nervous system. A thorough assessment is essential in planning and implementing appropriate patient care. The assessment includes a complete history, a physical examination, diagnostic testing, identification of modifiable and nonmodifiable risk factors, and information related to the psychosocial impact of the disorder on the patient.

Nursing diagnoses focus primarily on self-care deficits, ineffective cerebral tissue perfusion, and decreased intracranial adaptive capacity. Nursing interventions are geared to promote comfort, improve healing, and prevent complications. Patient teaching—a crucial nursing activity—involves information about medication regimens, providing a safe environment, signs and symptoms of possible complications, reducing modifiable risk factors (through weight control, activity and diet restrictions, stress management, and smoking cessation), and medical follow-up. With self-care deficits, consider the impact of neurologic dysfunction on self-esteem.

ANATOMY AND PHYSIOLOGY REVIEW

Key facts about the neuron

- Basic functional unit of the nervous system
- Components: cell body, dendrites, and axon

Key parts of the CNS

- Spinal cord
- Brain
- Cerebrum
- Corpus callosum
- Basal ganglia
- Diencephalon
- Brain stem
- Cerebellum

● **Neuron**
- The nerve cell, or neuron, is the basic functional unit of the nervous system
- The neuron consists of a cell body, dendrites, and an axon; some axons are surrounded by a myelin sheath (myelinated neuron)
- The neuron conducts impulses across a synapse to muscles, glands, and organs
- Neurotransmitters (anines, acetylcholine, serotonin), catecholamines (dopamine, norepinephrine), polypeptides (endorphins), and amino acids (gamma-aminobutyric acid) excite the next neuron in the chain
    - Produce an action potential
    - Some neurotransmitters inhibit; others excite

● **Central nervous system (CNS)**
- The CNS includes the brain and the spinal cord
    - Brain
        · The *cerebrum* is divided into two hemispheres, separated by a fissure and joined by the corpus callosum, that contain four lobes each (see *A close look at the cerebrum and its functions*)
            - The frontal lobe is the site of personality, intellectual functioning, motor speech, and abstract thought
            - The parietal lobe is the site of sensation, integration of sensory information, and spatial relationships
            - The temporal lobe is the auditory and visual receptive area, and the site of integration of somatization
            - The occipital lobe is the site of visual interpretation
        · The *corpus callosum* consists of nerve fibers that transmit nerve impulses from one hemisphere of the brain to the other

A close look at the cerebrum and its functions

The cerebrum is divided into four lobes, based on anatomic landmarks and functional differences. The lobes — parietal, occipital, temporal, and frontal — are named for the cranial bones that lie over them.

This illustration shows the locations of the cerebral lobes and explains their functions. It also shows the location of the cerebellum and sensory and motor cortexes.

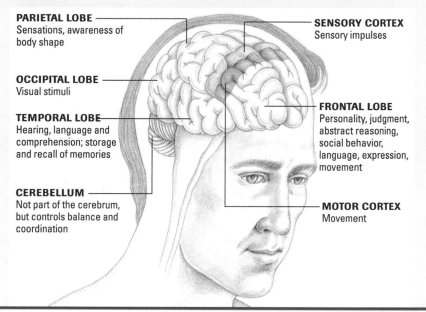

PARIETAL LOBE
Sensations, awareness of body shape

OCCIPITAL LOBE
Visual stimuli

TEMPORAL LOBE
Hearing, language and comprehension; storage and recall of memories

CEREBELLUM
Not part of the cerebrum, but controls balance and coordination

SENSORY CORTEX
Sensory impulses

FRONTAL LOBE
Personality, judgment, abstract reasoning, social behavior, language, expression, movement

MOTOR CORTEX
Movement

- The *basal ganglia,* located deep in the cerebral hemispheres, is responsible for fine motor movements
- The *diencephalon* consists of the thalamus and hypothalamus
  - The thalamus relays sensory impulses of pain, temperature, and sensation, and memory
  - The hypothalamus controls temperature regulation, emotional states, hunger and appetite, sleep-wake cycle, thirst, sexual behavior, autonomic nervous system (ANS), and endocrine functions
- The *brain stem* comprises the midbrain, pons, and medulla oblongata
  - The midbrain consists of the tectum and the cerebral peduncles; it serves as the nerve pathway between the cerebral hemispheres
  - The pons consists of the pons dorsalis and pons ventralis; portions of the pons control heart rate, blood pressure, and respirations
  - The medulla oblongata contains motor fibers from the brain to the spinal cord and sensory fibers from the spinal cord to the brain; these fibers affect vomiting, vasomotor, respiratory, and cardiac response

Four lobes of the cerebrum

- Frontal lobe: the site of personality, intellectual functioning, and motor speech
- Parietal lobe: the site of sensation, integration of sensory information, and spatial relationships
- Temporal lobe: the site of hearing, taste, smell, and speech
- Occipital lobe: the site of vision

Key facts about the thalamus and hypothalamus

- Components of the diencephalon
- The thalamus relays sensory impulses of pain, temperature, and touch to the cortex
- The hypothalamus controls temperature regulation, emotional states, appetite, sleep-wake cycle, thirst, ANS, and endocrine functions

Key components of the brain stem

- Midbrain: serves as the nerve pathway between the cerebral hemispheres
- Pons: portions control the respiratory system
- Medulla oblongata: contains the vomiting, vasometer, respiratory, and cardiac centers

Key functions of the cranial nerves

- CN I: Olfactory
  - Smell
- CN II: Optic
  - Vision
- CN III: Oculomotor
  - Most eye movement
  - Pupillary constriction
  - Upper eyelid elevation
- CN IV: Trochlear
  - Down and in eye movement
- CN V: Trigeminal
  - Chewing
  - Corneal reflex
  - Face and scalp sensations
- CN VI: Abducens
  - Lateral eye movement
- CN VII: Facial
  - Expressions in forehead, eye, and mouth
  - Taste
- CN VIII: Acoustic
  - Hearing
  - Balance
- CN IX: Glossopharyngeal
  - Swallowing
  - Salivating
  - Taste
- CN X: Vagus
  - Swallowing
  - Gag reflex
  - Talking
  - Sensations of the throat, larynx, and abdominal viscera
  - Activities of the thoracic and abdominal viscera
- CN XI: Accessory
  - Shoulder movement
  - Head rotation
- CN XII: Hypoglossal
  - Tongue movement

Key facts about the blood–brain barrier

- The endothelial cells within the capillaries of the brain
- Prevents substances in plasma from reaching the brain and CSF

Identifying cranial nerves

The cranial nerves have either sensory or motor function or both. They're assigned Roman numerals and are written this way: CN I, CN II, CN III, and so forth. This illustration lists the function of each cranial nerve.

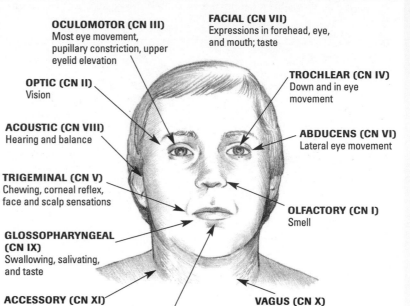

OCULOMOTOR (CN III)
Most eye movement, pupillary constriction, upper eyelid elevation

FACIAL (CN VII)
Expressions in forehead, eye, and mouth; taste

OPTIC (CN II)
Vision

TROCHLEAR (CN IV)
Down and in eye movement

ACOUSTIC (CN VIII)
Hearing and balance

ABDUCENS (CN VI)
Lateral eye movement

TRIGEMINAL (CN V)
Chewing, corneal reflex, face and scalp sensations

OLFACTORY (CN I)
Smell

GLOSSOPHARYNGEAL (CN IX)
Swallowing, salivating, and taste

ACCESSORY (CN XI)
Shoulder movement and head rotation

HYPOGLOSSAL (CN XII)
Tongue movement

VAGUS (CN X)
Swallowing, gag reflex, talking; sensations of throat, larynx, and abdominal viscera; activities of thoracic and abdominal viscera, such as heart rate and peristalsis

---

- Fibers decussate within the medulla oblongata
- The *cerebellum* coordinates muscle tone, movement, balance, posture, and position sense
- Blood is supplied to the brain via the internal carotid arteries, vertebral arteries, and circle of Willis (anterior and posterior cerebral and communicating arteries); these interconnecting arteries allow for collateral circulation
- The *reticular activating system* coordinates sensory input and regulates level of arousal, attention, sleep-wake cycles, consciousness, and response to stimuli
- The *blood-brain barrier* is a term for the endothelial cells within the capillaries of the brain that prevent substances in plasma from reaching the brain and cerebrospinal fluid (CSF)
- The *limbic system* stores recent memories and is involved in basic emotional drives, such as fear, hunger, and sexual drives, as well as the visceral response that accompanies them

- Spinal cord
  - The *spinal cord* consists of gray matter and white matter
    - Gray matter forms an H-shaped core in the center of the spinal cord
    - White matter includes the spinal cord's ascending (sensory) and descending (motor) tracts
  - The spinal cord's reflex arc is a chain of neural activity consisting of one synapse and two neurons (monosynaptic reflex)
- The CNS is covered and protected by the meninges, which comprise three membranous layers
  - Dura mater
  - Pia mater
  - Arachnoid membrane
- Four ventricles produce and circulate CSF
  - CSF surrounds and protects the brain and spinal cord
  - CSF exchanges nutrients and wastes at the cellular level
  - CSF delivers drugs
  - CSF regulates intracranial volume

● **Peripheral nervous system (PNS)**
- The PNS and the CNS together constitute the nervous system
- The PNS comprises 12 pairs of cranial nerves, 31 pairs of spinal nerves, and the ANS
  - The cranial nerves consist of the olfactory, optic, oculomotor, trochlear, trigeminal, abducent, facial, acoustic, glossopharyngeal, vagus, accessory, and hypoglossal nerves (see *Identifying cranial nerves*)
  - Spinal nerves carry mixed impulses (motor and sensory) to and from the spinal cord
  - The ANS regulates smooth muscle, cardiac muscle, and glands; it comprises the sympathetic and parasympathetic nervous systems
    - Sympathetic activity results in adrenergic responses
    - Parasympathetic activity results in cholinergic responses

ASSESSMENT FINDINGS

● **History**
- Memory impairment
- Inability to recognize objects (agnosia)
- Numbness and tingling
- Muscle weakness, twitching and spasm
- Ringing in the ears
- Difficulty chewing, swallowing, talking, and walking
- Headache
- Dizziness
- Fainting
- Loss of balance and coordination
- Nausea and vomiting

Key parts of the PNS
- Cranial nerves
- Spinal nerves
- ANS

Key functions of the ANS
- Regulates smooth muscle, cardiac muscle, and glands
- Comprises the sympathetic and parasympathetic nervous systems

Key history assessment findings in a patient with a nervous system disorder
- Memory impairment
- Numbness and tingling
- Muscle weakness, twitching and spasm
- Ringing in the ears

Key facts about the Glasgow Coma Scale

- Provides a quick, standardized account of neurologic status
- Assesses eye opening response, motor response, and verbal response
- A score of 7 or less indicates severe neurologic damage

Glasgow Coma Scale

To assess a patient's level of consciousness quickly and to uncover baseline changes, use the Glasgow Coma Scale. This assessment tool grades consciousness in relation to eye opening and motor and verbal responses. A decreased reaction score in one or more categories warns of an impending neurologic crisis. A patient scoring 7 or less is comatose and probably has severe neurologic damage.

TEST	PATIENT'S REACTION	SCORE
Best eye opening response	Open spontaneously	4
	Open to verbal command	3
	Open to pain	2
	No response	1
Best motor response	Obeys verbal command	6
	Localizes painful stimuli	5
	Flexion-withdrawal	4
	Flexion-abnormal (decorticate rigidity)	3
	Extension (decerebrate rigidity)	2
	No response	1
Best verbal response	Oriented and converses	5
	Disoriented and converses	4
	Inappropriate words	3
	Incomprehensible sounds	2
	No response	1
Total		3 to 15

- Pain
- Mental confusion or excitement
- Emotional lability
- Blurred or double vision
- Changes in vision
- Change in bowel and bladder patterns
- Sexual dysfunction
- Tremors
- Stiff neck
- Drooping eyelids
- Seizures
- Trauma

● Physical examination
- Paresthesia
- Loss of sensation
- Altered level of consciousness (LOC) (see *Glasgow Coma Scale*)
- Ataxic gait
- Dyskinesia
- Tinnitus
- Dysphagia

Key physical assessment findings in a patient with a nervous system disorder

- Altered LOC
- Abnormal pupil size and reaction
- Abnormal reflexes: Babinski's, plantar response
- Loss of cough, gag, corneal, oculocephalic, and oculovestibular reflexes

- Aphasia
- Seizures
- Diplopia
- Papilledema
- Change in visual fields
- Loss of vision
- Abnormal temperature
- Pulse changes
- Abnormal respirations
- Hypertension
- Weakness
- Spasticity, rigidity, flaccidity
- Abnormal pupil size and reaction
- Abnormal reflexes: Babinski's, plantar response, changes in muscle reflexes
- Loss of cough, gag, corneal, oculocephalic, and oculovestibular reflexes
- Ptosis

DIAGNOSTIC TESTS AND PROCEDURES

● **EEG**
  - Definition and purpose
    - Noninvasive test of the brain
    - Graphic representation of the brain's electrical activity
  - Nursing interventions before the procedure
    - Explain the procedure to the patient
    - Determine the patient's ability to lie still
    - Reassure the patient that electrical shock won't occur
    - Explain that the patient will be subjected to stimuli, such as lights and sounds
    - Withhold medications, stimulants, and depressants for 24 to 48 hours before the procedure

● **Computerized tomography (CT) scan**
  - Definition and purpose
    - Noninvasive scan
    - Contrast dye may be used
    - Visualization of the brain and its structures
  - Nursing interventions before the procedure
    - Explain the procedure to the patient
    - Obtain signed informed consent per facility policy
    - Note the patient's allergies to iodine, seafood, and radiopaque dyes, if a dye will be used
    - Allay the patient's anxiety and administer sedation, as ordered
    - Inform the patient about possible throat irritation and flushing of the face, if dye is used
    - Tell the patient that he must lie still during the test

Key facts about MRI

- Allows for visualization of the brain and its structures
- Interventions:
- Be aware that patients with pacemakers, surgical and orthopedic clips, bullet fragments, or shrapnel shouldn't be scanned
- Assess for history of claustrophobia
- Remove jewelry and metal objects from the patient

Key facts about cerebral angiography

- Invasive procedure using a radiopaque dye
- Allows for examination of the cerebral arteries
- Intervention: note the patient's allergies before the procedure

Key facts about lumbar puncture

- Invasive test
- Purposes:
- Collection of CSF from lumbar subarachnoid
- Measurement of CSF pressure
- Injection of radiopaque dye for myelogram
- Intervention: know that the procedure is contraindicated in the presence of increased ICP

– Tell the patient to remove hairpins

● **Magnetic resonance imaging (MRI)**
  - Definition and purpose
    – Noninvasive scan using magnetic and radio waves
    – Visualization of the brain and its structures
  - Nursing interventions before the procedure
    – Explain the procedure to the patient
    – Complete a pretest assessment per facility policy
    – Obtain signed informed consent
    – Be aware that a patient with a pacemaker, surgical or orthopedic clip, aneurysm clip, artificial heart valves, intrauterine device, bullet fragments, or shrapnel shouldn't be scanned
    – Assess for history of claustrophobia
    – Remove jewelry and metal objects from the patient
    – Determine the patient's ability to lie still
    – Administer sedation as prescribed

● **Cerebral angiography**
  - Definition and purpose
    – Fluoroscopic procedure using a radiopaque dye
    – Examination of the cerebral arteries
  - Nursing interventions before the procedure
    – Explain the procedure to the patient
    – Obtain signed informed consent
    – Note the patient's allergies to iodine, seafood, or radiopaque dyes
    – Inform the patient about possible throat irritation, flushing of the face, and a metallic taste in the mouth
  - Nursing interventions after the procedure
    – Monitor vital signs
    – Check the insertion site for bleeding
    – Maintain affected extremity in straight alignment for 6 hours, or as ordered to prevent a hematoma
    – Check pulses in affected extremity
    – Provide adequate hydration orally or I.V., as indicated
    – Monitor neurovital signs (see *Understanding neurovital signs*)
    – Allay the patient's anxiety
    – Assess for motor or sensory deficits

● **Lumbar puncture (LP)**
  - Definition and purpose
    – Invasive procedure
    – Collection of CSF from the lumbar subarachnoid space, measurement of CSF pressure, and injection of radiopaque dye for myelogram
  - Nursing interventions before the procedure
    – Explain the procedure to the patient
    – Obtain signed informed consent

Understanding neurovital signs

Neurologic vital signs supplement the routine measurement of temperature, pulse rate, and respirations by evaluating the patient's level of consciousness (LOC), pupillary activity, and orientation to place, time, date, and person. They provide a simple, indispensable tool for quickly checking the patient's neurologic status.

LOC, a measure of environmental awareness and self-awareness, reflects cortical function and usually provides the first sign of central nervous system (CNS) deterioration. Changes in pupillary activity (pupil size, shape, equality, and response to light) may signal increased intracranial pressure associated with a space-occupying lesion. Evaluating muscle strength and tone, reflexes, and posture also may help identify CNS damage.

Changes in vital signs alone rarely indicate neurologic compromise; therefore, evaluate any changes in light of a complete neurologic assessment. Because vital signs are controlled at the medullary level, changes related to neurologic compromise are ominous.

– Determine the patient's ability to lie still in a flexed, lateral, recumbent position
– Know that the presence of increased intracranial pressure (ICP) is a contraindication for having the test because brain herniation may develop when CSF is removed
- Nursing interventions after the procedure
  – Keep the patient flat in the prone position for 2 hours, then flat in the side-lying position for 2 to 3 hours, then in the prone or supine position for 6 or more hours
  – Administer analgesics as prescribed
  – Check the puncture site for bleeding
  – Monitor neurovital signs
  – Encourage fluids to offset CSF leakage
  – Monitor for headache

- **CSF analysis**
  - Definition and purpose
    – Laboratory test of CSF obtained via LP
    – Microscopic examination of CSF for blood, white blood cells (WBCs), immunoglobulins (Igs), bacteria, protein, glucose, specific gravity, pH, and electrolytes
  - Nursing interventions
    – Label specimens properly and send to the laboratory immediately
    – Adhere to nursing interventions after an LP

- **Electromyography (EMG)**
  - Definition and purpose
    – Noninvasive test of muscles

Key facts about myleography

- Invasive test involving an injection of dye via LP
- Allows for visualization of the subarachnoid space, spinal cord, and vertebrae
- Intervention: note the patient's allergies before the procedure

Key facts about brain scan

- Invasive test involving injection of a radiopaque dye
- Provides visual imaging of blood flow and distribution and brain structures
- Intervention: note the patient's allergies before the procedure

Key facts about skull X-rays

- Noninvasive test
- Radiographic picture of head and neck bones
- Intervention: determine the patient's ability to lie still during the procedure

– Graphic recording of the electrical activity of a muscle at rest and during contraction
- Nursing interventions
  – Explain that the patient must flex and relax his muscles during the procedure
  – Stress the importance of cooperation during the procedure
  – Explain that the patient will feel some discomfort, but not pain
  – Administer analgesics as prescribed, after the procedure

● Myelography
- Definition and purpose
  – Injection of radiopaque water-based dye by LP
  – Visualization of the subarachnoid space, spinal cord, and vertebrae under fluoroscopy
- Nursing interventions before the procedure
  – Explain the procedure to the patient
  – Obtain signed informed consent
  – Note the patient's allergies to iodine, seafood, and radiopaque dyes
  – Inform the patient about possible throat irritation and flushing of the face
- Nursing interventions after the procedure
  – Keep the patient flat in bed for at least 3 hours, with the head of the bed raised 30 to 45 degrees
  – Follow postprocedural management for specific dye used
  – Check the puncture site for bleeding
  – Monitor neurovital signs
  – Encourage fluids
  – Assess for photophobia

● Brain scan
- Definition and purpose
  – Procedure that involves injection of a radiopaque dye
  – Visual imaging of blood flow and distribution and brain structures
- Nursing interventions before the procedure
  – Explain the procedure to the patient
  – Note the patient's allergies to iodine, seafood, and radiopaque dyes
  – Inform the patient about possible throat irritation and flushing of the face
  – Determine the patient's ability to lie still during the procedure

● Skull X-rays
- Definition and purpose
  – Noninvasive examination
  – Radiographic picture of head and neck bones
- Nursing interventions before the procedure
  – Explain the procedure to the patient

– Determine the patient's ability to lie still during the procedure

– Explain the events that will occur during the procedure

● **Positron emission tomography (PET) scan**
  • Definition and purpose
    – Imaging that involves injection of a radioisotope
    – Visualization of oxygen uptake, blood flow, and glucose metabolism
  • Nursing interventions
    – Explain the procedure to the patient
    – Determine the patient's ability to lie still during the procedure
    – Withhold alcohol, tobacco, and caffeine for 24 hours before the procedure
    – Withhold medications as directed, before the procedure
    – Check the injection site for bleeding after the procedure

● **Blood chemistry**
  • Definition and purpose
    – Laboratory test of a blood sample
    – Analysis for potassium, sodium, calcium, phosphorus, protein, albumin, osmolality, glucose, bicarbonate, blood urea nitrogen (BUN), and creatinine
  • Nursing interventions
    – Explain the procedure to the patient
    – Monitor the site for bleeding after the procedure

● **Hematologic studies**
  • Definition and purpose
    – Laboratory test of a blood sample
    – Analysis for WBCs, red blood cells (RBCs), erythrocyte sedimentation rate (ESR), prothrombin time (PT), partial thromboplastin time (PTT), platelets, hemoglobin (Hb), and hematocrit (HCT)
  • Nursing interventions
    – Explain the procedure to the patient
    – Note current drug therapy before the procedure
    – Check the venipuncture site for bleeding after the procedure

PSYCHOSOCIAL IMPACT OF NERVOUS SYSTEM DISORDERS

● **Developmental impact**
  • Changes in body image
  • Loss of control over body functions
  • Fear of rejection
  • Embarrassment from changes in body structure and function
  • Decreased self-esteem
  • Fear of dying
  • Dependence

Key facts about PET scan
● Invasive test that involves injection of a radioisotope
● Provides visualization of oxygen uptake, blood flow, and glucose metabolism
● Intervention: withhold alcohol, tobacco, and caffeine for 24 hours before the procedure

Key facts about blood chemistry
● Blood test
● Analysis for potassium, sodium, calcium, phosphorus, protein, albumin, osmolality, glucose, bicarbonate, BUN, and creatinine
● Intervention: monitor the site for bleeding after the procedure

Key facts about hematologic studies
● Blood test
● Analysis for WBCs, RBCs, ESR, PT, PTT, Hb, and HCT
● Intervention: check the venipuncture site for bleeding after the procedure

Psychosocial impact of nervous system disorders
● Change in body image
● Loss of control over body functions
● Disruption or loss of employment to patient or caregiver
● Restrictions or changes in activity

Modifiable risk factors for a nervous system disorder

- Exposure to chemical or environmental pollutants
- Substance abuse
- Smoking
- Alcohol
- Participation in contact sports
- Hypertension

Nonmodifiable risk factors for a nervous system disorder

- Aging
- Family history of neurologic disease
- History of cardiac disease
- History of head injury
- Exposure to viral or bacterial infection

Key probable nursing diagnoses for a nervous system disorder

- Impaired physical mobility
- Feeding self-care deficit; bathing or hygiene self-care deficit; toileting self-care deficit
- Disturbed sensory perception
- Disturbed thought processes

● **Economic impact**
  - Disruption or loss of employment to patient or caregiver
  - Cost of hospitalizations and rehabilitation
  - Cost of home health care
  - Cost of special equipment

● **Occupational and recreational impact**
  - Restrictions or inability to continue work activity
  - Changes in leisure activity
  - Restrictions or loss of physical activity
  - Need for vocational training

● **Social impact**
  - Changes in communication ability
  - Changes in eating modes
  - Changes in elimination patterns and modes
  - Social isolation
  - Changes in sexual function
  - Changes in role performance

RISK FACTORS

● **Modifiable risk factors**
  - Exposure to chemical or environmental pollutants
  - Substance abuse
  - Smoking
  - Alcohol
  - Participation in contact sports
  - Hypertension
  - Diabetes

● **Nonmodifiable risk factors**
  - Aging
  - Family history of neurologic disease
  - History of cardiac disease
  - History of head injury
  - Exposure to viral or bacterial infection

NURSING DIAGNOSES

● **Probable nursing diagnoses**
  - Impaired physical mobility
  - Feeding self-care deficit
  - Bathing or hygiene self-care deficit
  - Dressing or grooming self-care deficit
  - Toileting self-care deficit
  - Disturbed sensory perception (visual)
  - Disturbed sensory perception (tactile)
  - Disturbed thought processes

- Social isolation
- Impaired home maintenance
- Unilateral neglect
- Disturbed body image
- Situational low self-esteem
- Risk for autonomic dysreflexia
- Risk for injury

● **Possible nursing diagnoses**
- Sexual dysfunction
- Impaired urinary elimination
- Impaired verbal communication
- Bowel incontinence
- Imbalanced nutrition: Less than body requirements
- Ineffective airway clearance
- Ineffective coping
- Ineffective tissue perfusion (cerebral)
- Powerlessness
- Risk for self-directed violence
- Insomnia
- Risk for aspiration

CRANIOTOMY

● **Description**
- Surgical opening of the cranium to excise a tumor, evacuate a blood clot, relieve ICP, or repair an aneurysm
- Classified as supratentorial, infratentorial, or transphenoidal

● **Preoperative nursing interventions**
- Complete patient and family preoperative teaching
  - Explian the procedure to the patient and his family
  - Describe the operating room, postanesthesia care unit (PACU), and preoperative and postoperative routines; demonstrate postoperative turning, coughing, deep breathing, and range-of-motion (ROM) exercises
  - Explain the postoperative need for monitoring devices, drainage tubes, surgical dressings, oxygen therapy, mechanical ventilation, I.V. therapy, medication, and pain control
- Complete a preoperative checklist: check that a signed informed consent is in the patient's chart
- Administer preoperative medications as prescribed
- Allay the patient's and his family's anxiety about surgery
- Document the patient's history and physical assessment database
- Explain that the patient's head will be shaved

● **Postoperative nursing interventions**
- Assess cardiac, respiratory, and neurologic status, including LOC

Key nursing interventions after a craniotomy

- Assess cardiac, respiratory, and neurologic status, including LOC.
- Assess pain and administer postoperative analgesics, as prescribed.
- Keep the patient's head in a neutral position.
- Reinforce turning, coughing, and deep breathing.
- Keep the patient in semi-Fowler's position.
- Monitor vital signs, urine specific gravity, I/O, CVP, laboratory studies, ECG, neurovital signs, neurovascular checks, ICP, ABG values, and pulse oximetry.
- Assess cough and gag reflexes.
- Check for signs of diabetes insipidus.
- Provide eye care and cold compresses, as indicated.
- Observe for signs of increasing ICP.
- Administer anticonvulsants as prescribed.
- Administer osmotic diuretics as prescribed.
- Maintain seizure precautions.

- Administer oxygen and maintain endotracheal (ET) tube to ventilator
- Monitor vital signs, intake and output (I/O), central venous pressure (CVP), laboratory studies, electrocardiogram (ECG), neurovital signs, neurovascular checks, ICP, arterial blood gas (ABG) values, and pulse oximetry
- Assess pain level, administer postoperative analgesics as prescribed, and note response
- Assess for return of peristalsis; give solid foods and liquids, as tolerated
- Administer I.V. fluids and total parenteral nutrition (TPN)
- Maintain the patient's head in a neutral position with the head of the bed elevated 45 degrees
- Provide emotional support to allay the patient's anxiety
- Provide wound care
- Assist with turning, coughing, and deep breathing
- Encourage incentive spirometry
- Maintain active or passive ROM exercises, as tolerated
- Monitor and maintain the position and patency of drainage tubes: nasogastric (NG), indwelling urinary catheter, and wound drainage
- Assess cough and gag reflexes
- Encourage the patient to express his feelings about changes in his body image or function
- Monitor for signs of diabetes insipidus
- Provide eye care as indicated
- Allow a rest period between each nursing activity
- **Monitor for signs of increasing ICP; maintain ICP monitoring and catheter**
- Administer corticosteroids as prescribed
- Administer anticonvulsants as prescribed
- Administer laxatives as prescribed
- Administer antacids as prescribed
- Administer osmotic diuretics as prescribed
- Maintain seizure precautions
- Individualize home care instructions
  - Know about the disorder and its implications
  - Follow instructions for medication use and be aware of possible adverse effects
  - Recognize the signs and symptoms of infection
  - Monitor for neurologic changes, including LOC
  - Demonstrate safety measures during seizure activity

● **Possible complications**
- Increased ICP
- Brain herniation
- Seizures
- Respiratory failure
- Diabetes insipidus
- Motor and sensory deficits

- Infection
- Meningitis
- Bleeding
- Fluid and electrolyte imbalance
- Hypovolemic shock

ENDARTERECTOMY

- **Description**
  - Surgical removal of artherosclerotic plaque or thrombosis from arteries with a patch graft repair of the vessel

- **Preoperative nursing interventions**
  - Complete patient and family preoperative teaching
    - Explain the procedure to the patient
    - Describe the operating room, PACU, and preoperative and postoperative routines
    - Demonstrate postoperative turning, coughing, deep breathing, and ROM exercises
    - Explain the postoperative need for monitoring devices, drainage tubes, surgical dressings, oxygen therapy, I.V. therapy, and pain control
  - Complete a preoperative checklist and obtain signed informed consent
  - Administer preoperative medications as prescribed
  - Allay the patient's and his family's anxiety about surgery
  - Document the patient's history and physical assessment database
  - Protect the surgical site from trauma
  - Perform a preoperative vascular assessment

- **Postoperative nursing interventions**
  - Check the surgical site for bleeding
  - Provide special care for carotid endarterectomy
    - **Check neck edema and airway patency**
    - Assess ability to swallow
  - Assess cardiac, respiratory, and neurologic status
  - Assess pain level, administer postoperative analgesics as prescribed, and evaluate response
  - Assess for return of peristalsis; give solid foods and liquids, as tolerated
  - Administer I.V. fluids
  - Allay the patient's anxiety
  - Provide wound care
  - Encourage turning, coughing, deep breathing, and use of incentive spirometry
  - Place the patient in semi-Fowler's position
  - Maintain the patient's head in a neutral position
  - Maintain activity: active or passive ROM and isometric exercises, as tolerated

Key facts about endarterectomy

- Removal of atheromas from arteries
- Patch graft repair of the vessel

Key nursing interventions before endarterectomy

- Demonstrate postoperative turning, coughing, deep breathing, and ROM exercises.
- Administer preoperative medications as prescribed.
- Perform a preoperative vascular assessment.

Key nursing interventions after endarterectomy

- Assess cardiac, respiratory, and neurologic status.
- Reinforce turning, coughing, deep breathing, and the use of incentive spirometer.
- Maintain the patient's head in a neutral position.
- Monitor vital signs, I/O, laboratory studies, neurovital signs, neurovascular checks, and pulse oximetry.
- Check the surgical site for bleeding.
- Provide special care for carotid endarterectomy.
- Administer anticoagulants.

- Administer oxygen
- Monitor vital signs, I/O, laboratory studies, neurovital signs, neurovascular checks, and pulse oximetry
- Monitor and maintain the position and patency of drainage tubes: NG, indwelling urinary catheter, and wound drainage
- Administer anticoagulants if prescribed
- Individualize home care instructions
  - Know about the disorder and its implications
  - Follow instructions for medication use and be aware of possible adverse effects
  - Protect the surgical site from trauma
  - Recognize the signs and symptoms of infection
  - Monitor for motor and sensory deficits

● **Possible surgical complications**
- Bleeding or hematoma at incision site
- Stroke
- Thrombosis
- Neurologic deficits
- Infection
- Cranial nerve injury

PARKINSON'S DISEASE

● **Definition**
- Progressive degenerative disease of the extrapyramidal system associated with dopamine deficiency

● **Causes**
- Unknown
- Imbalance of dopamine and acetylcholine in substantia nigra in basal ganglia
- Cerebrovascular disease
- Drug-induced: phentolamine (Regitine), reserpine (Serpasil), methyldopa (Aldomet)
- Dopamine deficiency
- Head trauma
- Viral infections

● **Pathophysiology**
- Nerve cells in the basal ganglia are destroyed, resulting in impaired muscular function
- Dopamine in the substantia nigra degenerates
- Lack of dopamine results in decreased inhibition of the synaptic transmitter for muscle tone and coordination

● **Assessment findings**
- "Pill rolling" tremors
- Shuffling gait

Key facts about Parkinson's disease

- Progressive degenerative disease of the extrapyramidal system
- Associated with dopamine deficiency

Common causes of Parkinson's disease

- Imbalance of dopamine and acetylcholine in basal ganglia
- Cerebrovascular disease
- Drugs
- Head trauma

- Stiff joints
- Masklike facial expression
- Dyskinesia
- Dysphagia
- Dysphonia
- Drooling
- "Cogwheel" rigidity
- Fatigue
- General weakness
- Stooped posture
- Tremors at rest
- Micrographia
- Difficulty in initiating voluntary activity
- Visual deficits
- Constipation
- Urinary hesitancy
- Orthostatic hypotension

● **Diagnostic test findings**
  - PET scan: identifies patterns of reduced uptake of 18F-DOPA
  - EEG: minimal slowing
  - CT scan: normal

● **Medical management**
  - Diet: high-residue, high-calorie, and high-protein; soft foods
  - Physical therapy
  - Activity: as tolerated
  - Monitoring: vital signs, I/O, and neurovital signs
  - Anticholinergics: trihexyphenidyl (Artane)
  - Antiparkinsonian agents: levodopa (Larodopa), carbidopa-levodopa (Sinemet), benztropine (Cogentin)
  - Antispasmodic: procyclidine (Kemadrin)
  - Antidepressant: amitriptyline (Elavil)
  - Antiviral: amantadine (Symmetrel)
  - Monoamine oxidase-B inhibitor: selegiline (Eldepryl)
  - Dopamine receptor agonists: pergolide (Permax), bromocriptine (Parlodel)

● **Nursing interventions**
  - Maintain the patient's diet
  - Assess neurovascular and respiratory status
  - Position the patient to prevent contractures
  - Monitor and record vital signs and I/O
  - Administer medications as prescribed
  - Encourage the patient to express his feelings about changes in his body image and function
  - Promote daily ambulation and mobility
  - Promote measures to prevent falls and maintain a safe environment
  - Change the patient's position slowly

Key signs and symptoms of Parkinson's disease

- "Pill rolling" tremors
- Shuffling gait
- Stiff joints
- Masklike facial expression
- Dyskinesia
- "Cogwheel" rigidity
- Stooped posture

Diagnosing Parkinson's disease

- EEG: minimal slowing
- CT scan: normal

Treating Parkinson's disease

- High-residue, high-calorie, and high-protein diet; soft foods
- Anticholinergics
- Antiparkinsonian agents
- Antispasmodic
- Antidepressant
- Dopamine receptor agonists

Key nursing interventions for a patient with Parkinson's disease

- Assess neurovascular and respiratory status.
- Promote measures to prevent falls.
- Maintain a patent airway.
- Reinforce gait training.
- Reinforce independence in care.

Key teaching topics for a patient with a nervous system disorder

- Smoking cessation
- Regular exercise
- Medication therapy
- Stress-reduction strategies
- Self-monitoring for infection
- Danger signs

TIME-OUT FOR TEACHING

Patients with nervous system disorders

Be sure to include the following topics in your teaching plan when caring for patients with neurologic disorders.

- Smoking cessation
- Optimal weight maintenance
- Regular exercise
- Medication therapy, including action, adverse effects, and scheduling of medications
- Dietary recommendations and restrictions
- Stress-reduction strategies
- Rest and activity patterns
- Frequent blood pressure monitoring
- Environmental safety
- Community resources
- Self-monitoring for infection
- Avoidance of alcohol
- Danger signs, including changes in mentation and level of consciousness
- Rehabilitation, including adaptive and assistive devices
- Coping mechanisms

- Maintain a patent airway
- Provide active and passive ROM exercises
- Provide skin care and assess skin integrity
- Provide oral hygiene
- Reinforce gait training
- Reinforce independence in activities of daily living (ADLs)
- Provide emotional support
- Provide information about the American Parkinson's Disease Association, Inc.; the Parkinson Disease Foundation; and the National Parkinson's Foundation
- Individualize home care instructions (for more information about patient teaching, see *Patients with nervous system disorders*)
  - Know about the disorder and its implications
  - Follow instructions for medication use and be aware of possible adverse effects
  - Recognize the signs and symptoms of respiratory distress
  - Alternate rest periods with activity
  - Promote a safe environment and prevent falls
  - Take measures to prevent choking
  - Maintain nutritional diet; increase intake of roughage and fluids to prevent constipation
  - Monitor weight
  - Know the location of local support services

Key complications of Parkinson's disease

- Depression
- Injury
- Aspiration

● **Complications**
- Depression
- Corneal ulceration
- Injury
- Aspiration
- Constipation
- Psychosis

- **Possible surgical interventions**
  - Stereotaxic thalamotomy to relieve tremor and rigidity
  - Deep brain stimulation

MULTIPLE SCLEROSIS (MS)

- **Definition**
  - Progressive immune-mediated demyelinating disease of motor and sensory neurons that has periods of remissions and exacerbation (see *Describing MS,* page 148)
- **Causes**
  - Unknown
  - Autoimmune disease
  - Viral
  - Genetic disposition
  - Environment exposure
- **Pathophysiology**
  - Scattered demyelination occurs in the brain and spinal cord (see *Demyelination in MS,* page 149)
  - Degeneration of myelin sheath results in patches of sclerotic tissue and impaired conduction of motor nerve impulses
- **Assessment findings**
  - Weakness
  - Fatigue
  - Pain
  - Nystagmus
  - Scanning speech
  - Ataxia
  - Diplopia
  - Paresthesia
  - Blurred vision
  - Impaired sensation
  - Feelings of euphoria
  - Depression
  - Paralysis
  - Bowel or bladder dysfunction
  - Intention tremor
  - Inability to sense or gauge body position
  - Optic neuritis
  - Intolerance to heat
  - Exacerbation and remission of symptoms
- **Diagnostic test findings**
  - MRI: normal except in chronic illness, when atrophy is found
  - CSF analysis: increased IgG, protein, WBCs
  - CT scan: normal except in chronic illness, when atrophy is found

Key facts about MS
- Progressive demyelinating disease of motor and sensory neurons
- Results in impaired conduction of motor nerve impulses
- Has periods of remissions and exacerbation

Common causes of MS
- Autoimmune disease
- Virus
- Genetic disposition

Key signs and symptoms of MS
- Weakness
- Nystagmus
- Diplopia
- Paresthesia
- Blurred vision
- Impaired sensation
- Paralysis
- Optic neuritis

Diagnosing MS
- CT scan: normal except in chronic illness, when atrophy is found
- MRI: normal except in chronic illness, when atrophy is found

Types of MS

- Relapsing-remitting
- Primary progressive
- Secondary progressive
- Progressive-relapsing

Treating MS

- Plasmapheresis
- Muscle relaxant
- Glucocorticoids
- Immunosuppressant
- Skeletal muscle relaxant

Key nursing interventions for a patient with MS

- Assess neurologic status.
- Encourage the patient to express his feelings about changes in his body image.
- Maintain active and passive ROM exercises.
- Establish bowel and bladder program.

Describing MS

Various types (or stages) of multiple sclerosis (MS) can be identified:

- Relapsing-remitting: Clear relapses (or acute attacks or exacerbations) with full recovery and lasting disability (Between attacks, the disease doesn't worsen.)
- Primary progressive: Steadily progressing or worsening with minor recovery or plateaus (This form is uncommon and may involve different brain and spinal cord damage from other forms.)
- Secondary progressive: Beginning as a pattern of clear-cut relapses and recovery but becoming steadily progressive and worsening between acute attacks
- Progressive-relapsing: Steadily progressing from the onset but also involving clear, acute attacks. (This form is rare.)

In addition, differential diagnosis must rule out spinal cord compression, foramen magnum tumor (which may mimic the exacerbations and remissions of MS), multiple small strokes, syphilis or another infection, thyroid disease, and chronic fatigue syndrome.

- Evoked potentials: slowing of nerve conduction
- Oligoclonal banding: positive
- EMG: abnormal

Medical management

- Diet: well-balanced
- Activity: as tolerated
- Monitoring: vital signs, I/O, and neurovital signs
- Speech therapy
- Plasmapheresis
- Muscle relaxant: baclofen (Lioresal)
- Physical therapy
- Corticosteroids: prednisone (Deltasone), methylprednisolone (Solu-Medrol)
- Immunomodulators: interferon beta-1a (Avonex), interferon beta-1b (Betaseron)
- Antiparkinson agent: amantadine (Symmetrel)
- CNS stimulant: modafinil (Provigil)
- Immunosuppressant: azathioprine (Imuran), cyclophosphamide (Cytoxan)
- Skeletal muscle relaxant: quinine sulfate (Quinamm)

Nursing interventions

- Assess neurologic status
- Monitor and record vital signs, I/O, and neurovital signs
- Administer medications as prescribed
- Maintain the patient's diet
- Encourage fluids

Demyelination in MS

Transverse section of cervical spine shows partial loss of myelin, characteristic of multiple sclerosis (MS). This degenerative process is called *demyelination*.

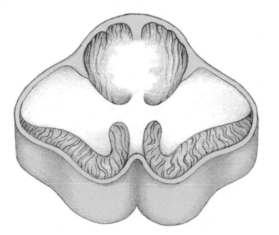

In this illustration, the loss of myelin is nearly complete. Clinical features of MS depend on the extent of demyelination.

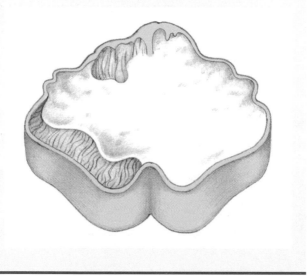

- Encourage the patient to express his feelings about changes in his body image and function
- Maintain active and passive ROM exercises
- Minimize effects of immobility
- Establish bowel and bladder program
- Maintain activity with adequate rest periods
- Assist in managing self-care
- Prevent injury
- Maintain a stress-free environment
- Provide emotional support

Key complications of MS

- UTI
- Respiratory tract infection
- Depression

Key facts about myasthenia gravis

- Neuromuscular disorder
- Results in weakness of voluntary muscles

Common causes of myasthenia gravis

- Insufficient acetylcholine
- Autoimmune disease

Key signs and symptoms of myasthenia gravis

- Muscle weakness that increases with activity and decreases with rest
- Dysphagia
- Dysarthria
- Dysphonia

- Provide information about the National Multiple Sclerosis Society
- Individualize home care instructions
  - Know about the disorder and its implications
  - Follow instructions for medication use and be aware of possible adverse effects
  - Identify ways to reduce stress
  - Recognize the signs and symptoms of exacerbation
  - Avoid exposure to people with infection
  - Alternate activity with rest periods
  - Maintain a safe environment
  - Use assistive devices in ADLs, such as specialized eating utensils and wheelchair ramps
  - Encourage independence
  - Avoid temperature extremes
  - Know the location of local support services

● **Complications**
- Urinary tract infection (UTI)
- Respiratory tract infection
- Contractures
- Depression
- Paraplegia
- Quadriplegia
- Pressure ulcer
- Deep vein thrombosis (DVT)

● **Possible surgical intervention**
- Contralateral thalamotomy

MYASTHENIA GRAVIS

● **Definition**
- Neuromuscular disorder that results in weakness of voluntary muscles

● **Causes**
- Insufficient acetylcholine
- Autoimmune disease
- Excessive cholinesterase

● **Pathophysiology**
- Disturbance occurs in transmission of nerve impulses at the myoneural junction
- Transmission defect results from deficiency in release of acetylcholine or deficient number of acetylcholine receptor sites
- Thymus gland may remain active, triggering autoimmune reaction

● **Assessment findings**
- Muscle weakness that increases with activity and decreases with rest
- Dysphagia

- Diplopia
- Dysarthria
- Dysphonia
- Ptosis
- Strabismus
- Impaired speech
- Respiratory distress
- Masklike expression
- Drooling

● **Diagnostic test findings**
- Neostigmine (Prostigmin) or edrophonium (Tensilon) test: relief from symptoms after medication administration
- EMG: decreased amplitude of evoked potentials
- Thymus scan: hyperplasia or thymoma

● **Medical management**
- Diet: high-calorie; soft foods
- Activity: as tolerated
- Monitoring: vital signs, I/O, and neurovital signs
- Glucocorticoids: prednisone (Deltasone), dexamethasone (Decadron), corticotropin (ACTH)
- Antacids: magnesium and aluminum hydroxide (Maalox), aluminum hydroxide gel (AlternaGEL)
- Anticholinesterase inhibitors: neostigmine (Prostigmin), pyridostigmine (Mestinon), ambenonium (Mytelase)
- Plasmapheresis
- Immunosuppressant: azathioprine (Imuran), cyclophosphamide (Cytoxan)

● **Nursing interventions**
- Maintain the patient's diet; encourage small, frequent meals
- Assess neurologic and respiratory status, including vital capacity and tidal volume
- Assess swallow and gag reflexes
- Monitor and record vital signs, I/O, neurovital signs, and blood glucose levels
- Administer medications, as prescribed, before meals to maximize muscles for swallowing
- Encourage the patient to express his feelings about changes in his body image and about difficulty in communicating verbally
- Determine the patient's activity tolerance
- Provide rest periods
- Provide oral hygiene
- Protect the patient from falls
- Watch the patient for choking while eating
- Provide information about the Myasthenia Gravis Foundation
- Individualize home care instructions

Diagnosing myasthenia gravis

- Neostigmine or edrophonium test: relief from symptoms after medication administration
- EMG: decreased amplitude of evoked potentials

Treating myasthenia gravis

- High-calorie diet
- Activity as tolerated
- Glucocorticoids, anti-cholinesterases, immunosuppressants
- Plasmopherisis

Key nursing interventions for a patient with myasthenia gravis

- Assess neurologic and respiratory status, including vital capacity and tidal volume.
- Assess swallow and gag reflexes.
- Administer medications, as prescribed, before meals to maximize muscles for swallowing.
- Watch the patient for choking while eating.

- Know about the disorder and its implications
- Follow instructions for medication use and be aware of possible adverse effects
- Identify ways to reduce stress
- Recognize the signs and symptoms of respiratory distress
- Recognize the signs and symptoms of myasthenic crisis
- Adhere to activity limitations
- Avoid hot foods and tonic preparations containing quinine
- Know the location of local support services

● **Complications**
- Myasthenic crisis
  - Increased symptoms of muscular weakness from undermedication or stress
  - Symptoms improve with edrophonium (Tensilon)
- Cholinergic crisis
  - Increased symptoms of muscular weakness and adverse effects of anticholinesterase medications from overmedication with cholinergic drugs
  - Symptoms worsen with edrophonium (Tensilon)

● **Possible surgical intervention**
- Thymectomy

GUILLAIN-BARRÉ SYNDROME (ACUTE INFECTIOUS POLYNEURITIS, POLYRADICULITIS)

● **Definition**
- Peripheral polyneuritis characterized by ascending paralysis

● **Causes**
- Unknown
- Virus
- Infection
- Autoimmune disease
- GI infection
- Vaccination
- Pregnancy

● **Pathophysiology**
- Preceding infection synthesizes lymphocytes, which attack the myelin sheath, causing demyelination
- Demyelination is followed by inflammation around nerve roots, veins, and capillaries
- Inflammatory process compresses nerve roots

● **Assessment findings**
- Acute onset of paresthesia and pain
- Generalized weakness
- Ascending paralysis (initiating in lower extremities)

- Tachycardia
- Hypertension
- Increased temperature
- Ptosis
- Visual disturbance
- Facial weakness
- Dysphagia
- Dysarthria

● Diagnostic test findings

- CSF analysis: increased protein
- EMG: slowed nerve conduction

● Medical management

- Diet: high-calorie, high-protein
- Position: semi-Fowler's
- Activity: bed rest, active and passive ROM and isometric exercises
- Monitoring: vital signs, I/O, pulse oximetry, vital capacity, and neurovital signs
- Plasmapheresis
- Nutritional support: enteral feedings
- Intubation and mechanical ventilation
- Physical therapy
- DVT prophylaxis
- Indwelling urinary catheter, chest physiotherapy, postural drainage, and suction
- Antibiotics: amoxicillin (Amoxil), ampicillin (Omnipen), gentamicin (Garamycin)
- Glucocorticoids: prednisone (Deltasone), dexamethasone (Decadron), corticotropin (ACTH)
- Antacids: magnesium and aluminum hydroxide (Maalox), aluminum hydroxide gel (AlternaGEL)
- IgG antibody: immune globulin I.V. (Gammagard)

● Nursing interventions

- Assess respiratory and neurologic status
- Monitor and record vital signs, I/O, vital capacity, neurovital signs, and pulse oximetry
- Assess muscle strength
- Assess gag and swallow reflexes
- Maintain the patient's nutritional intake
- Administer oxygen as needed
- Provide suction and turning; encourage coughing, deep breathing, and use of incentive spirometry
- Maintain the position and patency of NG and ET tubes
- Keep the patient in semi-Fowler's position
- Administer medications as prescribed

Diagnosing Guillain-Barré syndrome

- CSF analysis: increased protein
- EMG: slowed nerve conduction

Treating Guillain-Barré syndrome

- Plasmapheresis
- Nutritional support: gastrostomy feedings, NG tube feedings
- Intubation and mechanical ventilation
- Glucocorticoids

Key nursing interventions for a patient with Guillain-Barré syndrome

- Assess respiratory and neurologic status.
- Maintain the position and patency of NG and ET tubes.
- Monitor and record vital signs, I/O, vital capacity, neurovital signs, and pulse oximetry.
- Assess muscle strength.
- Assess gag and swallow reflexes.
- Assess for Homans' sign.
- Apply antiembolism stockings.
- Reposition the patient every 2 hours.

- Encourage the patient to express his feelings about powerlessness, changes in his body image and function, and difficulty in communicating verbally
- Provide eye and mouth care
- Establish alternate means of communicating with the patient
- Protect the patient from falls
- Provide skin care and assess skin integrity
- Provide ROM exercises
- Establish a bowel and bladder program
- Assess for Homans' sign
- Apply antiembolism stockings
- Reposition the patient every 2 hours
- Provide emotional support
- Provide information about the Guillain-Barré Foundation
- Individualize home care instructions
    - Know about the disorder and its implications
    - Follow instructions for medication use and be aware of possible adverse effects
    - Identify ways to reduce stress
    - Maintain a safe, quiet environment
    - Minimize environmental stress
    - Exercise hands, arms, and legs regularly
    - Know the location of local support services

● **Complications**
- Respiratory failure
- Contractures
- Cardiac arrhythmias
- DVT
- Aspiration
- Pneumonia
- Pressure ulcer

● **Possible surgical interventions**
- None

SEIZURE DISORDERS

● **Definition**
- Involuntary muscle contractions caused by abnormal discharge of electrical impulses from nerve cells
- Classification of seizures (see *Classifying seizures*)
    - Generalized seizures
        - Involvement of both hemispheres
        - Generalized absence (petit mal)
        - Clonic
        - Tonic

Classifying seizures

Seizures can take various forms depending on their origin and whether they're localized to one area of the brain, as occurs in partial seizures, or occur in both hemispheres, as happens in generalized seizures. This chart describes each type of seizure and lists common signs and symptoms.

TYPE	DESCRIPTION	SIGNS AND SYMPTOMS
Partial		
Simple partial	Symptoms confined to one hemisphere	May have motor (change in posture), sensory (hallucinations), or autonomic (flushing, tachycardia) symptoms; no loss of consciousness
Complex partial	Begins in one focal area, but spreads to both hemispheres (more common in adults)	Loss of consciousness; aura of visual disturbances; postictal symptoms
Generalized		
Absence (petit mal)	Sudden onset; lasts 5 to 10 seconds; can have 100 daily; precipitated by stress, hyperventilation, hypoglycemia, fatigue; differentiated from daydreaming	Loss of responsiveness, but continued ability to maintain posture control and not fall; twitching eyelids; lip smacking; no postictal symptoms
Myoclonic	Movement disorder (not a seizure); seen as child awakens or falls asleep; may be precipitated by touch or visual stimuli; focal or generalized; symmetrical or asymmetrical	No loss of consciousness; sudden, brief, shocklike involuntary contraction of one muscle group
Clonic	Opposing muscles contract and relax alternately in rhythmic pattern; may occur in one limb more than others	Mucus production
Tonic	Muscles are maintained in continuous contracted state (rigid posture)	Variable loss of consciousness; pupils dilate; eyes roll up; glottis closes; possible incontinence; may foam at mouth
Tonic-clonic (grand mal, major motor)	Violent total body seizure	Aura; tonic first (20 to 40 seconds); clonic next; postictal symptoms
Atonic	Drop and fall attack; needs to wear protective helmet	Loss of posture tone
Akinetic	Sudden brief loss of muscle tone or posture	Temporary loss of consciousness

(continued)

Types of partial seizures
- Simple partial: symptoms confined to one hemisphere
- Complex partial: begins in one focal area; spreads to both hemispheres

Types of generalized seizures
- Absence (petit mal): loss of responsiveness, but continued ability to maintain posture control and not fall
- Myoclonic: movement disorder (not a seizure)
- Clonic: opposing muscles contract and relax alternately in rhythmic pattern
- Tonic: muscles are maintained in continuous contracted state (rigid posture)
- Tonic-clonic (grand mal, major motor): violent total body seizure
- Atonic: drop and fall attack
- Akinetic: sudden brief loss of muscle tone or posture

- Generalized tonic-clonic (grand mal)
- Myoclonic
- Atonic
- Akinetic

Unclassified seizures

- Febrile: seizure threshold lowered by elevated temperature
- Status epilepticus: prolonged or frequent repetition of seizures without interruption

Classifying seizures *(continued)*

TYPE	DESCRIPTION	SIGNS AND SYMPTOMS
Unclassified		
Febrile	Seizure threshold lowered by elevated temperature; only one seizure per fever; common in 4% of population under age 5; occurs when temperature is rapidly rising	Lasts less than 5 minutes; generalized, transient, and nonprogressive; doesn't generally result in brain damage; EEG is normal after 2 weeks
Status epilepticus	Prolonged or frequent repetition of seizures without interruption; results in anoxia and cardiac and respiratory arrest	Consciousness not regained between seizures; lasts more than 30 minutes

- Partial seizures (focal seizures)
  - Involvement of one hemisphere
  - Simple partial
  - Complex partial
- Unclassified seizures
  - Febrile
  - Status epilepticus

Common causes of seizures

- Idiopathic
- Head injury
- Brain tumor

● **Causes**
- Idiopathic origin
- Head injury
- Hypoglycemia
- Brain tumor
- Infection
- Anoxia

● **Pathophysiology**
- Many neurons fire in a synchronous pattern, resulting in a transient physiologic disturbance
- Physiologic disturbances include abnormal movements, abnormal sensations, and a change in LOC

Key signs and symptoms of a seizure

- Aura
- Loss of consciousness
- Muscle twitches and spasms

● **Assessment findings**
- Aura
- Loss of consciousness
- Muscle twitches and spasms
- Dyspnea
- Fixed and dilated pupils
- Incontinence
- Deep sleep (postictal)

Diagnosing seizure disorders

- EEG: abnormal wave patterns
- MRI: pathologic changes

● **Diagnostic test findings**
- EEG: abnormal wave patterns, focus of seizure activity

- CT scan: a space-occupying lesion
- MRI: pathologic changes
- Brain mapping: identification of seizure areas

● **Medical management**
- Seizure precautions
- Diet: ketogenic
- I.V. therapy: saline lock
- Activity: bed rest
- Monitoring: vital signs, I/O, and neurovital signs
- Laboratory studies: glucose, potassium, and anticonvulsant drug levels, if applicable
- Anticonvulsants: phenytoin (Dilantin), ethosuximide (Zarontin), phenobarbital (Luminal), carbamazepine (Tegretol), valproic acid (Depakote), gabapentin (Neurontin), lamotrigine (Lamictal), topiramate (Topamax)
- Diazepam (Valium) or lorazepam (Ativan), for status epilepticus

● **Nursing interventions**
- Assess neurologic and respiratory status
- Maintain a patent airway
- Monitor and record vital signs, I/O, neurovital signs, and laboratory studies
- Administer medications as prescribed
- Maintain seizure precautions
- Protect the patient from injury during seizure activity
- Observe and record seizure activity
    - Initial movement
    - Respiratory pattern
    - Duration of seizure
    - Loss of consciousness
    - Aura
    - Incontinence
    - Pupillary changes
- Assess postictal state
- Encourage the patient to express his feelings about powerlessness
- Maintain the patient's diet
- Provide information about the Epilepsy Foundation of America; the National Epilepsy League, Inc.; and the National Association to Control Epilepsy
- Individualize home care instructions
    - Know about the disorder and its implications
    - Follow instructions for medication use and be aware of possible adverse effects
    - Recognize the signs and symptoms of seizure onset
    - Avoid drinking alcohol
    - Promote a safe environment
    - Wear a medical identification bracelet
    - Identify and time seizure activity
    - Prevent injury during seizure activity

Treating seizure disorders

- Seizure precautions
- Anticonvulsants
- Diazepam for status epilepticus

Key nursing interventions for a patient with a seizure disorder

- Maintain a patent airway.
- Protect the patient from injury.
- Observe and record seizure activity.
- Assess postictal state.
- Maintain seizure precautions.

Key complications of seizure disorders

- Musculoskeletal injury
- Hypoxia

Key facts about increased ICP

- Elevated ICP beyond the normal pressure exerted by blood, brain, and CSF within the skull
- Results in decreased cerebral circulation and anoxia
- May lead to permanent brain damage

Common causes of increased ICP

- Brain tumor
- Edema
- Hemorrhage
- Hydrocephalus

Key signs and symptoms of increased ICP

- Restlessness
- Hypertension
- Bradycardia
- Pupillary changes
- Altered LOC
- Widening pulse pressure
- Abnormal posturing

● **Complications**
  - Musculoskeletal injury
  - Hypoxia
  - Status epilepticus

● **Possible surgical intervention**
  - Excision of epileptogenic area (rare)

INCREASED INTRACRANIAL PRESSURE

● **Definition**
  - ICP elevated beyond the normal pressure exerted by blood, brain, and CSF within the skull

● **Causes**
  - Brain tumor
  - Abscess
  - Space-occupying lesion
  - Edema
  - Hemorrhage
  - Hydrocephalus
  - Head injury
  - Infection
  - Congenital abnormality

● **Pathophysiology**
  - Because the skull can't expand, an increase in brain tissue, CSF, or blood results in increased ICP
  - Increased ICP results in compromised cerebral circulation and anoxia, which can lead to brain injury

● **Assessment findings**
  - Restlessness
  - Anxiety
  - Hypertension
  - Bradycardia
  - Pupillary changes
    - Sluggish reaction
    - Dilation
  - Weakness
  - Altered LOC
  - Widening pulse pressure
  - Abnormal posturing
    - Decortication
    - Decerebration
  - Headache
  - Vomiting
  - Papilledema

Diagnostic test findings
- Glasgow Coma Scale: calculates neurologic impairment
- ICP measurement via ventriculostomy, epidural sensor, and subarachnoid screw: increased pressure
- LP: contraindicated

Medical management
- Monitoring: vital signs, I/O, ECG, ICP, neurovital signs, cerebral perfusion pressure (CPP), and arterial pressure
- ICP monitoring: ventriculostomy, subarachnoid screw, epidural sensor
- Diet: withhold food and fluids, as ordered
- I.V. therapy: electrolyte replacement, minimal fluid administration
- Oxygen therapy
- Intubation and mechanical ventilation with hyperventilation
- GI decompression: NG tube
- Position: semi-Fowler's
- Activity: bed rest, passive ROM exercises
- Laboratory studies: potassium, sodium, glucose, osmolality, BUN, serum osmolarity, and creatinine levels
- Indwelling urinary catheter
- Diuretics: mannitol (Osmitrol), furosemide (Lasix)
- Antacids: magnesium and aluminum hydroxide (Maalox)
- CSF drainage via ventriculostomy
- Anticonvulsant: phenytoin (Dilantin)
- Glucocorticoid: dexamethasone (Decadron)
- Histamine antagonist: ranitidine (Zantac)
- Barbiturate-induced coma or sedation
- Seizure precautions
- Pulse oximetry
- Mucosal barrier fortifier: sucralfate (Carafate)

Nursing interventions
- Assess neurologic and respiratory status
- Monitor and record vital signs, I/O, ICP, neurovital signs, laboratory studies, CPP, and pulse oximetry
- Maintain neutral alignment of the patient's neck with his body
- Maintain fluid restrictions
- Administer I.V. fluids
- Administer oxygen
- Suction only as needed
- Assist with turning, coughing, and deep breathing
- Maintain the position and patency of the NG tube; provide low suctioning
- Maintain the position and patency of the ET tube and indwelling urinary catheter
- Keep the patient in semi-Fowler's position
- Maintain a quiet and dimly lit room
- Administer medications as prescribed

Diagnosing increased ICP
- ICP measurement via ventriculostomy, epidural sensor, and subarachnoid screw: increased pressure
- LP: contraindicated

Treating increased ICP
- Oxygen therapy
- Intubation and mechanical ventilation with hyperventilation
- Position: semi-Fowler's
- Monitoring: vital signs, I/O, ECG, ICP, neurovital signs, CPP, and arterial pressure
- Laboratory studies: potassium, sodium, glucose, osmolality, BUN, serum osmolarity, and creatinine levels
- Diuretics
- CSF drainage via ventriculostomy
- Anticonvulsant
- Glucocorticoid
- Seizure precautions

Key nursing interventions for a patient with increased ICP
- Maintain fluid restrictions.
- Suction only as needed.
- Assess neurologic and respiratory status.
- Keep the patient in semi-Fowler's position.
- Monitor and record vital signs, I/O, ICP, neurovital signs, laboratory studies, CPP, and pulse oximetry.
- Maintain neutral alignment of the patient's neck with his body.
- Prevent jugular vein constriction.
- Maintain seizure precautions.

- Provide emotional support to allay the patient's anxiety
- Reposition the patient every 2 hours
- Provide rest periods between each nursing activity
- Maintain a quiet environment
- Enforce bed rest
- Prevent Valsalva's maneuver
- Provide mouth and skin care
- Provide appropriate sensory input and stimuli with frequent reorientation
- Assist with ADLs; make referrals to appropriate community agencies
- Maintain seizure precautions
- Individualize home care instructions
  - Know about the disorder and its implications
  - Follow instructions for medication use and be aware of possible adverse effects
  - Recognize the signs and symptoms of altered LOC
  - Recognize the signs and symptoms of seizures
  - Minimize environmental stress
  - Set limits for impulsive behavior
  - Continue fluid restrictions

● **Complications**
- Brain herniation
- Coma
- Seizure
- Death

● **Possible surgical intervention**
- Craniotomy for surgical decompression

HEAD INJURY

● **Definition**
- Classified by the type of fracture, hemorrhage, or trauma to the brain
- Fractures
  - Depressed
  - Comminuted
  - Linear
  - Basilar skull fracture
- Hemorrhages
  - Epidural
  - Subdural hematoma
  - Intracerebral
  - Subarachnoid
  - Ruptured cerebral aneurysm or arteriovenous malformation (AVM)
- Trauma
  - Concussion
  - Contusion
  - Scalp injury

Key complications of increased ICP

- Seizure
- Coma
- Death

Key types of head injuries

- Fracture
- Hemorrhage
- Trauma

Causes
- Motor vehicle accidents
- Falls
- Assaults
- Blunt trauma
- Penetrating trauma

Pathophysiology
- Brain injury or bleeding within the brain results in edema and hypoxia to cerebral tissue

Assessment findings
- Disorientation to time, place, or person
- Paresthesia
- Positive Babinski's reflex
- Altered LOC
- Otorrhea
- Rhinorrhea
- Headache
- Dysarthria, aphasia
- Decreased response to tactile stimuli
- Altered gag reflex
- Change in motor function
- Unequal pupil size
- Loss of pupil reaction

Diagnostic test findings
- Skull X-ray: skull fracture
- CT scan: hemorrhage, cerebral edema, or shift of midline structures
- MRI: hemorrhage, cerebral edema, or shift of midline structures
- Cerebral angiography: intracerebral, subdural, epidural hematoma, aneurysm, or AVM
- Echoencephalogram: shift of midline structures

Medical management
- Neurovascular, cardiovascular, and respiratory assessment
- Reflex checks: oculocephalic, oculovestibular, corneal, cough, and gag
- Monitoring: vital signs, I/O, ECG, hemodynamic variables, ICP, CVP, neurovital signs, and arterial line
- Diet: restricted fluids
- I.V. therapy: electrolyte replacement, saline lock
- Oxygen therapy
- Intubation and mechanical ventilation with hyperventilation
- GI decompression: NG tube
- Position: semi-Fowler's
- Activity: bed rest, active and passive ROM exercises
- Laboratory studies: potassium, sodium, osmolality, ABG analysis, Hb, and HCT

- Indwelling urinary catheter
- Analgesic: codeine (Paveral)
- Diuretics: mannitol (Osmitrol), furosemide (Lasix)
- Antacids: magnesium and aluminum hydroxide (Maalox), aluminum hydroxide gel (AlternaGEL)
- Anticonvulsant: phenytoin (Dilantin)
- Benzodiazepines
- Glucocorticoid: dexamethasone (Decadron)
- Histamine antagonists: cimetidine (Tagamet), ranitidine (Zantac)
- Cervical collar
- Mucosal barrier fortifier: sucralfate (Carafate)
- Pulse oximetry

● Nursing interventions
- Assess neurologic and respiratory status
- Monitor and record vital signs, I/O, hemodynamic variables, ICP, CVP, laboratory studies, and pulse oximetry
- Check cough and gag reflexes
- Observe for signs of increasing ICP
- Assess for CSF leak: otorrhea, rhinorrhea
- Administer oxygen
- Maintain position and patency of ET tube
- Elevate the head of the bed to reduce cerebral edema
- Maintain seizure precautions
- Administer medications as prescribed
- Restrict fluids
- Administer I.V. fluids
- Encourage coughing and deep breathing
- Maintain position, patency, and low suction of NG tube
- Encourage the patient to express feelings about changes in body image and function
- Assess pain
- Check for signs of diabetes insipidus
- Provide appropriate sensory input and stimuli with frequent reorientation
- Provide means of communication
- Provide eye, skin, and mouth care
- Reposition the patient every 2 hours
- Assist with ADLs
- Provide emotional support
- Provide information about the National Head Injury Foundation
- Individualize home care instructions (for patient and family)
  - Know about the disorder and its implications
  - Follow instructions for medication use and be aware of possible adverse effects
  - Recognize the signs and symptoms of decreased LOC
  - Recognize seizure activity and how to provide safety
  - Set limits for impulsive behavior

Key interventions in nursing care for a patient with a head injury

- Administer oxygen.
- Assess neurologic and respiratory status.
- Elevate the head of the bed to reduce cerebral edema.
- Maintain seizure precautions.
- Assess for CSF leak: otorrhea, rhinorrhea.
- Check for signs of diabetes insipidus.
- Check cough and gag reflexes.
- Observe for signs of increasing ICP.

        – Adhere to fluid restrictions

        – Know the location of local support services

● **Complications**
- Shock
- Meningitis
- Increased ICP
- Stress ulcer
- Diabetes insipidus
- Infection
- Depression
- Brain death
- Hematoma

● **Possible surgical intervention**
- Craniotomy for evacuation of hematomas

STROKE

● **Definition**
- Disruption of cerebral circulation due to ischemia or hemorrhage that results in motor and sensory deficits

● **Causes**
- Thrombosis
- Embolism
- Hemorrhage
- Vasospasm
- Risk factors
    - Age: increased risk after age 55
    - Family history
    - Race: African Americans at higher risk
    - Gender: men at higher risk
    - Prior stroke, transient ischemic attack (TIA), or heart attack
    - Hypertension
    - Cigarette smoking
    - Diabetes mellitus
    - Atherosclerosis
    - Atrial fibrillation
    - Sickle cell disease
    - High blood cholesterol level
    - High-fat diet
    - Obesity
    - Physical inactivity
    - Use of hormonal contraceptives or hormone replacement therapy
    - Migraines
    - Clotting disorder

Key complications of head injury
- Shock
- Increased ICP
- Brain death

Key facts about stroke
- Disruption of cerebral circulation
- Results in motor and sensory deficits

Common causes of stroke
- Thrombosis
- Embolism
- Hemorrhage
- Top risk factors for stroke
- Hypertension
- Smoking
- Prior stroke, TIA, or heart attack
- Atrial fibrillation

Key signs and symptoms of stroke

- Sudden numbness or weakness on one side of body
- Sudden confusion or trouble speaking
- Sudden visual disturbance
- Sudden difficulty walking
- Sudden severe headache

Diagnosing stroke

- CT scan: intracranial bleeding, infarct, or shift of midline structures
- MRI: intracranial bleeding, infarct, or shift of midline structures
- Digital subtraction angiography: occlusion or narrowing of vessels

Treating stroke

- Maintain airway, breathing, and circulation
- Reperfusion agent: tissue plasminogen activator if within 3 hours of symptom onset
- Antihypertensives
- Physical therapy, speech therapy, occupational therapy

Pathophysiology

- Disruption of cerebral blood flow causes cerebral anoxia
- Cerebral anoxia results in cerebral infarction
- Infarction results in edema and deficits

Assessment findings

- Sudden numbness or weakness on one side of the body
- Sudden confusion or trouble speaking
- Sudden visual disturbance
- Sudden difficulty with walking, balancing, coordination, or dizziness
- Sudden severe headache
- Syncope
- Change in LOC
- Seizures

Diagnostic test findings

- CT scan: intracranial bleeding, infarct, or shift of midline structures
- MRI: intracranial bleeding, infarct, or shift of midline structures
- LP: increased pressure, bloody CSF
- EEG: focal slowing in area of lesion
- Brain scan: decreased perfusion
- Digital subtraction angiography: occlusion or narrowing of vessels

Medical management

- Maintenance of airway, breathing, and circulation
- Neurologic, cardiovasular, and respiratory assessment
- Reperfusion agent: tissue plasminogen activator (Activase), if symptoms are recognized within 3 hours of onset
- Oxygen therapy
- Intubation and mechanical ventilation
- Monitoring: vital signs, I/O, cardiac rhythm, and pulse oximetry
- Seizure precautions
- Analgesic: codeine (Paveral)
- Diet: low-sodium, increased potassium; tube feedings or TPN, as indicated
- I.V. therapy
- Position: semi-Fowler's
- Activity: active and passive ROM and isometric exercises
- Laboratory studies: sodium, potassium, glucose, ABG analysis, PT, and PTT
- Indwelling urinary catheter
- Antiplatelet agent: aspirin, ticlopidine (Ticlid)
- Diuretics: mannitol (Osmitrol), furosemide (Lasix)
- DVT prophalaxis
- Anticonvulsant: phenytoin (Dilantin)
- Glucocorticoid: dexamethasone (Decadron)
- Histamine antagonists: ranitidine (Zantac)
- Antihypertensives: nitroglycerin (Nitrostat), nitroprusside (Nipride)
- Anticoagulants: warfarin (Coumadin), heparin; use with caution

- Antiarrhythmic: diltiazem (Cardizem)
- Physical therapy, speech therapy, and occupational therapy

● **Nursing interventions**
- Assess neurovascular, cardiac, and respiratory status
- Monitor and record vital signs, I/O, ICP, laboratory studies, and pulse oximetry
- Administer oxygen and assist with ET intubation, if indicated
- Monitor for signs of complications if tissue plasminogen activator (TPA) was administered
- Maintain the patient's nutritional status
- Administer I.V. fluids
- Reposition the patient every 2 hours; provide skin care and assess skin integrity
- Encourage coughing, deep breathing, and use of incentive spirometry
- Administer medications as prescribed
- Encourage the patient to express his feelings about changes in his body image and function and about difficulty in communicating
- Maintain a quiet environment
- Assess for receptive and expressive aphasia
- Assess for hemianopsia
- Protect the patient from falls and injury
- Apply antiembolism stockings
- Monitor the patient's swallowing ability, and maintain aspiration precautions
- Maintain seizure precautions
- Provide passive ROM exercises
- Provide a means of communication
- Assist with ADLs
- Provide emotional support
- Provide information about the American Heart Association and the National Stroke Foundation
- Individualize home care instructions
  - Know about the disorder and its implications
  - Follow instructions for medication use and be aware of possible adverse effects
  - Recognize the signs and symptoms of seizures
  - Reinforce established methods of communication (aphasic patient)
  - Monitor blood pressure
  - Use assistive devices in ADLs
  - Continue physical therapy, speech therapy, and occupational therapy
  - Know the location of local support services

● **Complications**
- Cerebral edema
- Hydrocephalus
- Vasospasm

Key facts about cerebral aneurysm
- Dilation or localized weakness of the middle layer of an artery
- Three types: saccular (berry), fusiform, and mycotic

Common causes of cerebral aneurysm
- Atherosclerosis
- Congenital weakness
- Hypertension

Key signs and symptoms of cerebral aneurysm
- Severe headache
- Altered LOC
- Vomiting

- Aspiration
- Pneumonia
- Increased ICP
- Motor and sensory deficits
- Speech deficits
- Depression
- Problems from immobility

● **Possible surgical interventions**
- Carotid endarterectomy
- Craniotomy for evacuation of a clot or for superior temporal artery—middle cerebral artery anastomosis

CEREBRAL ANEURYSM

● **Definition**
- Dilation or localized weakness of the middle layer of an artery (see *Most common sites of cerebral aneurysm*)
- Classified by aneurysm type
  - Saccular (berry)
  - Fusiform
  - Mycotic

● **Causes**
- Atherosclerosis
- Trauma
- Congenital weakness
- Hypertension
- Connective tissue disorders
- Sickle cell anemia
- Infection
- Neoplasm
- Vasculopathies

● **Pathophysiology**
- Enlargement of aneurysm compresses nerves
- Enlargement of the aneurysm finally results in dissolution of the wall and rupture of the aneurysm
- Rupture of the aneurysm results in subarachnoid hemorrhage
- Release of serotonin, prostaglandins, and catecholamines from blood precipitates vasospasm

● **Assessment findings**
- Diplopia
- Ptosis
- Severe headache
- Hemiparesis
- Nuchal rigidity
- Altered LOC

Most common sites of cerebral aneurysm

Cerebral aneurysms usually arise at arterial bifurcations in the Circle of Willis and its branches. This illustration shows the most common aneurysm sites around this circle.

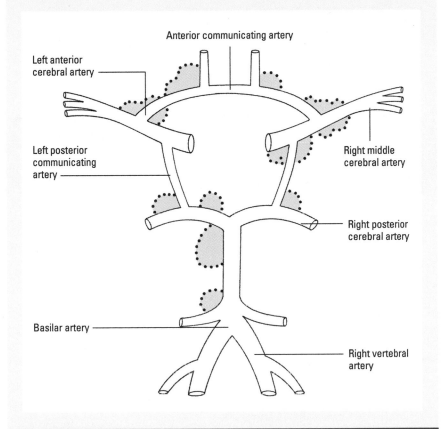

Anterior communicating artery

Left anterior cerebral artery

Left posterior communicating artery

Right middle cerebral artery

Right posterior cerebral artery

Basilar artery

Right vertebral artery

Where cerebral aneurysms arise

- Arterial bifurcations in the Circle of Willis and its branches

- Seizure activity
- Blurred vision
- Vomiting
- **Diagnostic test findings**
  - CT scan: shift of intracranial midline structures, blood in subarachnoid space
  - MRI: shift of intracranial midline structures, blood in subarachnoid space
  - Cerebral angiogram: identification of vasospasm and vasculature associated with aneurysm
  - LP (contraindicated with increased ICP): increased pressure, protein, WBCs; bloody and xanthochromic CSF
- **Medical management**
  - Neurovascular, cardiovascular, and respiratory assessment

Diagnosing cerebral aneurysm

- CT scan: shift of intracranial midline structures, blood in subarachnoid space
- Cerebral angiogram: identification of vasospasm and vasculature associated with aneurysm

Treating cerebral aneurysm

- Neurovascular, cardiovascular, and respiratory assessment
- Clipping or wrapping of aneurysm
- Antihypertensives

Key nursing interventions for a patient with a cerebral aneurysm

- Keep the patient in semi-Fowler's position.
- Maintain a quiet, darkened environment.
- Assess pain.
- Assess for signs of increased ICP.
- Maintain seizure and aneurysm precautions.
- Prevent constipation.
- Assess for meningeal irritation.

- Monitoring: vital signs, pulse oximetry, I/O (fluid restrictions), ICP, neurovital signs, and arterial line
- Intubation and mechanical ventilation
- I.V. therapy: minimal fluids
- Oxygen therapy
- Position: semi-Fowler's
- Activity: bed rest, passive ROM exercises
- Precautions: aneurysm and seizure
- Antacids: magnesium and aluminum hydroxide (Maalox), aluminum hydroxide gel (AlternaGEL)
- Anticonvulsant: phenytoin (Dilantin), fosphenytoin (Cerebyx)
- Glucocorticoid: dexamethasone (Decadron)
- Histamine antagonist: ranitidine (Zantac)
- Stool softener: docusate (Colace)
- Antifibrinolytic: aminocaproic acid (Amicar)
- Antihypertensives: labetalol (Normodyne), hydralazine (Apresoline)
- Analgesic: morphine sulfate
- Ergot alkaloid: methysergide (Sansert)
- Calcium channel blocker: nimodipine (Nimotop)
- Mucosal barrier fortifier: sucralfate (Carafate)

● Nursing interventions

- Assess neurologic, cardiovascular, and respiratory systems
- Monitor and record vital signs, I/O, ICP, and pulse oximetry
- Administer oxygen
- Assess pain level
- Assess for signs of increased ICP
- Maintain seizure and aneurysm precautions
- Restrict fluids
- Keep the patient in semi-Fowler's position
- Administer medication as prescribed
- Encourage the patient to express his feelings about a fear of dying
- Provide emotional support to allay the patient's anxiety
- Maintain a quiet, darkened environment
- Allow a rest period between nursing activities
- Maintain bed rest
- Prevent Valsalva's maneuver
- Provide passive ROM exercises
- Provide skin care
- Assist with ADLs
- Assess for meningeal irritation
- Individualize home care instructions
  - Know about the disorder and its implications
  - Follow instructions for medication use and be aware of possible adverse effects
  - Recognize the signs and symptoms of altered LOC
  - Minimize environmental stress

    – Alter ADLs to compensate for neurologic deficits

    – Prevent constipation

- **Complications**
  - Vasospasm
  - Rebleeding of the aneurysm
  - Increased ICP
  - Rupture of the aneurysm
  - Hydrocephalus
  - Brain herniation
  - Brain death
- **Possible surgical interventions**
  - Clipping or wrapping of an aneurysm
  - Proximal or Hunterian ligation
  - Electrolytically detachable platinum coils
  - Craniotomy to evaluate hematoma
  - Endovascular therapy

BRAIN TUMOR

- **Definition**
  - Malignant or benign tumor of the brain that may be primary or metastatic
- **Causes**
  - Genetic
  - Environmental
- **Pathophysiology**
  - Unregulated cell growth and uncontrolled cell division result in the development of a neoplasm
  - Tumors are classified according to tissue of origin
    - Angiomas
    - Gliomas
    - Meningiomas
    - Neuromas
    - Metastatic lesions
    - Developmental (congenital) tumors
  - Tumors can be infiltrative and destroy surrounding tissue or be encapsulated and displace brain tissue
  - Presence of lesion and compression of blood vessels produces ischemia, edema, and increased ICP
- **Assessment findings**
  - Tumor in any brain area
    - Headache
    - Projectile vomiting
    - Papilledema
  - Tumor in the frontal lobe

Key complications of cerebral aneurysm

- Vasospasm
- Rupture
- Brain herniation

Key facts about a brain tumor

- Malignant or benign tumor of the brain
- May be primary or metastatic

Common causes of a brain tumor

- Genetic
- Environmental

Key signs and symptoms of a brain tumor

- Headache
- Vomiting
- Seizures
- Visual impairment

– Personality changes
– Aphasia (expressive)
– Memory loss
• Tumor in the temporal lobe
– Seizures
– Aphasia (receptive)
• Tumor in the parietal lobe
– Motor seizures
– Sensory impairment
• Tumor in the occipital lobe
– Visual impairment
– Homonymous hemianopia
– Visual hallucinations
• Tumor in the cerebellum
– Impaired equilibrium
– Impaired coordination

Diagnostic test findings
• MRI or CT scan: location and size of tumor
• Skull X-ray: location and size of tumor
• Angiography: location and size of tumor
• EEG: seizure activity
• LP (contraindicated with increased ICP): increased protein

Medical management
• Radiation therapy
• Antineoplastics: vincristine (Oncovin), lomustine (CeeNU), carmustine (BiCNU)
• Monitoring: vital signs, I/O, ICP, and neurovital signs
• Diet: high-protein, high-calorie; TPN if indicated
• I.V. therapy: fluids as ordered
• Oxygen therapy
• Position: semi-Fowler's
• Activity: bed rest
• Laboratory studies: sodium, potassium, and glucose levels
• Antiemetic: ondansetron (Zofran)
• Analgesic: morphine sulfate
• Diuretics: mannitol (Osmitrol), furosemide (Lasix)
• Anticonvulsant: phenytoin (Dilantin)
• Glucocorticoid: dexamethasone (Decadron)
• Seizure precautions
• Stereotaxic brachytherapy
• Stereotaxic radiosurgery (Roentgen knife)
• Mucosal barrier fortifier: sucralfate (Carafate)

Nursing interventions
• Assess neurologic and respiratory status
• Monitor and record vital signs, I/O, pulse oximetry, and laboratory studies

Diagnosing a brain tumor
• EEG: seizure activity
• MRI or CT scan: location and size of tumor
• Skull X-ray: location and size of tumor

Treating a brain tumor
• Radiation therapy
• Antineoplastics
• Diuretics
• Anticonvulsant
• Glucocorticoid
• Seizure precautions

- Assess pain
- Assess for increased ICP
- Maintain seizure precautions
- Maintain the patient's diet; administer TPN
- Administer I.V. fluids
- Administer oxygen
- Keep the patient in semi-Fowler's position
- Administer medications as prescribed
- Encourage the patient to express his feelings about his diagnosis
- Provide postchemotherapeutic and postradiation nursing care
  - Provide prophylactic skin and mouth care
  - Monitor dietary intake
  - Administer antiemetics and antidiarrheals, as prescribed
  - Monitor the patient for bleeding, infection, and electrolyte imbalance
  - Provide rest periods
- Provide emotional support
- Provide information about the National Head Injury Foundation and the Association for Brain Tumor Research
- Individualize home care instructions
  - Know about the disorder and its implications
  - Follow instructions for medication use and be aware of possible adverse effects
  - Recognize the signs and symptoms of altered LOC
  - Maintain a safe, quiet environment
  - Make quality-of-life decisions
  - Make referrals for hospice care
  - Know the location of local support services

● **Complications**
- Increased ICP
- Brain herniation
- Seizures
- Metastasis
- Death

● **Possible surgical intervention**
- Craniotomy for surgical excision of a tumor

SPINAL CORD INJURY

● **Definition**
- Traumatic injury to the spinal cord that results in sensory and motor deficits
- Two types of spinal cord injury
  - Paraplegia: paralysis of the lower extremities
  - Quadriplegia: paralysis of all four extremities

Common causes of spinal cord injury

- Motor vehicle accidents
- Falls
- Penetrating wounds
- Trauma

Key signs and symptoms of spinal cord injury

- Paralysis below the level of the injury
- Paresthesia below the level of the injury
- Loss of bowel and bladder control

Diagnosing spinal cord injury

- CT scan: spinal cord edema, vertebral fracture, spinal cord compression
- MRI: spinal cord edema, vertebral fracture, spinal cord compression

Treating spinal cord injury

- Position: flat, neck immobilized
- Glucocorticoids
- Cervical collar
- Maintenance of vertebral alignment: Stryker turning frame, Crutchfield tongs, Halo brace
- Muscle relaxant
- Specialized bed: rotation (Rotorest, Tilt and Turn, Paragon)

● **Causes**
- Motor vehicle accidents
- Falls
- Penetrating wounds
- Trauma
- Infection
- Tumor
- Congenital anomaly

● **Pathophysiology**
- Injury may result in complete transection of the spinal cord
- Associated edema and hemorrhage from the injury cause ischemia
- Necrosis and scar tissue form in the area of the traumatized cord
- Injury may result in paraplegia or quadriplegia

● **Assessment findings**
- Paralysis below the level of the injury
- Paresthesia below the level of the injury
- Neck pain
- Loss of bowel and bladder control
- Respiratory distress
- Numbness and tingling
- Flaccid muscle
- Absence of reflexes below the level of the injury
- Loss of perspiration below level of the injury

● **Diagnostic test findings**
- Spinal X-rays: vertebral fracture
- CT scan: spinal cord edema, vertebral fracture, spinal cord compression
- MRI: spinal cord edema, vertebral fracture, spinal cord compression

● **Medical management**
- Position: flat, neck immobilized with cervical collar
- Monitoring: vital signs, I/O, ECG, ICP, pulse oximetry, and neurovital signs
- Intubation and mechanical ventilation
- Oxygen therapy
- Maintenance of vertebral alignment: Stryker turning frame, Crutchfield tongs, Halo brace
- DVT prophalaxis
- Diet: low-calcium, high-protein
- I.V. therapy
- GI decompression: NG tube
- Activity: bed rest, passive ROM exercises
- Laboratory studies: sodium, potassium, and glucose levels and WBC count
- Indwelling urinary catheter
- Anticonvulsant: phenytoin (Dilantin)
- Corticosteroids: dexamethasone (Decadron), methylprednisolone (Solu-Medrol)

- Laxative: bisacodyl (Dulcolax)
- Antianxiety agent: diazepam (Valium)
- Antihypertensives: diazoxide (Hyperstat), hydralazine (Apresoline)
- Muscle relaxant: dantrolene (Dantrium)
- Specialized bed: rotation (Rotorest, Tilt and Turn, Paragon)
- Mucosal barrier fortifier: sucralfate (Carafate)
- Physical and occupational therapy

Nursing interventions

- Assess neurologic and respiratory status
- Monitor and record vital signs, I/O, laboratory studies, and pulse oximetry
- Assess for spinal shock
- Administer oxygen
- Provide suction and turning; encourage coughing and deep breathing
- Keep the patient flat as directed
- Encourage fluids
- Administer I.V. fluids
- Administer medications as prescribed
- Encourage the patient to express his feelings about his diagnosis
- Reposition the patient every 2 hours using the logrolling technique
- Maintain body alignment
- Initiate bowel and bladder retraining
- Provide passive ROM exercises
- Check for autonomic dysreflexia
- Provide skin care and assess skin integrity
- Apply antiembolism stockings
- Provide emotional support
- Provide information about the National Spinal Cord Injury Association
- Individualize home care instructions
    - Know about the disorder and its implications
    - Follow instructions for medication use and be aware of possible adverse effects
    - Exercise regularly to strengthen muscles
    - Recognize the signs and symptoms of autonomic dysreflexia, UTI, and upper respiratory infection
    - Continue bowel and bladder program
    - Maintain acidic urine with cranberry juice
    - Consume adequate fluids: 3 qt (3 L)/day
    - Use assistive devices for ADLs
    - Maintain skin integrity
    - Reinforce independence
    - Know the location of local support services

Complications

- Spinal shock
- Autonomic dysreflexia
- Respiratory failure

Key nursing interventions for a patient with spinal cord injury

- Assess neurologic and respiratory status.
- Keep the patient flat.
- Monitor and record vital signs, I/O, laboratory studies, and pulse oximetry.
- Reposition the patient every 2 hours using the logrolling technique.
- Check for autonomic dysreflexia.
- Assess for spinal shock.
- Provide skin care.

Key complications of spinal cord injury

- Autonomic dysreflexia
- Respiratory failure
- Depression

- Pressure ulcers
- Pneumonia
- Depression

● **Possible surgical interventions**
- Laminectomy
- Spinal fusion

AMYOTROPHIC LATERAL SCLEROSIS (ALS)— LOU GEHRIG DISEASE

● **Definition**
- Progressive degenerative neurologic disease resulting in decreased motor function in the upper and lower motor neuron systems (see *Motor neuron disease*)

● **Causes**
- Unknown cause
- Genetic predisposition
- Viral infection
- Excess of glutamate

● **Pathophysiology**
- Myelin sheaths are destroyed and replaced with scar tissue, resulting in distorted or blocked nerve impulses
- Nerve cells die and muscle fibers have atrophic changes

● **Assessment findings**
- Fatigue
- Awkwardness of fine finger movements
- Dysphagia
- Muscle weakness of hands and arms
- Fasciculations of face
- Spasticity
- Emotional lability
- Muscle incoordination

● **Diagnostic test findings**
- No one specific diagnostic test used
- Diagnosis based on assessment findings
- EMG: decreased amplitude of evoked potentials
- Laboratory values: elevated creatine kinase

● **Medical management**
- Focused on symptomatic relief
- Activity: as tolerated
- Monitoring: vital signs, I/O, neurovital signs
- Mechanical ventilation: negative-pressure ventilators
- Enteral feedings
- Antispasmodics: baclofen (Lioresal), tizanidine (Zanaflex)
- Investigational: thyrotropin-releasing hormone, interferon

Key facts about ALS

- Progressive degenerative neurologic disease
- Results in decreased motor function in the upper and lower motor neuron systems

Common causes of ALS

- Genetic predisposition
- Virus

Key signs and symptoms of ALS

- Fatigue
- Awkwardness of fine finger movements
- Dysphagia
- Muscle weakness of hands and arms

Diagnosing ALS

- No one specific diagnostic test used
- Diagnosis based on assessment findings

Treating ALS

- Focus on symptomatic relief
- Antispasmodics

Motor neuron disease

In its final stages, motor neuron disease affects both upper and lower motor neuron cells. However, the site of initial cell damage varies according to the specific disease.

- *Progressive bulbar palsy:* degeneration of upper motor neurons in the medulla oblongata
- *Progressive muscular atrophy:* degeneration of lower motor neurons in the spinal cord
- *Amyotrophic lateral sclerosis:* Degeneration of upper motor neurons in the medulla oblongata and lower motor neurons in the spinal cord.

- Glutamate antagonist: riluzole (Rilutek)
- Physical therapy

● **Nursing interventions**
- Assess neurologic and respiratory status
- Monitor and record vital signs and I/O
- Assess swallow and gag reflexes; maintain aspiration precautions
- Maintain the patient's diet
- Administer medications as prescribed
- Provide information regarding advanced directives or a "living will"
- Suction oral pharynx as necessary
- Encourage active ROM or assist with passive ROM exercises
- Assist the patient to maintain as much independence as possible
- Provide emotional support for the patient and his family
- Provide information about the ALS Foundation
- Individualize home care instructions
    - Know about the disorder and its implications
    - Follow instructions for medication use and be aware of possible adverse effects
    - Maintain tucked chin position while eating or drinking
    - Use tonsillar suction tip to clear oral pharynx
    - Use prosthetic devices to assist with ADLs

● **Complications**
- Depression
- Respiratory failure
- Pneumonia
- Death

● **Possible surgical intervention**
- Tracheostomy for respiratory failure

INTERVERTEBRAL DISK HERNIATION

● **Definition**
- All or part of the nucleus pulposus is forced through the disk's outer ring (annulus fibrosus)

Common causes of intervertebral disk herniation

- Degenerative disk changes
- Trauma

Key signs and symptoms of intervertebral disk herniation

- Lumbosacral:
- Acute, intermittent pain in the lower back
- Pain on ambulation
- Weakness, numbness, and tingling of the foot and leg
- Cervical:
- Weakness of the affected upper extremity
- Neck pain that radiates down the arm to the hand
- Thoracic:
- Bandlike pain around chest

Diagnosing intervertebral disk herniation

- MRI: herniation of spine and degenerative changes
- Myelogram: degree of injury and level of herniation

Treating intervertebral disk herniation

- Nonsteroidal anti-inflammatory drugs
- Corticosteroids
- Analgesics
- Orthopedic devices, including back brace, cervical collar, or traction

● **Causes**
- Degenerative disk changes
- Trauma
- Physical stress
- Scoliosis/kyphosis
- Spondylosis

● **Pathophysiology**
- The extruded disk may impinge on spinal nerve roots as they exit from the spinal canal or on the spinal cord itself
- The result is back pain and other signs of nerve root irritation

● **Assessment findings**
- In lumbosacral area
  - Acute, intermittent pain in the lower back radiating across the buttock and down the leg
  - Pain on ambulation
  - Weakness, numbness, and tingling of the foot and leg
  - Diminished reflexes of the affected extremity
- In cervical area
  - Weakness of the affected upper extremity
  - Neck pain that radiates down the arm to the hand
  - Sensory loss of the hand
  - Diminished or absent reflexes of the arm
- In thoracic area
  - Bandlike pain around chest

● **Diagnostic test findings**
- MRI: herniation of affected area of spine, degenerative changes, and condition of the canal and nerve root
- Myelogram: degree of injury and level of herniation
- CT scan: outlines bone and soft tissue structures
- Lasegue's sign and straight-leg-raising test: positive

● **Medical management**
- Monitoring: vital signs, I/O, laboratory studies, and neurovascular checks
- Position: bed rest in semi-Fowler's position with hip and knee flexion and passive ROM exercises, as indicated
- Heating pad and moist, warm compresses
- Analgesics: propoxyphene (Darvon), oxycodone and acetaminophen (Percocet, Tylox), hydrocodone (Vicodin), oxycodone hydrochloride (OxyContin)
- Nonsteroidal anti-inflammatory drugs: indomethacin (Indocin), ibuprofen (Motrin), sulindac (Clinoril), piroxicam (Feldene), flurbiprofen (Ansaid), diclofenac (Voltaren), naproxen (Naprosyn), diflunisal (Dolobid)
- Muscle relaxants: diazepam (Valium), cyclobenzaprine (Flexeril), methocarbamol (Robaxin), metaxalone (Skelaxin)
- Physical therapy
- Diet: increased fiber and fluids

- Corticosteroids: oral or epidural
- Orthopedic devices, including back brace, cervical collar,, or traction
- Transcutaneous electrical nerve stimulation

● **Nursing interventions**
- Monitor neurovascular status, vital signs, I/O, and laboratory values
- Assess level of pain and administer analgesics, as necessary
- Administer medications as prescribed
- Maintain traction, braces, or cervical collar
- Maintain the patient's diet
- Encourage fluids
- Maintain bed rest with proper body alignment; immobilize neck with cervical collar if indicated
- Encourage the patient to express his feelings about his diagnosis
- Reposition the patient every 2 hours using the logrolling technique
- Promote independence in ADLs
- Individualize home care instruction
    - Know about the disorder and its implications
    - Follow instructions for medication use and be aware of possible adverse effects
    - Exercise regularly, according to physical therapist's guidelines, to strengthen and stretch the muscles
    - Avoid heavy lifting
    - Avoid flexion, extension, or rotation of the neck, if cervical
    - Use a back brace or cervical collar
    - Practice relaxation techniques
    - Use proper body mechanics

● **Complications**
- Persistent neurologic deficits
- Bowel and bladder dysfunction

● **Possible surgical interventions**
- Microdiscectomy
- Percutaneous discectomy
- Laminotomy or discectomy, with or without the use of instrumentation

MENINGITIS

● **Definition**
- Inflammation of the brain and spinal cord meninges

● **Causes**
- Bacterial infection, such as *Neisseria meningitides* and *Streptococcus pneumoniae*, most common cause
- *Haemophilus influenzae* is a common bacterial cause in children ages 2 months to 7 years
- Beta-hemolytic streptococci and *Listeria monocytogenes* are common causes in infants

---

Key nursing interventions for a patient with intervertebral disk herniation

- Maintain bed rest with proper body alignment.
- Monitor neurovascular status, vital signs, I/O, and laboratory values.
- Assess level of pain and administer analgesics, as necessary.
- Reposition the patient every 2 hours using the logrolling technique.
- Maintain traction, braces, and cervical collar.

Key complications of intervertebral disk herniation

- Neurologic deficits
- Bowel and bladder dysfunction

Key fact about meningitis

- Inflammation of the brain and spinal cord meninges

Common causes of meningitis

- Bacterial infection
- Viral infection
- Fungal infection

Key signs and symptoms of meningitis

- Fever
- Chills
- Tachycardia
- Petechial rash
- Severe throbbing headache
- Photophobia
- Nuchal rigidity
- Positive Kernig's sign
- Positive Brudzinski's sign
- Decreased LOC
- Ataxia
- Seizures

Diagnosing meningitis

- Cultures: identify source of infection in blood, urine, and nose and throat secretions
- LP: elevated CSF pressure; cloudy, turbid, or clear in appearance; normal or increased protein; glucose decreased or normal; culture and sensitivity tests identify bacteria, unless viral cause

Treating meningitis

- I.V. therapy: electrolyte replacement, saline lock
- Oxygen therapy
- Antibiotics
- Anticonvulsants
- Diuretic

- Enteroviruses, mumps, and herpes simplex are common causes of viral meningitis (aseptic meningitis)
- Cryptococcosis, candidiasis, histoplasmosis, and coccidioidomycosis are common causes of fungal meningitis
- Tuberculosis meningitis is a bacterial infection caused by *Mycobacterium tuberculosis*

● **Pathophysiology**
- Infecting organisms gain entry through basilar skull fractures with dural tears, chronic otitis media or sinusitis, neurosurgical contamination, penetrating head wounds, or septicemia
- Infecting organisms produce an inflammatory response
- Exudate formation causes meningeal irritation and increased ICP

● **Assessment findings**
- Severe throbbing headache
- Nuchal rigidity
- Fever
- Tachycardia
- Chills
- Petechial rash
- Photophobia
- Positive Kernig's sign (see *Important signs of meningitis*)
- Positive Brudzinski's sign
- Altered LOC
- Cranial nerve palsies, most commonly ptosis, diplopia, facial weakness, tinnitus, vertigo, and deafness
- Focal motor weakness
- Ataxia
- Seizures

● **Diagnostic test findings**
- LP: elevated CSF pressure; cloudy, turbid, or clear in appearance; normal or increased protein; glucose decreased or normal; culture and sensitivity tests identify bacteria, unless viral cause
- Cultures: identify source of infection in blood, urine, and nose and throat secretions
- X-rays: assesses for fractures, abscesses, or signs of infection in chest, skull, and sinuses
- WBC count: elevated

● **Medical management**
- Monitoring: vital signs, I/O, cardiac rhythm, pulse oximetry, and laboratory values
- Antibiotics: penicillin, ampicillin (Omnipen), or chloramphenicol (Chloromycetin), or one of the cephalosporins (ceftriaxone [Rocephin], cefotaxime [Claforan]); vancomycin (Vancocin) alone or in combination with rifampin (Rifadin), for resistant strains
- Antipyretics and analgesics: aspirin, acetaminophen (Tylenol)

Important signs of meningitis

Brudzinski's sign: Place the patient in a dorsal recumbent position, put your hands behind her neck, and bend it forward. Pain and resistance may indicate meningeal inflammation, neck injury, or arthritis. If the patient also flexes her hips and knees in response to this manipulation, chances are she has meningitis.

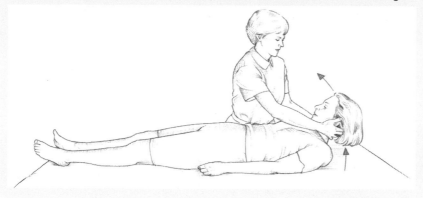

Kernig's sign: Place the patient in a supine position. Flex her leg at the hip and knee and then straighten the knee. Pain or resistance points to meningitis.

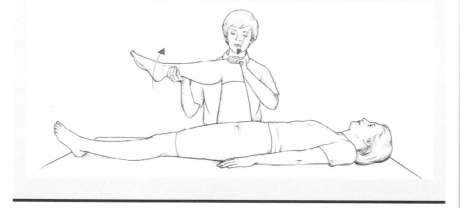

- Oxygen therapy
- I.V. therapy: electrolyte replacement
- Diet: withhold food and fluids, as ordered; enteral or parenteral feeding, as indicated
- Position: semi-Fowler's
- Activity: bed rest in darkened room
- Anticonvulsants: phenytoin (Dilantin), phenobarbital (Luminal)
- Glucocorticoid: dexamethasone (Decadron)
- Diuretic: mannitol (Osmitrol)
- Isolation
- Seizure precautions

● **Nursing interventions**
- Assess neurologic, cardiovascular, and respiratory status

- Monitor and record vital signs, I/O, ICP, laboratory studies, and pulse oximetry
- Implement isolation techniques if necessary
- Administer medications as ordered
- Administer I.V. fluids
- Administer oxygen
- Keep the patient on bed rest in the semi-Fowler's position
- Provide emotional support to allay the patient's anxiety
- Reposition the patient every 2 hours; provide ROM exercises
- Maintain a quiet, dimly lit environment
- Maintain seizure precautions
- Use a cooling blanket or tepid bath to control temperature
- Assess for headache and administer analgesics, as appropriate
- Provide nutrition as appropriate
- Provide skin care
- Report meningococcal meningitis to local health authorities
- Individualize home care instruction
  - Know about the disorder and its implications
  - Follow instructions for medication use and be aware of possible adverse effects
  - Recognize signs and symptoms of meningitis
  - Recognize signs and symptoms of ICP
  - Prevent meningitis from recurring by seeking proper medical treatment for chronic sinusitis or other chronic infections

● **Complications**
- Visual impairment
- Optic neuritis
- Deafness
- Personality changes
- Seizures
- Paresis
- Death

● **Possible surgical intervention**
- None

ALZHEIMER'S DISEASE

● **Definition**
- Irreversible, chronic degenerative disorder of the cerebral cortex characterized by progressive dementia

● **Causes**
- Exact cause unknown
- Neurotransmitter deficiencies
- Virus
- Trauma

Stages of Alzheimer's disease

EARLY STAGE	INTERMEDIATE STAGE	END STAGE
• Recent memory loss • Inability to learn and retain new information • Difficulty finding words • Personality changes and mood swings • Progressive difficulty performing activities of daily living (ADLs)	• Inability to learn and recall new information • Reduced ability to remember past events • Increased need for assistance with ADLs • Wandering • Agitation, hostility, or physical aggressiveness • Lack of orientation to time and place • Bladder and bowel incontinence	• Inability to walk • Total incontinence • No recent or remote memory • Inability to swallow and eat • No intelligible speech

- Genetics

Pathophysiology
- Neurofibrillary tangles, which are a twisting and distortion of the protein in the neuron
- Neuritic plaques that represent areas of degeneration and granulovascular changes
- Senile plaques, which are the result of dying nerve cells that accumulate around protein

Assessment findings
- Altered behavior and memory may include recent memory loss and impaired judgment (see *Stages of Alzheimer's disease*)
- Muscle rigidity, myoclonic jerks, and restlessness
- Obsessive behaviors
- Anomia (inability to remember one's name)
- Aphasia (impaired ability to communicate verbally or in writing)
- Loss of self-care skills (late finding)
- Loss of speech (late finding)
- Loss of voluntary movement (late finding)

Diagnostic test findings
- Diagnosed when other dementia-producing conditions have been ruled out; diagnosis confirmed at autopsy
- EEG: may be normal early in disease
- MRI: structural and neurologic changes; decrease in size of hippocampus occurs in late stages
- PET scan: Evaluates metabolic activity of the brain; may identify the disease earlier
- Neuropsychologic testing: a series of tests to evaluate cognitive status

Stages of Alzheimer's disease
- Early stage
- Intermediate stage
- End stage

Key signs and symptoms of Alzheimer's disease
- Altered behavior and memory
- Restlessness
- Loss of self-care skills (late)

Diagnosing Alzheimer's disease
- Diagnosed when other dementia-producing conditions have been ruled out
- Diagnosis confirmed at autopsy

● **Medical management**
- Monitor: vital signs, I/O, and laboratory values
- Maintain patient safety
- Diet: individualized according to the patient's needs
- Provide hydration, I.V. or orally
- Activity as tolerated
- Anticholinesterase agents: tacrine (Cognex), donepezil (Aricept), rivastigmine (Exelon), and galantamine (Reminyl)
- N-methyl-D-aspartate antagonist: memantine (Axura)
- Free-radical scavenger: tocophersolan (vitamin E)
- Physical and occupational therapy

● **Nursing interventions**
- Monitor neurologic status, including emotional state, mental status, and motor function
- Monitor and record vital signs, I/O, and laboratory values
- Provide a safe environment
- Provide small, frequent feedings, and stay with the patient to encourage him to eat
- Assess ability to swallow; maintain aspiration precautions
- Use feeding aids when necessary
- Encourage fluid intake
- Administer medications as ordered
- Provide skin and mouth care
- Provide for repetitive activity and exercise
- Assess ability to perform self-care and assist when necessary
- Obtain physical and occupational therapy consults
- Provide emotional support to patient and his family
- Provide information about the Alzheimer's Association
- Individualize home care instructions
  - Know about the disorder and its implications
  - Follow instructions for medication use and be aware of possible adverse effects
  - Refer family members or caregivers to local support groups
  - Discuss power of attorney and advance directives with family
  - Review safety measures
  - Learn stress-relief measures

● **Complications**
- Malnutrition or dehydration
- Pressure ulcers
- Muscle contractions
- Physical injuries
- Abuse
- Depression
- Infection
- Death

- **Possible surgical intervention**
  - None

BELL'S PALSY

- **Definition**
  - Disease of the seventh cranial nerve that produces unilateral facial weakness or paralysis
- **Causes**
  - Infection
  - Hemorrhage
  - Tumor
  - Meningitis
  - Local trauma
  - Stress
  - Pregnancy (third trimester)
- **Pathophysiology**
  - The seventh cranial nerve, which is responsible for motor innervation of the muscles of the face, is blocked
  - The conduction block is due to an inflammatory reaction around the nerve (usually at the internal auditory meatus)
- **Assessment findings**
  - Eye rolls upward and tears excessively when the patient attempts to close it
  - Inability to close eye completely on the affected side
  - Pain around the jaw or ear
  - Ringing in the ears
  - Taste distortion on the affected anterior portion of the tongue
  - Unilateral facial weakness
  - Speech difficulties
- **Diagnostic test findings**
  - Based on clinical presentation
  - EMG: predicts level of expected recovery
- **Medical management**
  - Corticosteroid: prednisone (Deltasone)
  - Moist heat
  - Physical therapy
  - Electrotherapy
  - Diet: soft, nutritionally balanced
  - I.V. therapy: saline lock
  - Position: semi-Fowler's
  - Activity: ad lib as tolerated
  - Monitoring: vital signs, I/O

Key facts about Bell's palsy
- Blocked seventh cranial nerve
- Results in unilateral facial weakness or paralysis

Key signs and symptoms of Bell's palsy
- Inability to close eye completely on the affected side
- Pain around the jaw or ear
- Unilateral facial weakness

Diagnosing Bell's palsy
- No specific diagnostic test
- EMG predicts level of expected recovery

Treating Bell's palsy
- Corticosteroid
- Moist heat

Key nursing interventions for a patient with Bell's palsy

- Arrange for privacy at mealtimes to avoid embarrassment.
- Provide massage therapy.
- Protect eye with patch, as indicated.
- Apply moist heat to affected side of face to reduce pain.

Key complications of Bell's palsy

- Facial paralysis
- Depression

TOP 10

Items to study for your next test on the nervous system

1. Structures and functions of the brain and spinal cord
2. The 12 cranial nerves and their functions
3. How the Glasgow Coma Scale is used
4. Probable nursing diagnosis for a nervous system disorder
5. Preoperative and postoperative care for a patient with surgery for a nervous system disorder
6. Teaching topics for a patient with a neurologic disorder
7. Management and nursing interventions for progressive neurologic disorders, such as Parkinson's disease, MS, Alzheimer's disease, Guillian-Barré, and ALS
8. Safety precautions for the patient experiencintg seizures
9. What happens with increased ICP
10. Key signs and symptoms of stroke

● **Nursing interventions**
- Maintain the patient's diet
- Avoid hot foods and fluids
- Arrange for privacy at mealtimes to avoid embarrassment
- Apply facial sling to improve lip alignment
- Provide frequent mouth care
- Administer medication as ordered
- Provide massage therapy
- Encourage active facial exercises
- Protect eye with patch, as indicated
- Apply moist heat to affected side of face to reduce pain
- Encourage the patient to verbalize feelings of altered body image
- Individualize home care instructions
  - Know about the disorder and its implications
  - Follow instructions for medication use and be aware of possible adverse effects
  - Perform facial exercise
  - Use moist heat to relieve pain
  - Perform massage and facial exercise
  - Take corticosteroids as instructed
  - Chew on unaffected side of mouth
  - Protect eye with patch

● **Complications**
- Facial contractures
- Facial paralysis
- Depression

● **Possible surgical intervention**
- None

NCLEX CHECKS

It's never too soon to begin your NCLEX preparation. Now that you've reviewed this chapter, carefully read each of the following questions and choose the best answer. Then compare your responses to the correct answers.

1. Brudzinski's sign and Kernig's sign are two tests that help diagnose which neurologic disorder?
- ☐ **1.** Alzheimer's disease
- ☐ **2.** Epilepsy
- ☐ **3.** Stroke
- ☐ **4.** Meningitis

2. A nurse is caring for a comatose client who has suffered a closed head injury. Which intervention should the nurse implement to prevent an increase in ICP?

☐ **1.** Suctioning the airway every hour
☐ **2.** Elevating the head of the bed 15 to 40 degrees
☐ **3.** Turning the client and changing his position every 2 hours
☐ **4.** Maintaining a well-lit room

3. A nurse explains to the client's family that which disorder is characterized by progressive degeneration of the cerebral cortex?

☐ **1.** Alzheimer's disease
☐ **2.** Epilepsy
☐ **3.** Guillain-Barré syndrome
☐ **4.** Stroke

4. To encourage adequate nutritional intake for a client with Alzheimer's disease, the nurse should:

☐ **1.** stay with the client and encourage him to eat.
☐ **2.** help the client fill out his menu.
☐ **3.** give the client privacy during meals.
☐ **4.** fill out the menu for the client.

5. A nurse is teaching a client and his family about dietary practices related to Parkinson's disease. A priority for the nurse to address is the risk of:

☐ **1.** fluid overload and drooling.
☐ **2.** aspiration and anorexia.
☐ **3.** choking and diarrhea.
☐ **4.** dysphagia and constipation.

6. A nurse is assessing a client with a brain tumor in the occipital lobe. She should expect which possible assessment findings? Select all that apply.

☐ **1.** Visual impairment
☐ **2.** Memory loss
☐ **3.** Aphasia
☐ **4.** Visual hallucinations
☐ **5.** Homonymous hemianopia
☐ **6.** Personality changes

7. A client undergoes an LP for a myelography. Shortly after the procedure, he reports a severe headache. What should the nurse do?

☐ **1.** Increase the client's fluid intake.
☐ **2.** Administer prescribed antihypertensives.
☐ **3.** Dim the lights in the room.
☐ **4.** Place cool packs over the LP site.

8. The nurse is caring for a client with increased ICP. Which procedure is contraindicated in this case?

☐ **1.** EEG
☐ **2.** Skull X-rays
☐ **3.** LP
☐ **4.** CT scan

9. A nurse is teaching a client about her newly diagnosed condition of MS. Which possible complication of MS should the nurse describe to the client?

☐ **1.** UTI
☐ **2.** Excessive bleeding
☐ **3.** Increasing confusion
☐ **4.** Tremors

10. A client is admitted to the hospital with Alzheimer's disease. Which nursing intervention is most important for the nurse to perform?

☐ **1.** Adjust environment for safety.
☐ **2.** Monitor bowel activity.
☐ **3.** Stimulate the client frequently.
☐ **4.** Allow as many visitors as possible.

ANSWERS AND RATIONALES

1. CORRECT ANSWER: 4
A positive response to one or both of these tests indicates meningeal irritation. Brudzinski's sign and Kernig's sign aren't used in the diagnosis of Alzheimer's disease, epilepsy, or stroke.

2. CORRECT ANSWER: 2
To facilitate venous drainage and avoid jugular compression, the nurse should elevate the head of the bed to 15 to 40 degrees. Suctioning increases ICP and should be avoided, if possible. Turning from side to side increases the risk of jugular compression and increased ICP. The room should be kept quiet and dimly lit.

3. CORRECT ANSWER: 1
Alzheimer's disease is characterized by progressive degeneration of the cerebral cortex leading to symptoms ranging from recent memory loss to debilitating dementia. Epilepsy is characterized by involuntary muscle contractions caused by abnormal discharge of electrical impulses from nerve cells. Guillain-Barré syndrome is characterized by ascending paralysis caused by demyelination and inflammation. Stroke is characterized by sensory and motor deficits caused by a disruption of cerebral circulation.

4. CORRECT ANSWER: 1
Staying with the client and encouraging him to feed himself will ensure adequate food intake. A client with Alzheimer's disease can forget to eat. Filling out the client's menu, helping the client to fill out his menu, or allowing privacy during meals doesn't ensure adequate nutritional intake.

5. CORRECT ANSWER: 4
Eating problems associated with Parkinson's disease include aspiration, choking, constipation, and dysphagia. Fluid overload isn't specifically related to Parkinson's disease and, although drooling occurs with Parkinson's disease, it

doesn't take priority. Anorexia and diarrhea aren't specifically associated with Parkinson's disease.

6. CORRECT ANSWER: 1, 4, 5

Because the occipital lobe is the site of vision, a brain tumor in that area may cause such visual disturbances as visual impairment, visual hallucinations, and homonymous hemianopia. Memory loss, aphasia, and personality changes typically occur in clients with tumors in the frontal lobe, the site of personality, motor speech, and intellectual functioning. Aphasia may also occur with tumors in the temporal lobe, the site of hearing, taste, smell, and speech.

7. CORRECT ANSWER: 1

Headache following an LP is usually caused by a CSF leak. Increased fluid intake will help restore CSF volume. Antihypertensives don't address the problem. Dimming the lights and putting ice packs on the site don't address the problem of reduced CSF volume, which caused the headache.

8. CORRECT ANSWER: 3

An LP, the removal of CSF from the subarachnoid space in the lumbar region, is contraindicated in the presence of increased ICP. Removing CSF could decrease pressure within the spinal column, causing the client's brain to herniate downward. ICP isn't affected by an EEG, skull X-rays, or a CT scan.

9. CORRECT ANSWER: 1

Complications of MS may include UTI, respiratory infection, contractures, depression, and paraplegia or quadraplegia.

10. CORRECT ANSWER: 1

The client with Alzheimer's disease may experience muscle rigidity, myoclonic jerks, and restlessness, which place the client at an increased risk for injury. Adjusting the client's environment for safety decreases the risk of injury. Reorienting the client frequently, providing familiar objects from home, and establishing a familiar routine may also help decrease the risk of injury.

Sensory system: Eyes and ears

PRETEST

1. The process of contraction and relaxation of the lens to allow it to focus light on the retina is called:

☐ 1. accommodation.

☐ 2. constriction.

☐ 3. image formation.

☐ 4. adaptation.

CORRECT ANSWER: 1

2. The external ear is separated from the middle ear by which structure?

☐ 1. Cochlea

☐ 2. Vestibule

☐ 3. Tympanic membrane

☐ 4. Auricle

CORRECT ANSWER: 3

3. Tonometry is an eye test that measures intraocular pressure. It's useful in diagnosing which ocular disorder?

☐ 1. Cataract

☐ 2. Glaucoma

☐ 3. Myopia

☐ 4. Retinal detachment

CORRECT ANSWER: 2

4. Teaching for a client after eye surgery should include:

- [ ] 1. avoidance of high-fat foods.
- [ ] 2. remaining flat in bed for 24 hours.
- [ ] 3. proper instillation of eyedrops.
- [ ] 4. wearing an eye shield at all times.

CORRECT ANSWER: 3

5. Hearing loss that occurs from interrupted passage of sound from the external ear to the inner ear is known as:

- [ ] 1. sensorineural hearing loss.
- [ ] 2. mixed hearing loss.
- [ ] 3. mechanical hearing loss.
- [ ] 4. conductive hearing loss.

CORRECT ANSWER: 4

LEARNING OBJECTIVES

After studying this chapter, you should be able to:

- Describe the psychosocial impact of sensory disorders.
- Differentiate between the modifiable and nonmodifiable risk factors in the development of a sensory disorder.
- List three probable and three possible nursing diagnoses for a patient with a sensory disorder.
- Identify nursing interventions for a patient with a sensory disorder.
- Identify three teaching topics for a patient with a sensory disorder.

CHAPTER OVERVIEW

Caring for the patient with a sensory disorder requires a sound understanding of eye and ear anatomy and physiology as well as the psychological impact of sight and hearing loss. A thorough assessment is essential to planning and implementing appropriate patient care. The assessment includes a complete history, physical examination, diagnostic testing, identification of modifiable and non-modifiable risk factors, and information related to the psychosocial impact of the disorder on the patient.

Nursing diagnoses focus primarily on sensory and perceptual disturbances, social isolation, and deficient knowledge. The goal of nursing interventions is to improve the patient's safety and decrease his anxiety about body image changes. Patient teaching—a crucial nursing activity—involves instructing the patient about diagnosis and treatment, medication regimens, signs and symptoms of complications, how to reduce modifiable risk factors, safety precautions to protect the eyes and ears, and medical follow-up.

ANATOMY AND PHYSIOLOGY REVIEW

● **Eyes**
- External structures
  - Eyelids—two movable, musculofibrous folds that protect the eye by opening and closing; distribute tears across the eyelid when blinking
  - Palpebral fissure—space between the open lids
  - Conjunctiva—thin, transparent mucous membrane that lines the lid
  - Extraocular muscles—focus muscles abduct, adduct, elevate, or depress; two muscles direct the eye laterally, inferiorly, or superiorly
  - Eyeball—spherical organ surrounded by orbital fat and positioned in orbit; three layers include the sclera, uvea, and retina
- Internal structures (see *Cross section of the eye*)
  - Sclera—dense, white, fibrous protective coating of the eye; optic nerve and central retinal vessel pass through posterior opening; anterior opening serves as a refracting window; provides structural strength to the front of the eye
  - Choroid—highly vascular posterior portion of the uveal tract that nourishes the retina
  - Iris—thin, circular, pigmented muscular structure in the eye; gives color to the eye; divides the space between the cornea and lens into the anterior and the posterior chamber; peripheral border attaches to the ciliary body
  - Ciliary body—muscular fibers in the middle pigmented layer of the eye that contract and relax the lens zonules; maintain intraocular pressure (IOP) by secreting aqueous humor
  - Schlemm's canal—system of channels responsible for drainage of aqueous humor

External structures of the eyes

- Eyelids
- Palpebral fissure
- Conjunctiva
- Extraocular muscles
- Eyeball

Internal structures of the eyes

- Sclera
- Choroid
- Iris
- Ciliary body
- Schlemm's canal
- Pupil
- Lens
- Vitreous humor
- Retina
- Lens zonules
- Retinal cones
- Retinal rods
- Macula lutea
- Optic nerve
- Optic disk

Cross section of the eye

This cross section details important anatomic structures of the eye.

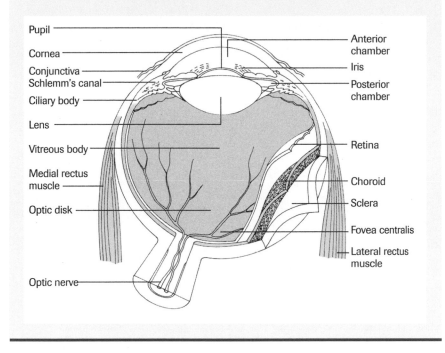

Key functions of the retina

- It lines the eye wall.
- Rods and cones respond to light energy and initiate the neural response that's interpreted in the brain.

The difference between rods and cones

- Rods are responsible for peripheral vision under decreased light conditions.
- Cones are responsible for visual acuity and color discrimination.

- Pupil—circulation aperture in the iris that changes size as the iris adapts to the amount of light entering the eye
- Lens—biconvex, avascular, colorless, and transparent structure suspended behind the iris by the zonules
- Vitreous humor—clear, transparent, avascular, gelatinous fluid that fills the space in the posterior portion of the eye; bounded by the lens, retina, and optic disk; maintains transparency and form of the eye
- Retina—thin, semitransparent layer of nerve tissue that lines the eye wall; rods and cones respond to light energy and initiate the neural response that's interpreted in the brain
- Lens zonules—suspend the lens; contraction and relaxation of zonules changes the shape of the lens and allows it to focus light on the retina
- Retinal cones—responsible for visual acuity and color discrimination
- Retinal rods—responsible for peripheral vision under decreased light conditions
- Macula lutea—center of the posterior retina with fovea centralis for acute vision, color vision, and resolution of image
- Optic nerve—convergence of the nerve fibers of the retina
- Optic disk—head of the optic nerve known as the blind spot

External ear structures

- External auditory canal
- Auricle
- Helix
- Anthelix
- Concha
- Antitragus
- Lobule

Middle ear structures

- Malleus
- Incus
- Stapes
- Tympanic membrane

Inner ear structures

- Vestibule
- Cochlea
- Semicircular canals
- Eustachian tube
- Acoustic nerve branches

How an image is formed

- Light rays enter the eye through the cornea and pass through the pupil, lens, and vitreous humor to the retina.
- Light rays stimulate the retinal sensory receptors to send impulses through the optic nerve to the occipital cortex, where the impulses are registered as visual sensations.

A close look at the ear

Use this illustration to review the structures of the ear.

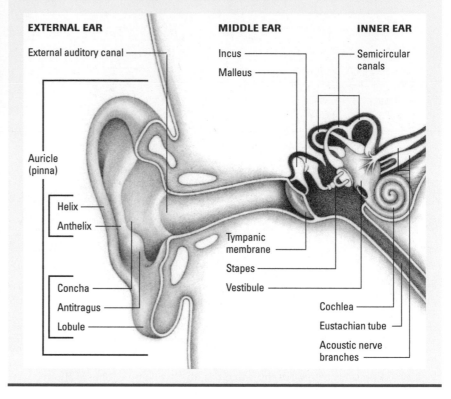

- Image formation
  - Light rays enter the eye through the cornea and pass through the pupil, lens, and vitreous body to the retina
  - Light rays stimulate the retinal sensory receptors to send impulses through the optic nerve to the occipital cortex, where the impulses are registered as visual sensations
- Aqueous humor formation
  - Watery, transparent liquid that flows through the anterior and posterior chambers and exits through Schlemm's canal
  - Serves a circulatory function for avascular tissues of the eye
  - Responsible for maintaining IOP
- Accommodation—the process of contraction and relaxation of the lens zonules that changes the shape of the lens and allows it to focus light on the retina

● **Ears**
  - External ear
    - Portion of ear that includes the pinna (auricle) and external auditory canal (see *A close look at the ear*)
    - Separated from the middle ear by the tympanic membrane

- Middle ear
  - Air-filled cavity in the temporal bone
  - Contains three small bones (malleus, incus, and stapes)
  - Opens to the eustachian tube or auditory tube, which connects to the nasopharynx
- Inner ear
  - Portion of the ear that consists of the cochlea, vestibule, and semicircular canals
  - Also known as the labyrinth
- Sound transmission—airborne vibrations are transformed to sound through mechanical stimulation of the endolymphatic fluids
- Equilibrium—position changes of the head are detected by maculae or cristae

ASSESSMENT FINDINGS

● History
- Eyes
  - Blurred vision
  - Difficulty focusing while reading
  - Headaches
  - Dizziness or vertigo
  - Eye or brow pain
  - Scratchy or itchy eye
  - Inflamed eye
  - Watery eye
  - Puffy eyelids
  - Crossed eyes
  - Unequal pupils
  - Squinting
  - Increased blinking
  - Reddened or bloodshot eyes
  - Eye secretions
  - Burning sensation
  - Double vision
  - Spots before the eye
  - Photophobia
  - Difficulty differentiating colors
  - Difficulty driving at night
  - Flashes of light
  - Sensation of a veil or curtain across the field of vision
  - Sudden change in vision
- Ears
  - Tinnitus
  - Decreased ability to hear in a crowd
  - Need to turn up volume on television and radio

Key warning signs for eye disorders
- Eye or brow pain
- Unequal pupils
- Spots before the eye
- Flashes of light
- Sensation of a veil or curtain across the field of vision
- Sudden change in vision

Key warning signs for ear disorders
- Tinnitus
- Decreased ability to hear in a crowd
- Need to turn up volume on television and radio

– Pain from the outer ear
– Head pain
– Feeling of fullness or water in the ear
– Redness or inflammation of the ear
– Drainage from the ear
– Fatigue

● **Physical examination**
  • Eyes
    – Visual acuity changes
    – Eye discharge
    – Sty
    – Presbyopia
    – Ptosis
    – Nystagmus
    – Optic atrophy
    – Myopia
    – Hyperopia
    – Anisometropia
    – Astigmatism
    – Loss of red reflex
    – Corneal sensitivity
  • Ears
    – Speech deterioration
    – Ear pain
    – Ear deformities
    – Ear lesions
    – Ear canal discharge
    – Mastoid pain
    – Cerumen accumulation
    – Ear canal inflammation
    – Foreign body in ear canal
    – Change in landmarks and color of tympanic membrane

DIAGNOSTIC TESTS AND PROCEDURES

● **Visual acuity**
  • Definition and purpose
    – A screening test of central vision
    – Tests clarity of vision using letter chart (Snellen) placed 20′ (6.1 m) from the patient (see *Visual acuity charts*)
    – Expressed in a ratio
      • Top number (20) is the distance between the patient and the chart
      • Bottom number is the distance from which a person with normal vision could read the line
  • Nursing interventions
    – Explain the procedure to the patient

Key eye examination findings

• Visual acuity changes
• Loss of red reflex
• Corneal sensitivity

Key ear examination findings

• Speech deterioration
• Ear pain
• Ear canal inflammation
• Change in landmarks and color of tympanic membrane

Key facts about visual acuity testing

• A screening test of central vision
• Tests clarity of vision using a letter chart placed 20′ from the patient
• Intervention: remind the patient to bring eyeglasses or contact lenses, if currently prescribed

Visual acuity charts

The most commonly used charts for testing vision are the Snellen alphabet chart (left) and the Snellen E chart (right)—the latter of which is used for young children and adults who can't read. Both charts are used to test distance vision and measure visual acuity. The patient reads each chart at a distance of 20′ (6.1 m).

RECORDING RESULTS

Visual acuity is recorded as a fraction. The top number (20) is the distance in feet between the patient and the chart. The bottom number is the distance in feet from which a person with normal vision could read the line. The larger the bottom number is, the poorer the patient's vision.

AGE DIFFERENCES

In adults and children age 6 and older, normal vision is measured as 20/20. For children younger than age 6, normal vision varies. For children age 3 and younger, normal vision is 20/50; for children age 4, 20/40; and for children age 5, 20/30.

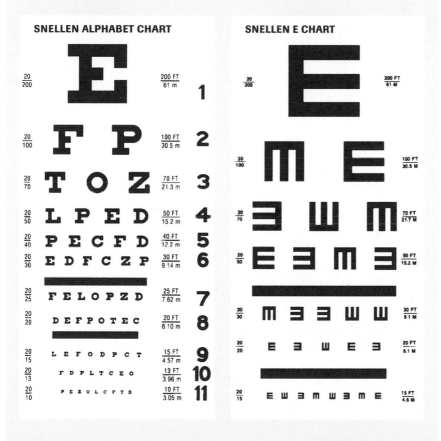

- Answer the patient's questions
- Remind the patient to bring eyeglasses or contact lenses, if currently prescribed
- Advise the examiner if the patient can't read alphabet letters

Types of visual acuity charts

- Snellen alphabet chart
- Snellen E chart

How to record visual acuity

- Record as a fraction
- Top number is the distance in feet between the patient and the chart (20)
- Bottom number is the distance in feet from which a person with normal vision can read the line

Normal vision measurement by age-group

- Adults and children age 6 and older: 20/20
- Children age 5: 20/30
- Children age 4: 20/40
- Children age 3 and younger: 20/50

Key facts about extraocular eye muscle testing

- Tests parallel alignment of the eyes
- Tests integrity of the nervous control of eye muscles (cranial nerves III, IV, and VI)
- Intervention: the patient follows a pencil or finger as it moves in the shape of the letter "H"

Key facts about visual field testing

- Test of the entire area seen by an eye
- Tests degree of peripheral vision of each eye by confrontation
- Intervention: advise the examiner if the patient has difficulty hearing or following directions

Key facts about tonometry

- Test used to measure IOP
- Intervention: advise that a puff of air or the instrument may be felt touching the eye and that he will need to remain still

Key facts about ophthalmoscopy

- Test to visualize the internal structure of the eye
- Intervention: ask the patient to focus on a point behind the examiner

– Advise the examiner if the patient has difficulty hearing or following directions

- **Extraocular eye muscle testing**
  - Definition and purpose
    – Tests parallel alignment of the eyes and integrity of nervous control of the eye muscles (cranial nerves III [oculomotor], IV [trochlear], and VI [abducens])
    – The patient follows a pencil or finger as it moves in the shape of the letter "H"
    – Correlated action of the extraocular muscles results in parallel gaze
  - Nursing interventions
    – Explain the procedure to the patient
    – Advise the examiner if the patient has difficulty hearing or following directions

- **Visual field testing**
  - Definition and purpose
    – Test of the entire area seen by the eye while focused on a central point
    – Tests degree of peripheral vision of each eye by confrontation
    – Examiner and patient sit 2' (0.6 m) apart, directly facing each other; the patient covers one eye while looking directly at the examiner's nose; the examiner covers one eye; the examiner moves an object along a horizontal plane into central view from peripheral points about one-half the distance between them
  - Nursing interventions
    – Explain the procedure to the patient
    – Answer the patient's questions
    – Advise the examiner if the patient has difficulty hearing or following directions

- **Tonometry**
  - Definition and purpose
    – Test to measure IOP with the use of a contact or noncontact tonometer
  - Aids in the evaluation of ocular conditions such as glacoma
  - Nursing interventions
    – Explain the procedure to the patient
    – Ask the patient to remain still
    – Depending on the method of examination, advise the patient that a puff of air or the instrument may be felt touching the eye

- **Ophthalmoscopy**
  - Definition and purpose
    – Test to visualize the internal structure of the eye through use of an ophthalmoscope (see *A close look at the retina*)
  - Nursing interventions
    – Explain the procedure to the patient
    – Have the patient remove contact lenses or glasses

A close look at the retina

This illustration shows the complex anatomy of the retina and its structures.

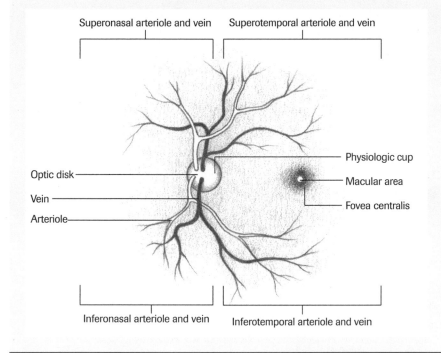

Superonasal arteriole and vein   Superotemporal arteriole and vein

Physiologic cup

Optic disk

Macular area

Vein

Fovea centralis

Arteriole

Inferonasal arteriole and vein   Inferotemporal arteriole and vein

– Darken the room
– Ask the patient to focus on a point behind the examiner

● **Ultrasound of the eye**
  • Definition and purpose
    – High-frequency sound waves are recorded to determine eye structure and function
    – May be used to detect tumors or lesions of the eye or retinal detachment
  • Nursing interventions before the procedure
    – Explain the procedure to the patient
    – Answer the patient's questions
    – Administer topical anesthetic eyedrops
  • Nursing interventions after the procedure
    – Advise the patient not to rub his eyes
    – Place the patient on eye rest

● **Otoscopic examination**
  • Definition and purpose
    – Use of an otoscope to visualize the external auditory canal
    – Used to help diagnose infection, a foreign body presence, or the condition of the tympanic membrane

Key facts about ultrasound of the eye

• Test used to detect tumors or lesions of the eye
• High-frequency pulses of ultrasound are emitted from a small probe placed on the eye
• Intervention: advise the patient not to rub his eyes

Key facts about otoscopic examination

• Test used to visualize the tympanic membrane
• Uses an otoscope
• Intervention: explain to the patient that he'll feel a gentle pull and slight pressure in his ear

Key facts about audiometry

- Test to measure the degree of hearing of different sound frequencies
- Examiner uses pure-tone or speech methods
- Intervention: explain to the patient that he must signal when he hears a tone while sitting in a soundproof room

Key facts about auditory acuity

- Assesses the patient's ability to hear a whispered phrase or ticking watch
- Provides a general estimate of the patient's hearing
- Intervention: advise the examiner if the patient has difficulty following directions

Psychosocial impact of sensory disorders

- Difficulty in school
- Decreased self-esteem
- Disruption or loss of job
- Restrictions in physical activity
- Social isolation

- Nursing interventions
  - Advise the patient to hold still
  - Explain to the patient that he'll feel a gentle pull on his auricle and a slight pressure in his ear
- **Audiometry**
  - Definition and purpose
    - Test to measure the degree of hearing of different sound frequencies
    - Examiner uses pure-tone or speech methods
  - Nursing interventions
    - Explain the procedure to the patient
    - Explain to the patient that he needs to wear earphones for the procedure
    - Explain to the patient that he needs to signal when he hears a tone while sitting in a soundproof room
- **Auditory acuity**
  - Definition and purpose
    - General estimation of the patient's hearing
    - Assesses the patient's ability to hear a whispered phrase or ticking watch
  - Nursing interventions
    - Explain the procedure to the patient
    - Answer the patient's questions
    - Advise the examiner if the patient has difficulty following directions

PSYCHOSOCIAL IMPACT OF SENSORY DISORDERS

- **Developmental impact**
  - Difficulty in school
  - Changes in body image
  - Fear of rejection
  - Decreased self-esteem
  - Potential developmental delays
- **Economic impact**
  - Cost of adaptive equipment
  - Disruption or loss of job
  - Cost of hospitalization and follow-up care
  - Cost of medications
- **Occupational impact**
  - Limited job opportunities
  - Restrictions in physical activity
- **Social impact**
  - Social isolation
  - Changes in role performance
  - Changes in leisure activity

RISK FACTORS

● **Modifiable risk factors**
  • Eyes
    – Work environment
    – Leisure activities
    – Sports activities
    – Exposure to airborne irritants
    – Sun exposure
  • Ears
    – Work environment
    – Use of earphones
    – Exposure to loud noises
    – Use of ototoxic drugs, such as streptomycin, neomycin, or aspirin

● **Nonmodifiable risk factors**
  • Eyes
    – Glaucoma
    – Diabetes
    – Hypertension
    – Eye trauma
    – Eye surgery
    – Family history
    – Cataracts
    – Aging
  • Ears
    – Diabetes
    – Aging
    – Congenital or genetic abnormalities
    – Ear trauma

NURSING DIAGNOSES

● **Probable nursing diagnoses**
  • Eyes
    – Disturbed sensory perception: visual
    – Fear
    – Anxiety
    – Deficient knowledge (specify)
    – Disturbed body image
  • Ears
    – Disturbed sensory perception: auditory
    – Social isolation
    – Deficient knowledge (specify)
    – Fear
    – Anxiety
    – Acute pain

Modifiable risk factors for sensory disorders

● Work environment
● Exposure to sun (eye)
● Exposure to loud noise (ear)

Nonmodifiable risk factors for sensory disorders

● Aging
● Diabetes
● Trauma

Probable nursing diagnoses for sensory disorders

● Disturbed sensory perception
● Fear
● Anxiety
● Deficient knowledge (specify)
● Disturbed body image

Possible nursing diagnoses for sensory disorders

- Acute pain
- Social isolation
- Risk for injury

Types of eye surgery

- Cataract surgery
  - Intracapsular
  - Extracapsular
- Corneal transplantation
- Retinal reattachment
- Glaucoma surgery
  - Laser iridotomy
  - Laser gonioplasty
  - Trabeculectomy

Key nursing interventions before eye surgery

- Complete preoperative teaching.
- Complete preoperative checklist.
- Administer preoperative medications.
- Document history and physical assessment data.

● Possible nursing diagnoses

- Eyes
  - Dressing or grooming self-care deficit
  - Acute pain
  - Social isolation
  - Risk for injury
- Ears
  - Acute pain
  - Risk for injury
  - Risk for infection

EYE SURGERIES

● Description

- Cataract surgery
  - Intracapsular—removal of the entire intact lens as a unit using a cryoprobe
  - Extracapsular—removal of the anterior capsule by expressing the lens nucleus and aspirating the remaining soft and cortical fragments using a special irrigation aspiration machine
- Corneal transplantation—microsurgical, full-thickness replacement of the cornea with tissue from a deceased donor
- Retinal reattachment—transscleral cryotherapy (scleral buckling) is applied around the retinal tear, producing a chorioretinal adhesion that seals the break so that liquid vitreous can no longer pass through the subretinal space
- Glaucoma surgery
  - Laser iridotomy—creation of an opening in the iris to allow aqueous humor to travel to the anterior chamber and trabecular meshwork to decrease intraocular pressure
  - Laser gonioplasty—creation of a stromal burn in the peripheral iris to cause iris contraction and deepen the anterior chamber angle
  - Trabeculectomy—a flap of sclera is dissected and a section of trabecular meshwork is removed to allow outflow of aqueous humor

● Preoperative nursing interventions

- Complete patient and family preoperative teaching
  - Explain the procedure to the patient
  - Describe the operating room, postanesthesia care unit, and preoperative and postoperative routines
  - Demonstrate postoperative turning and deep breathing
  - Explain the postoperative need for surgical eye bandages, oxygen therapy, I.V. therapy, and pain control, as appropriate
  - Explain that most surgeries are outpatient; the patient is usually discharged within 2 hours of the procedure
- Complete the preoperative checklist
- Administer the preoperative medications, as prescribed

• Allay the patient's and his family's anxiety about surgery
• Document the patient's history and physical assessment data
• Confirm that the patient has transportation home after surgery

Postoperative nursing interventions
• Assess the patient's pain level, administer postoperative analgesics as prescribed, and evaluate effect
• Administer I.V. fluids, as prescribed
• Monitor and record vital signs
• Inspect the surgical eye bandages and change them, as directed
• Encourage the patient to express his feelings about the surgery, and provide emotional support
• Assess the patient's ability to complete activities of daily living and self-care
• Provide for patient safety
• Administer antibiotics, as prescribed
• Orient the patient to time, place, and surroundings
• Assess the patient's eye for drainage, redness, swelling, cloudy vision, halos around lights, and impaired vision
• Individualize home care instructions
  – Know about the disorder and its treatment
  – Follow instructions for medication use, and be aware of possible adverse effects
  – Maintain eye rest as prescribed
  – Use an eye shield or patch, as prescribed, such as during sleep
  – Use dark glasses in bright light
  – Avoid reading and close-up vision
  – Apply cold or warm compresses, as prescribed
  – Don't rub or wipe eyes
  – Instill eyedrops correctly
  – Make environmental adjustments for safety
  – Observe driving restrictions
  – Avoid coughing, sneezing, lifting, constipation, squeezing eyes shut, and fast head movements
  – Avoid smoking
  – Comply with medical follow-up

Possible surgical complications
• Cataract surgery
  – Corneal endothelial damage
  – Pupillary block
  – Glaucoma
  – Hemorrhage
  – Wound fistula
  – Choroidal detachment
  – Uveitis
  – Infection

Key nursing interventions after eye surgery
• Assess pain level and administer analgesics.
• Monitor and record vital signs.
• Provide for the patient's safety.
• Assess the eye for drainage, redness, swelling, cloudy vision, halos around lights, and impaired vision.
• Provide home care instructions.

Key complications after eye surgery
• Vision loss
• Hemorrhage
• Infection

- Corneal transplant
  - Hemorrhage
  - Epithelial defects
  - Wound leaks
  - Glaucoma
  - Graft rejection
- Retinal reattachment
  - Increased IOP
  - Glaucoma
  - Infection
  - Choroidal detachment
  - Diplopia
- Glaucoma surgery
  - Vision loss

EAR SURGERIES

● Description
- Tympanoplasty—procedure to repair tympanic membrane rupture
- Cochlear implant—placement of an electronic device that delivers electrical signals to the cochlear nerve to create sound

● Preoperative nursing interventions
- Complete patient and family preoperative teaching
  - Explain the procedure to the patient
  - Describe preoperative and postoperative routines
  - Explain the postoperative need for drainage tubes, surgical dressings, oxygen therapy, I.V. therapy, and pain control, as appropriate
- Complete the preoperative checklist
- Administer preoperative medications, as prescribed
- Allay the patient's and his family's anxiety about surgery
- Document the patient's history and physical assessment data

● Postoperative nursing interventions
- Assess the patient's pain level, administer postoperative analgesics as prescribed, and evaluate effect
- Administer I.V. fluids, as prescribed
- Monitor and record vital signs, intake and output (I/O), laboratory studies, and pulse oximetry
- Inspect the surgical dressing and change it, as directed
- Monitor and maintain the position and patency of wound drainage tubes
- Encourage the patient to express his feelings about the surgery, and provide emotional support
- Assess the patient for dizziness, nystagmus, and nausea
- Administer antibiotics, as prescribed
- Administer antivertigo agent, as prescribed
- Administer antiemetic, as prescribed

Types of ear surgery

- Tympanoplasty
- Cochlear implant

Key nursing interventions before ear surgery

- Complete preoperative teaching.
- Complete the preoperative checklist.
- Administer preoperative medications.
- Document history and physical assessment data.

- Advance the patient's diet, as tolerated
- Individualize home care instructions
    - Know about the disorder and its treatment
    - Follow instructions for medication use, and be aware of possible adverse effects
    - Avoid blowing the nose, sneezing, or coughing
    - Watch for signs and symptoms of complications
    - Avoid sudden head movements
    - Follow bathing instructions
    - Decrease environmental noise
    - Avoid people with infections
    - Cover ears when outside
    - Perform wound care, as directed
    - Observe activity restrictions
    - Comply with medical follow-up

● **Possible surgical complications**
- Infection
- Tissue rejection of graft or prosthesis
- Facial nerve paralysis

SENILE CATARACTS

● **Definition**
- Gradual, progressive opacification of the normally clear, transparent crystalline lens
- Three types: nuclear, cortical, and posterior subcapsular

● **Causes**
- Aging
- Blunt or penetrating trauma
- Long-term steroid treatment
- Diabetes mellitus
- Hypertension
- Hypoparathyroidism
- Radiation exposure
- Anterior uveitis
- Ultraviolet light and sunlight exposure
- Congenital

● **Pathophysiology**
- Progressive oxidation to the lens occurs with aging
- The nucleus of the lens takes on a yellowish brown hue
- Surrounding opacities are spokelike, white densities anterior and posterior to the nucleus

● **Assessment findings**
- Change in visual acuity
- Diplopia

Key nursing interventions after ear surgery
- Assess pain level and administer analgesics.
- Monitor and record vital signs.
- Assess the patient for dizziness, nystagmus, and nausea.
- Provide home care instructions.

Key facts about senile cataracts
- Opacification of the normally clear, transparent crystalline lens
- Three types: nuclear, cortical, posterior subcapsular

Common causes of senile cataracts
- Aging
- Diabetes mellitus
- Hypertension
- Ultraviolet light and sunlight exposure

Key teaching points for a patient with a sensory disorder

- The disorder and treatment plan
- Medication therapy
- Changes in lifestyle and activities
- Activity limitation
- Follow-up

Key signs and symptoms of senile cataracts

- Change in visual acuity
- Disabling glare
- Yellow, gray, or white pupil
- Loss of red reflex

Diagnosing cataracts

- Ophthalmoscopy: dark area in normally homogenous red reflex
- Ultrasound: areas of increased density around the nucleus of the lens

Treating senile cataracts

- Intracapsular cataract extraction
- Extracapsular cataract extraction

Key nursing interventions for a patient with senile cataracts

- Assess vision status.
- Provide for the patient's safety.
- Provide home care instructions.

TIME-OUT FOR TEACHING

Patients with a sensory disorder

Be sure to include these topics in your teaching plan for the patient with a sensory disorder.

- Explanation of the disorder and treatment plan
- Medication therapy, including the dosage, adverse effects, and scheduling
- Feelings about changes in lifestyle and activities of daily living (ADLs)
- Signs and symptoms of infection, hearing loss, and decreased vision
- Activity limitations
- Activities that prevent social isolation
- Environment adaptations
- Independence with ADLs and any modifications and assistive devices needed to compensate for limited sensory input
- Community agencies and resources for supportive services
- Follow-up appointments

PREVENTIVE CARE

- Eye: protection from injury, bright sun, and chemicals; need for eye rest; work in well-lighted areas
- Ear: wear protective devices during work, leisure, and sports; avoid exposure to high-frequency sounds

---

- Disabling glare
- Dimmed or blurred vision
- Distorted images
- Poor night vision
- Yellow, gray, or white pupil
- Loss of red reflex

● Diagnostic test findings

- Ophthalmoscopy or slit lamp: reveals a dark area in the normally homogenous red reflex
- Ultrasound of eye: areas of increased density around the nucleus of the lens
- Maddox rod test: evaluates macular function

● Medical management

- No specific medical treatment
- Laboratory studies: IOP, endothelial cell counter, A-scan ultrasound

● Nursing interventions

- Assess vision status
- Provide information about preventing cataracts, cataract progression, and surgery
- Provide for the patient's safety
- Individualize home care instructions (for more information about teaching, see *Patients with a sensory disorder*)
    - Know about the disorder and its treatment
    - Wear dark glasses in bright light
    - Avoid sitting in direct sunlight

- **Complications**
  - Glaucoma
  - Blindness
  - Severe vision loss
  - Infection
- **Surgical interventions**
  - Intracapsular cataract extraction
  - Extracapsular cataract extraction

GLAUCOMA

- **Definition**
  - A group of diseases that differ in pathophysiology, clinical presentation, and treatment
  - Characterized by visual field loss because of damage to the optic nerve caused by increased IOP
  - The increased IOP results from pathologic changes that prevent normal circulation and outflow of aqueous humor
- **Causes/Risk factors**
  - Aging
  - Obesity
  - Smoking
  - Diabetes mellitus
  - Black race (increases risk)
  - Family history of glaucoma
  - Previous eye trauma or surgery
  - Long-term steroid treatment
  - Uveitis
  - Congenital defects
  - Hyperopia
  - Plateau iris
  - Hypertension
  - Cardiovascular disease
- **Pathophysiology**
  - Open-angle glaucoma: increased IOP is caused by increased resistance to aqueous humor drainage, resulting in neuronal and optic nerve degeneration
  - Acute angle-closure glaucoma: increased resistance to aqueous humor flow caused by blockage of trabecular meshwork by the peripheral iris
- **Assessment findings**
  - Primary open-angle glaucoma
    - Begins in one eye and progresses to the other eye
    - Decreased peripheral vision
    - Atrophy and cupping of the optic nerve head
    - Increased IOP

Key signs and symptoms of glaucoma

- Primary open-angle
- Begins in one eye and progresses to other eye
- Decreased peripheral vision
- Increased IOP
- Acute angle-closure
- Unilateral
- Acute eye or facial pain
- Halo vision
- Increased IOP
- Nausea and vomiting

Diagnosing glaucoma

- Tonometry: increased IOP
- Ophthalmoscopy: edema of the optic disc or excavation

Treating glaucoma

- Topical beta-adrenergic blocker
- Topical adrenergic agonist
- Carbonic anhydrase inhibitor
- Miotic agent
- Sodium restriction
- Surgery

- – Mild headaches
- – Halos around lights
- Acute angle-closure glaucoma
  - – Typically unilateral
  - – Feeling of fullness in the eye
  - – Acute eye or facial pain
  - – Halo vision
  - – Blurred vision
  - – Redness in the eye
  - – Increased IOP
  - – Atrophy and cupping of optic nerve head
  - – Dilated pupil
  - – Abrupt decrease in visual acuity
  - – Nausea and vomiting

Diagnostic test findings

- Tonometry: increased IOP
- Visual field test: decreased field of vision
- Gonioscopy: occluded anterior chamber angle
- Ophthalmoscopy: edema of the optic disc (acute attack) or excavation (chronic episodes)

Medical management

- Dietary restrictions: sodium and fluid
- Activity: as tolerated
- Monitoring: vital signs and I/O
- Topical beta-adrenergic blocker: levobunolol (Betagan)
- Topical adrenergic agonist: brimonidine (Alphagan)
- Carbonic anhydrase inhibitor: acetazolamide (Diamox)
- Beta-adrenergic blocker/carbonic anhydrase inhibitor combination: dorzolamide HCl/timolol (Cosopt)
- Prostaglandin analog: latanoprost (Xalatan)
- Miotic agent: pilocarpine (Pilocar)
- Avoid such drugs as atropine, anticholinergics, or others with pupil-dilating effects

Nursing interventions

- Maintain the patient's diet and fluid restrictions
- Assess vision status
- Monitor and record vital signs, I/O, and laboratory studies
- Administer medications, as prescribed
- Encourage the patient to express his feelings about his disorder, and provide emotional support
- Assess eye pain
- Individualize home care instructions
  - – Know about the disorder and its treatment
  - – Follow instructions for medication use, and be aware of possible adverse effects

 – Be sure to instill eyedrops correctly
 – Avoid rubbing the eyes
 – Wear protective glasses or goggles while participating in sports or swimming
 – Monitor the eyes for redness, discharge, watering, blurred or cloudy vision, halos, flashes of light, and floaters
 – Comply with medical follow-up

● **Complications**
 • Blindness
 • Infection

● **Surgical interventions**
 • Laser iridectomy
 • Laser gonioplasty
 • Trabeculectomy

RETINAL DETACHMENT

● **Definition**
 • Separation of the sensory layers of the retina from the underlying retinal pigment epithelium

● **Causes**
 • Aging
 • Diabetic neovascularization
 • Familial tendency
 • Hemorrhage
 • Inflammatory process
 • Myopia
 • Trauma
 • Tumor
 • Intraocular surgery

● **Pathophysiology**
 • Vitreous body traction causes retinal tears or holes
 • Vitreous fluid leaks through holes or tears behind the retina
 • Retinal separation occurs

● **Assessment findings**
 • Floating spots
 • Recurrent flashes of light (photopsia)
 • With progression of detachment, painless vision loss may be described as a veil, curtain, or cobweb that eliminates part of the visual field

● **Diagnostic tests**
 • Ophthalmoscopy: gray or opaque retina; in severe detachment, retinal folds and ballooning out of the area
 • Indirect ophthalmoscopy: retinal tear or detachment
 • Ultrasound: retinal tear or detachment in the presence of a cataract

Treating retinal detachment

- Complete bed rest with the retinal hole or tear at the lowest point of eye
- Eye patch
- Surgical repair

Key nursing interventions for a patient with retinal detachment

- Position the patient according to the surgical procedure.
- Tell the patient to avoid activities that increase IOP.
- Protect the eye with a shield or glasses.
- Administer eyedrops as ordered.

Key complications of retinal detachment

- Blindness
- Infection

● **Medical management**
- Activity: complete bed rest with the retinal hole or tear at the lowest point of the eye
- Restrict eye movement until surgical reattachment

● **Nursing interventions**
- Monitor and record vital signs, I/O, and laboratory studies
- Provide preoperative care
  - Maintain bed rest with the retinal hole or tear at the lowest position of the eye
  - Apply an eye patch
  - Provide emotional support
  - Explain the procedure and what to expect postoperatively
  - Administer preoperative antibiotics as ordered
  - Wash the face with no-tear shampoo
  - Administer cycloplegic-mydriatic eyedrops as ordered
- Provide postoperative care
  - Position the patient as ordered
  - Tell the patient to avoid activities that increase IOP, such as coughing, sneezing, vomiting, lifting, straining during bowel movements, bending from the waist, and rapidly moving the head
  - Administer antiemetics, as indicated
  - Protect the eye with a shield or glasses
  - Apply cold compresses as ordered
  - Assess for pain, administer analgesics as needed, and evaluate effect
  - Administer cycloplegic and steroid-antibiotic eyedrops as ordered
- Individualize home care instructions
  - Know about the disorder and its treatment
  - Follow instructions for medication use, and be aware of possible adverse effects
  - Instill eyedrops, as prescribed
  - Notify the physician if experiencing floaters, flashes of light, blurred vision, or pain unrelieved by analgesics
  - Report fever, yellow or green eye discharge, increased redness or puffiness of the eye, or reduced vision
  - Perform dressing changes
  - Wear an eye shield at night
  - Wear prescribed eye goggles while participating in contact sports
  - Follow activity restrictions and head positioning
  - Comply with medical follow-up

● **Complications**
- Blindness
- Infection

● **Surgical interventions**
- Cryothermy
- Laser therapy
- Scleral buckling procedure

MÉNIÈRE'S DISEASE

● **Definition**
  - Condition of the inner ear in which there's an increase in volume and pressure of the endolymph of the inner ear. Characterized by recurrent and usually progressive symptoms, including vertigo, tinnitus, a sensation of pressure in the ears, and neurosensory hearing loss

● **Causes**
  - Exact mechanism unknown
  - Possible causes
    - Abnormal hormonal influence on blood flow to the labyrinth
    - Excess labyrinth fluid (endolymph)
    - Injury
    - Allergic response
    - Autoimmune disorder
    - Abnormal metabolites

● **Pathophysiology**
  - Distention and increased fluid in the ear occur because of the increased volume of endolymph

● **Assessment findings**
  - Paroxysmal whirling vertigo with nausea and vomiting
  - Tinnitus followed by decreased hearing
  - Fluctuating unilateral neurosensory hearing loss of low tones
  - Sense of pressure or fullness in the ear
  - Nystagmus
  - Ataxia

● **Diagnostic test findings**
  - Audiogram: hearing loss
  - Electrocholeography: increased inner ear pressure due to excess fluid
  - Magnetic resonance imaging: rules out acoustic neuroma
  - Electronystagmography: labyrinth dysfunction
  - Auditory dehydration test: positive audiometric fluctuation

● **Medical management**
  - Diet: low-salt, low-sugar; avoidance of chocolate, coffee, and alcohol
  - I.V. hydration
  - Activity: as tolerated
  - Monitoring: vital signs and I/O
  - Adrenergic agonist: ephedrine (Pretz-D)
  - Corticosteroid: prednisone (Deltasone)
  - Benzodiazepine: diazepam (Valium)
  - Anticholinergic: scopolamine (Isopto)
  - Antihistamine: meclizine (Antivert)
  - Diuretic: spironolactone (Aldactone)
  - Antiemetic: prochlorperazine (Compazine), promethazine (Phenergan)
  - Smoking cessation

Key nursing interventions for a patient with Ménière's disease

- Assess hearing status.
- Provide for the patient's safety.
- Administer medication.
- Provide home care instructions.

Key complications of Ménière's disease

- Injury
- Hearing loss

Key facts about hearing loss

- Mechanical or nervous impediment to the transmission of sound waves
- Types: conductive hearing loss, sensorineural hearing loss, and mixed loss

Common causes of hearing loss

- Conductive: the interrupted passage of sound from the external ear to the inner ear
- Sensorineural: impaired cochlea or acoustic nerve transmission of sound impulses within the inner ear or brain

● **Nursing interventions**
- Maintain the patient's diet
- Assess hearing status, especially after an attack
- Monitor and record vital signs, I/O, and laboratory studies
- Administer medications, as prescribed
- Allay the patient's anxiety and provide emotional support
- Provide for the patient's safety
- Individualize home care instructions
  - Know about the disorder and its treatment
  - Follow instructions for medication use, and be aware of possible adverse effects
  - Follow safety measures for vertigo events
  - Use hearing-assistive devices, if appropriate
  - Practice stress reduction
  - Comply with medical follow-up

● **Complications**
- Injury
- Hearing loss

● **Surgical interventions**
- Endolymphatic sac decompression
- Endolymphatic mastoid shunt
- Ultrasonic surgery
- Labyrinthectomy
- Vestibular neurectomy

HEARING LOSS

● **Definition**
- A mechanical or nervous impediment to the transmission of sound waves
- Major forms are classified as conductive loss, sensorineural loss, or mixed loss

● **Causes**
- Conductive hearing loss
  - Obstruction of the external ear canal, such as from impacted cerumen, edema of the ear canal, neoplasms, or stenosis
  - Congenital malformations
  - Disruption or fixation of the middle ear ossicles
  - Fluid behind the eardrum or within the middle ear
  - Perforated tympanic membrane
  - Scar tissue in the ear canal or eardrum
  - Trauma to the tympanic membrane or inner ear
  - Tumors of the tympanic membrane
- Sensorineural hearing loss
  - Congenital factors
  - Hereditary factors

– Noise trauma
– Aging (presbycusis)
– Ménière's disease
– Ototoxicity
– Systemic disease, such as certain collagen diseases, diabetes, syphilis, and Paget's disease

Pathophysiology

- Conductive hearing loss results from the interrupted passage of sound from the external ear to the inner ear
- Sensorineural hearing loss is caused by impaired cochlea or acoustic nerve (CN VIII) transmission of sound impulses within the inner ear or brain
- Mixed loss is a combined dysfunction of conduction and sensorineural transmission

Assessment findings

- Congenital hearing loss
  – Lack of response to auditory stimulation
  – Impaired speech development
- Gradual hearing loss or following acute infection
  – Altered hearing at all frequencies and decibel levels
- Presbycusis
  – Tinnitus
  – Inability to understand the spoken word
- Hearing loss caused by neoplasm or fluid
  – Feeling of fullness in the ear

Diagnostic test findings

- Whisper test: reduced ability or inability to hear
- Rinne test: air conduction greater than bone conduction in sensorineural hearing loss; bone conduction greater than air conduction suggests conductive loss
- Weber's test: sound lateralizes to the better-functioning ear in sensorineural hearing loss; sound lateralizes to the ear with the poorest hearing in conductive hearing loss
- Audiometry: hearing loss
- Tympanometry: impaired compliance

Medical management

- Rehabilitation: speech and hearing
- Sound amplification: hearing aid, pocket talker
- Treating the cause of hearing loss: wax removal or infection control

Nursing interventions

- Provide information on hearing aids or other assistive devices
- Assess the patient's degree of hearing loss
- Speak slowly and distinctly
- Approach within the patient's visual range
- Develop alternative means of communication
- Provide emotional support, and encourage verbalization of fears

---

Key signs and symptoms of hearing loss

- Altered hearing at all frequencies and decibel levels
- Lack of response to auditory stimulation
- Tinnitus

Diagnosing hearing loss

- Rinne test: air conduction greater than bone conduction (sensorineural); bone conduction greater than air conduction (conductive)
- Weber's test: sound lateralizes to the better-functioning ear (sensorineural) or to the poorest-hearing ear (conductive)
- Audiometry: hearing loss

Treating hearing loss

- Sound amplification
- Treatment of the cause of hearing loss
- Surgery

Key nursing interventions for a patient with hearing loss

- Stand in front of the patient when speaking.
- Speak slowly and distinctly.
- Develop alternative means of communication.

- Individualize home care instructions
  - Know about the disorder and its treatment
  - Maintain the hearing aid or assistive device
  - Replace batteries when appropriate
  - Use alternative means of communication
  - Engage in social activities
  - Comply with medical follow-up

● **Complications**
  - Deafness
  - Speech impairment
  - Developmental delays

● **Surgical interventions**
  - Stapedectomy
  - Tympanoplasty
  - Cochlear implant

Key complications of hearing loss

- Deafness
- Speech impairment

TOP 10

Items to study for your next test on the eyes and ears

1. Structures of the eyes and ears
2. The difference between rods and cones
3. The bones of the middle ear
4. How to record visual acuity using a Snellen chart
5. How to test extraocular eye muscle function
6. Key signs and symptoms of cataracts, glaucoma, and retinal detachment
7. Types of hearing loss
8. Nursing interventions for the patient having eye or ear surgery
9. Teaching topics for the patient with a sensory disorder
10. Probable nursing diagnoses that apply to the patient with a sensory disorder

NCLEX CHECKS

It's never too soon to begin your NCLEX preparation. Now that you've reviewed this chapter, carefully read each of the following questions and choose the best answer. Then compare your responses to the correct answers.

1. A nurse is teaching a client being discharged after cataract removal and intraocular lens insertion. Which statement by the client indicates that further teaching is necessary?
- ☐ **1.** "I'll rest by reading a book."
- ☐ **2.** "I'll wear sunglasses when I'm outside during the day."
- ☐ **3.** "I'll wear an eye shield when I sleep."
- ☐ **4.** "I'll administer eyedrops as I have been instructed."

2. A client with retinal detachment is most likely to report which symptoms?
- ☐ **1.** Eye pain, halo vision, and redness in the eye
- ☐ **2.** Light flashes and floaters
- ☐ **3.** A recent driving accident while changing lanes
- ☐ **4.** Disabling glare

3. A nurse is assessing a client's extraocular eye movements as part of the neurologic examination. Which cranial nerves is the nurse assessing? Select all that apply.
- ☐ **1.** Cranial nerve II
- ☐ **2.** Cranial nerve III
- ☐ **3.** Cranial nerve IV
- ☐ **4.** Cranial nerve V
- ☐ **5.** Cranial nerve VI
- ☐ **6.** Cranial nerve VIII

4. A nurse is teaching a client with early glaucoma. The nurse should instruct the client to:

☐ **1.** wear an eye patch at night.

☐ **2.** avoid constipation.

☐ **3.** administer eyedrops.

☐ **4.** use cold compresses to relieve eye pain.

5. Which drug reported during a health history should concern a nurse most about ototoxicity?

☐ **1.** Acetaminophen

☐ **2.** Penicillin

☐ **3.** Aspirin

☐ **4.** Oxycodone

6. A client has an absence of the red reflex on ophthalmoscopic examination. The nurse knows that this finding is most likely associated with which disorder?

☐ **1.** Open-angle glaucoma

☐ **2.** Cataract

☐ **3.** Retinal detachment

☐ **4.** Acute angle-closure glaucoma

7. A characteristic symptom of Ménière's disease may be:

☐ **1.** paroxysmal whirling vertigo.

☐ **2.** blurred vision.

☐ **3.** headache.

☐ **4.** feeling of fullness in the ears.

8. During a Weber's test for hearing loss, sensorineural hearing loss would be indicated with which result?

☐ **1.** Sound lateralizing to the better-functioning ear

☐ **2.** Sound lateralizing to the ear with the poorest hearing

☐ **3.** No sound heard

☐ **4.** Sound heard equally in both ears

9. A modifiable risk factor for both eye and ear health would be:

☐ **1.** family history of a sensory disorder.

☐ **2.** work environment.

☐ **3.** diabetes mellitus.

☐ **4.** aging.

10. A probable nursing diagnosis for clients experiencing hearing loss would be:

☐ **1.** *Ineffective health maintenance*

☐ **2.** *Adult failure to thrive*

☐ **3.** *Complicated grieving*

☐ **4.** *Social isolation*

ANSWERS AND RATIONALES

1. CORRECT ANSWER: 1

Following cataract surgery, the client shouldn't read until his vision stabilizes. The client should protect his eyes by wearing sunglasses in sunlight and an eye shield at night. The client should administer eyedrops as prescribed.

2. CORRECT ANSWER: 2

Light flashes and floaters are characteristic of a detached retina. Eye pain, halo vision, and redness in the eye are findings of acute angle-closure glaucoma. Difficulty seeing cars in another lane suggests a loss of peripheral vision, which may indicate glaucoma. Disabling glare is a symptom of cataracts.

3. CORRECT ANSWER: 2, 3, 5

Assessing extraocular eye movements helps evaluate the function of cranial nerves III (oculomotor), IV (trochlear), and VI (abducens). The oculomotor nerve originates in the brainstem and controls the movement of the eyeball up, down, and inward; raises the eyelid; and constricts the pupil. The trochlear nerve rotates the eyeball downward and outward. The abducens nerve originates in the pons and rotates the eyeball laterally. Assessing the client's vision helps evaluation of cranial nerve II. Cranial nerve V, the trigeminal nerve, has three branches that require assessment: the ophthalmic branch, the maxillary branch, and the mandibular branch. Assessing hearing (cochlear) and balance (vestibular) helps evaluation of cranial nerve VIII, the acoustic nerve.

4. CORRECT ANSWER: 3

Administering eyedrops is a critical component of self-care for a client with glaucoma. An eye patch, avoiding constipation, and applying cold compresses aren't necessary unless the client has undergone eye surgery.

5. CORRECT ANSWER: 3

Aspirin, as well as streptomycin and neomycin, is associated with ototoxicity. Acetaminophen, penicillin, and oxycodone are not.

6. CORRECT ANSWER: 2

A loss of the red reflex, the reflection of light on the vascular retina, is characteristic of a cataract. It isn't associated with open-angle glaucoma, retinal detachment, or acute angle-closure glaucoma.

7. CORRECT ANSWER: 1

A characteristic assessment finding for Ménière's disease is paroxysmal vertigo, usually accompanied by nausea and vomiting. Blurred vision or headache may be a sign of many disorders. A feeling of fullness in the ears may be a sign of fluid in the ear or ear infection.

8. CORRECT ANSWER: 1

During a Weber's test, sound lateralizing to the better-functioning ear indicates sensorineural hearing loss. Sound lateralizing to the ear with the poorest hearing indicates conductive hearing loss. No sound heard would indicate complete hearing loss. Equal sounds may indicate no hearing loss.

9. CORRECT ANSWER: 2
The work environment may be altered to prevent eye and ear injury. Family history, diabetes mellitus, and aging are nonmodifiable risk factors.

10. CORRECT ANSWER: 4
Clients experiencing hearing loss may have difficulty integrating themselves into social situations. The other nursing diagnoses aren't indicated for hearing loss.

5

Gastrointestinal system

1. Esophageal varices are a possible complication of which GI disorder?

☐ 1. Irritable bowel syndrome

☐ 2. Peritonitis

☒ 3. Cirrhosis

☐ 4. Crohn's disease

CORRECT ANSWER: 3

2. Which laboratory study results are important findings in the diagnosis of pancreatitis?

☒ 1. Elevated amylase and lipase levels

☐ 2. Decreased hemoglobin and hematocrit levels

☐ 3. Elevated ammonia levels and decreased albumin levels

☐ 4. Decreased sodium and chloride levels

CORRECT ANSWER: 1

3. A classic symptom of cholecystitis is:

☐ 1. psoas sign.

☒ 2. Murphy's sign.

☐ 3. Cullen's sign.

☐ 4. Turner's sign.

CORRECT ANSWER: 2

4. Teaching for the client with irritable bowel syndrome should focus on:

☒ 1. avoidance of dietary irritants.

☐ 2. decreased sodium intake.

☐ 3. nutritional supplements.

☐ 4. increased potassium intake.

CORRECT ANSWER: 1

5. A probable nursing diagnosis for a client with a GI disorder is:

☐ 1. *Excess fluid volume*

☐ 2. *Impaired parenting*

☐ 3. *Adult failure to thrive*

☒ 4. *Imbalanced nutrition: Less than body requirements*

CORRECT ANSWER: 4

LEARNING OBJECTIVES

After studying this chapter, you should be able to:

- Describe the psychosocial impact of GI disorders.
- Differentiate between modifiable and nonmodifiable risk factors in the development of a GI disorder.
- List three probable and three possible nursing diagnoses for a patient with a GI disorder.
- Identify nursing interventions for a patient with a GI disorder.
- Identify three teaching goals for a patient with a GI disorder.

CHAPTER OVERVIEW

Caring for the patient with a GI disorder requires a sound understanding of GI anatomy, physiology, and function. A thorough assessment is essential to planning and implementing appropriate patient care. The assessment includes a complete history, physical examination, diagnostic testing, identification of modifiable and nonmodifiable risk factors, and information related to the psychosocial impact of GI dysfunction on the patient.

Nursing diagnoses focus primarily on a change in bowel habits (constipation or diarrhea), imbalanced nutrition, and body image. Patient teaching—a crucial nursing activity—involves teaching patients about the disorder, treatment plan, medication regimens, signs and symptoms of possible complications, reduction of modifiable risk factors (decreased alcohol consumption, diet restrictions, stress management, and smoking cessation), and medical follow-up. The psychosocial impact of changes in body image and decreased self-esteem is also an important aspect of nursing care.

ANATOMY AND PHYSIOLOGY REVIEW

● **Mouth** (see *Parts of the GI system*)
  - Mechanical and chemical digestion originate here
  - Tongue and teeth are accessory organs of digestion
  - Salivary glands secrete saliva, which is slightly acidic and combines with food during mastication to begin its chemical breakdown

● **Pharynx**
  - Connects the mouth and larynx to the esophagus
  - Doesn't participate in the digestive process but aids in swallowing

● **Esophagus**
  - This organ, located behind the trachea and ending at the stomach, provides for the transfer of food from the oropharynx to the stomach
  - Closure of the epiglottis prevents food from entering the trachea
  - Closure of the cardiac sphincter prevents reflux of gastric contents

● **Stomach**
  - A hollow, C-shaped, 1-qt (1-L) muscular pouch located under the diaphragm
  - Secretes pepsin, renin, lipase, mucus, and hydrochloric acid for digestion
  - Mixes and stores chyme
  - Secretes intrinsic factor necessary for absorption of cyanocobalamin (vitamin B_{12})
  - Upper portion connects to the esophagus, and the lower portion connects to the duodenum

● **Small intestine**
  - Consists of the duodenum, jejunum, and ileum
    – Chyme, in liquid or semiliquid form, enters the duodenum through the pyloric sphincter

---

Key functions of the mouth

- Where mechanical and chemical digestion originate
- Tongue and teeth are accessory organs of digestion
- Salivary glands secrete saliva

Key function of the esophagus

- Provides for the transfer of food from the oropharynx to the stomach

Key functions of the stomach

- Secretes pepsin, renin, lipase, mucus, and hydrochloric acid for digestion
- Mixes and stores chyme
- Secretes intrinsic factor necessary for absorption of cyanocobalamin

Key functions of the intestines

- Small intestine: digests food and absorbs nutrients
- Large intestine: absorbs fluids and electrolytes; synthesizes vitamin K using intestinal bacteria; and stores fecal material

Parts of the GI system

This illustration shows the GI system's major anatomic structures. Knowing these structures will help you conduct an accurate physical assessment.

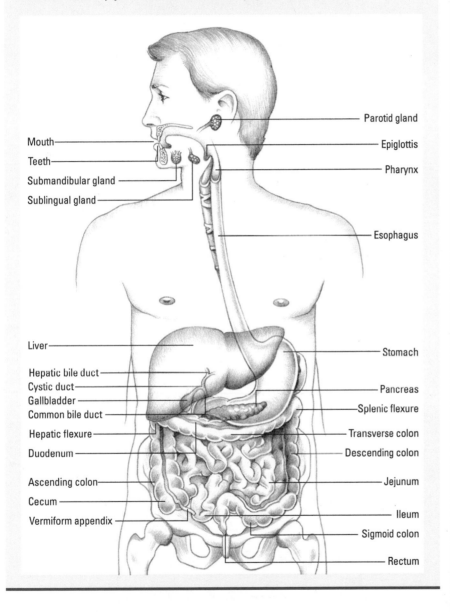

Mouth
Teeth
Submandibular gland
Sublingual gland

Parotid gland
Epiglottis
Pharynx

Esophagus

Liver
Hepatic bile duct
Cystic duct
Gallbladder
Common bile duct
Hepatic flexure
Duodenum
Ascending colon
Cecum
Vermiform appendix

Stomach
Pancreas
Splenic flexure
Transverse colon
Descending colon
Jejunum
Ileum
Sigmoid colon
Rectum

Parts of the GI system

- Parotid gland
- Mouth
- Teeth
- Epiglottis
- Submandibular gland
- Sublingual gland
- Pharynx
- Esophagus
- Liver
- Stomach
- Hepatic bile duct
- Cystic duct
- Gallbladder
- Pancreas
- Common bile duct
- Splenic flexure
- Hepatic flexure
- Transverse colon
- Descending colon
- Duodenum
- Jejunum
- Ascending colon
- Cecum
- Vermiform appendix
- Ileum
- Sigmoid colon
- Rectum

    – Bile and pancreatic secretions enter the duodenum through the common bile duct at the ampulla of Vater
- Digestion occurs here, and nutrients and fluids are absorbed
- Lined with villi
- Motor activity includes mixing and peristalsis
- Connects to the stomach at the upper end at the pyloric sphincter and to the large intestine at the lower end at the iliocecal sphincter

- **Large intestine**
  - Consists of the cecum, colon, rectum, and anus
  - Segments of the colon are the cecum, ascending colon, transverse colon, descending colon, and sigmoid colon
  - Chyme enters the cecum through the ileocecal valve
  - Has several functions
    - Absorbs fluid and electrolytes
    - Synthesizes vitamin K using intestinal bacteria
    - Stores fecal material
  - Chyme becomes more solid as the intestinal wall of the colon absorbs water
  - Defecation is the movement of waste material (feces) from the rectum through the anal sphincter

- **Liver**
  - Largest internal organ in the body
  - Produces bile (main function), which emulsifies fats and stimulates peristalsis
  - Conveys bile from the gallbladder, where it's stored, until it enters the duodenum at Oddi's sphincter through the common bile duct
  - Metabolizes carbohydrates, fats, and proteins
  - Synthesizes coagulation factors VII, IX, X, and prothrombin
  - Stores fat-soluble vitamins A, D, E, K, B$_{12}$, copper, and iron
  - Detoxifies chemicals (such as drugs)
  - Excretes bilirubin
  - Obtains dual blood supply from the portal vein and hepatic artery
  - Produces and stores glycogen
  - Promotes erythropoiesis when bone marrow production is insufficient

- **Gallbladder**
  - Hollow, pear-shaped organ that stores bile and is located below the liver
  - Secretes bile via the cystic duct that travels to the common bile duct

- **Pancreas**
  - Accessory gland of digestion located horizontally along the posterior curvature of the stomach
  - Exocrine function: secretes three digestive enzymes
    - Amylase
    - Lipase
    - Trypsin
  - Endocrine function: secretes hormones from the islets of Langerhans
    - Insulin
    - Glucagon
    - Somatostatin
  - Main pancreatic duct joins the common bile duct and empties into the duodenum at the ampulla of Vater
  - Responsible for secreting large amounts of sodium bicarbonate, which neutralizes acid chyme

ASSESSMENT FINDINGS

● **History**
- Inadequate diet
- Change in bowel pattern
  - Constipation
  - Diarrhea
  - Flatus
- Complaints of indigestion
- Nausea and vomiting
- Abdominal pain (for more information, see *Abdominal pain: Determining the possible causes,* pages 222 and 223)
- Dysphagia
- Loss of appetite, anorexia
- Weight loss or gain

● **Physical examination**
- Abnormal color and consistency of stool
  - Melena
  - Clay-colored stools
  - Frothy stools
  - Steatorrhea
  - Occult blood in stool
- Abdominal tenderness
- Guarding
- Abdominal mass
- Abnormal bowel sounds
- Abdominal distention
- Rectal bleeding
- Jaundice
- Edema
- Hematemesis
- Anorexia
- Hepatomegaly
- Splenomegaly

DIAGNOSTIC TESTS AND PROCEDURES

● **Upper GI series**
- Definition and purpose
  - Fluoroscopic procedure using barium as a contrast medium
  - Examination of the esophagus, stomach, duodenum, and other portions of the small bowel after swallowing barium
- Nursing interventions before the procedure
  - Explain the procedure to the patient
  - Withhold food and fluids
  - Administer fluids, cathartics, and enemas, as prescribed

(Text continues on page 224.)

Key signs and symptoms of a GI disorder

- Weight changes
- Rectal bleeding
- Jaundice
- Hematemesis
- Abdominal pain
- Nausea and vomiting

Stool abnormalities associated with GI disorders

- Melena
- Clay-colored stools
- Frothy stools
- Steatorrhea
- Occult blood in stool

Key facts about an upper GI series

- Fluoroscopic procedure that allows for examination of the esophagus, stomach, duodenum, and other portions of the small bowel after swallowing barium
- Intervention: before the procedure, administer fluids, cathartics, and enemas, as prescribed

Key signs and symptoms of a possible abdominal problem

- Abdominal tenderness
- Fever
- Abdominal rigidity
- Abdominal mass
- Urine frequency
- Anorexia, nausea, vomiting
- Bowel sound changes
- Amenorrhea
- Abdominal distention
- Weight changes
- Weakness
- Costovertebral angle tenderness
- Bowel sound changes

GO WITH THE FLOW

Abdominal pain: Determining the possible causes

This flowchart highlights the decision-making process used to determine the possible causes of a patient's abdominal pain.

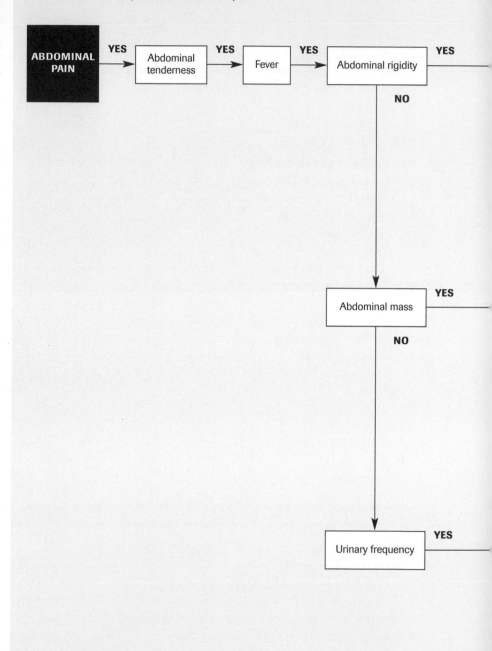

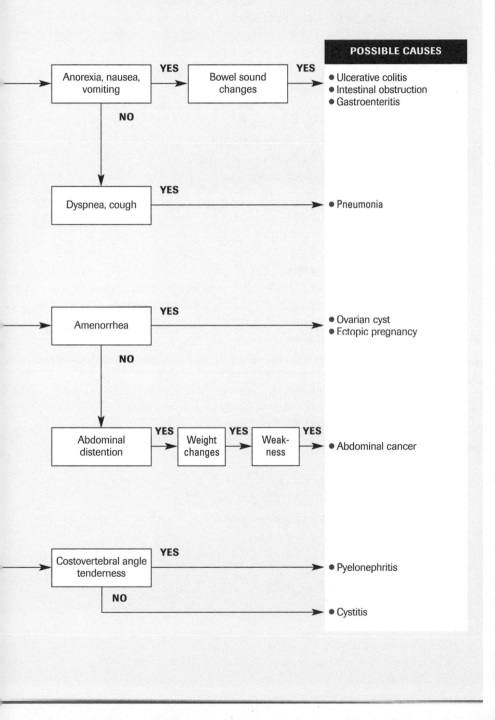

POSSIBLE CAUSES

Anorexia, nausea, vomiting — YES → Bowel sound changes — YES →
- Ulcerative colitis
- Intestinal obstruction
- Gastroenteritis

Dyspnea, cough — YES →
- Pneumonia

Amenorrhea — YES →
- Ovarian cyst
- Ectopic pregnancy

Abdominal distention — YES → Weight changes — YES → Weakness — YES →
- Abdominal cancer

Costovertebral angle tenderness — YES →
- Pyelonephritis

NO →
- Cystitis

Possible causes of abdominal pain

- Ulcerative colitis
- Intestinal obstruction
- Gastroenteritis
- Pneumonia
- Ovarian cyst
- Ectopic pregnancy
- Abdominal cancer
- Pyelonephritis
- Cystitis

Key facts about a lower GI series

- Fluoroscopic procedure that allows for examination of the large intestine after administration of a barium enema
- Intervention: before the procedure, withhold food and fluids

Key facts about endoscopy

- Provides direct visualization of the esophagus and stomach
- Intervention: withhold food and fluids 6 to 12 hours before the test

Key facts about the fecal occult blood test

- Analysis of the stool for blood
- Intervention: advise the patient to avoid red meat, iron, and high fiber for 1 to 3 days prior to the procedure

Key facts about the fecal fat test

- Analysis of the stool for fat
- Intervention: advise the patient to restrict alcohol intake and maintain a high-fat diet for 72 hours before examination

- Nursing interventions after the procedure
  - Inform the patient that stool will be light-colored for several days
  - Administer cathartics, fluids, and enemas, as prescribed

● **Lower GI series (barium enema)**
- Definition and purpose
  - Fluoroscopic procedure using barium as a contrast medium
  - Examination of the large intestine after administration of barium via an enema
- Nursing interventions before the procedure
  - Explain the procedure to the patient
  - Withhold food and fluids
  - Administer bowel preparation (laxatives and enemas), as prescribed
- Nursing interventions after the procedure
  - Encourage fluids, unless contraindicated
  - Administer enemas and laxatives, as prescribed
  - Monitor color, consistency, and amount of stool

● **Endoscopy**
- Definition and purpose
  - Procedure using an endoscope
  - Direct visualization of the esophagus and stomach
- Nursing interventions before the procedure
  - Explain the procedure to the patient
  - Withhold food and fluids for 6 to 12 hours before the test
  - Check that an informed consent form has been signed
  - Obtain baseline vital signs
  - Administer sedatives, as prescribed
- Nursing interventions after the procedure
  - Withhold food and fluids until the gag and cough reflex returns
  - Monitor vital signs
  - Assess vasovagal response

● **Fecal occult blood test**
- Definition and purpose
  - Laboratory test using a reagent
  - Analysis of stool for blood
- Nursing interventions before the procedure
  - Explain the procedure to the patient
  - Advise the patient to avoid red meat, iron, and high fiber for 1 to 3 days
  - Document the administration of aspirin, vitamin C, and anti-inflammatory drugs

● **Fecal fat test**
- Definition and purpose
  - Laboratory test using a stain
  - Analysis of stool for fat
- Nursing interventions before the procedure

- Explain the procedure to the patient
- Advise the patient to restrict alcohol intake and maintain a high-fat diet 72 hours before the examination
- Refrigerate the specimen until it can be sent to the laboratory
- Document current medications

● **Proctosigmoidoscopy**
- Definition and purpose
  - Procedure using a lighted scope
  - Direct visualization of the sigmoid colon, rectum, and anal canal
- Nursing interventions before the procedure
  - Explain the procedure to the patient
  - Administer bowel preparation, as prescribed
  - Place an obtained written informed consent in the patient's chart
  - Document iron intake
- Nursing interventions after the procedure
  - Check the patient for bleeding
  - Monitor the patient's vital signs

● **Barium swallow**
- Definition and purpose
  - Procedure using barium as a contrast medium
  - Fluoroscopic examination of the pharynx and esophagus after administration of barium
- Nursing interventions before the procedure
  - Explain the procedure to the patient
  - Withhold food and fluids for 6 to 12 hours before the test
- Nursing interventions after the procedure
  - Encourage fluids, unless contraindicated
  - Administer laxatives, as prescribed
  - Assess bowel function

● **Cholangiography**
- Definition and purpose
  - Procedure using an injection of a radiopaque dye through an intravenous catheter
  - Radiographic examination of the biliary duct system
- Nursing interventions before the procedure
  - Explain the procedure to the patient
  - Encourage a low-residue, high–simple fat diet 1 day before the examination
  - Withhold food and fluids after midnight
  - Note the patient's allergies to iodine, seafood, and radiopaque dyes
  - Inform the patient about possible throat irritation and flushing of the face
- Nursing interventions after the procedure
  - Check the injection site for bleeding
  - Monitor the patient's vital signs

Key facts about liver scan

- Invasive procedure using an I.V. injection of a radioisotope
- Provides an image of blood flow distribution in the liver
- Intervention: after the procedure, assess the patient for signs of delayed allergic reaction

Key facts about gastric analysis

- Aspiration of the contents of the stomach through an NG tube
- Measures the acidity of gastric secretions
- Intervention: instruct the patient not to smoke for 8 to 12 hours before the test

Key facts about ultrasonography

- Noninvasive procedure that uses echoes from sound waves
- Provides visualization of body organs
- Intervention: withhold food and fluids for 8 to 12 hours before the procedure

Key facts about blood chemistry

- Laboratory test of a blood sample
- Analysis for potassium, sodium, calcium, glucose, BUN, and other substances
- Intervention: check the site for bleeding after the procedure

● **Liver scan**
- Definition and purpose
  - Procedure using an I.V. injection of a radioisotope
  - Visual imaging of the distribution of blood flow in the liver
- Nursing interventions before the procedure
  - Explain the procedure to the patient
  - Determine the patient's ability to lie still during the procedure
  - Check the patient for possible allergies
- Nursing interventions after the procedure
  - Assess the I.V. insertion site for bleeding, bruising, or hematoma
  - Assess the patient for signs of delayed allergic reaction to the radioisotope, such as itching and hives

● **Gastric analysis**
- Definition and purpose
  - Procedure that aspirates the contents of the stomach through a nasogastric (NG) tube
  - Fasting analysis to measure the acidity of gastric secretions
- Nursing interventions before the procedure
  - Explain the procedure to the patient
  - Insert an NG tube
  - Withhold food and fluids after midnight
  - Instruct the patient not to smoke for 8 to 12 hours before the test
  - Withhold medications that can affect gastric secretions for 24 hours before the procedure
- Nursing interventions after the procedure
  - Obtain the patient's vital signs
  - Note reactions to gastric acid stimulant, if used

● **Ultrasonography**
- Definition and purpose
  - Noninvasive procedure that uses echoes from sound waves
  - Visualization of body organs
- Nursing interventions before the procedure
  - Explain the procedure to the patient
  - Withhold food and fluids for 8 to 12 hours
  - Determine the patient's ability to lie still during the procedure
  - Ask the patient not to smoke or chew gum for 8 to 12 hours before the test
  - Administer enemas, as prescribed

● **Blood chemistry**
- Definition and purpose
  - Laboratory test of a blood sample
  - Analysis for potassium, sodium, calcium, phosphorus, glucose, bicarbonate, blood urea nitrogen (BUN), creatinine, protein, albumin, osmolality, amylase, lipase, alkaline phosphatase, ammonia, bilirubin, lactate dehydrogenase (LD), sulfobromophthalein test, aspartate

aminotransferase (AST), serum alanine aminotransferase (ALT), hepatitis-associated antigens, carcinoembryonic antigen (CEA), and alpha-fetoprotein
- Nursing interventions
  - Explain the procedure to the patient
  - Check the site for bleeding after the procedure

Hematologic studies
- Definition and purpose
  - Laboratory test of a blood sample
  - Analysis for red blood cells (RBCs), white blood cells (WBCs), platelets, prothrombin time (PT), partial thromboplastin time (PTT), hemoglobin (Hb), and hematocrit (HCT)
- Nursing interventions
  - Explain the procedure to the patient
  - Note current drug therapy before the procedure
  - Check the site for bleeding after the procedure

Liver biopsy
- Definition and purpose
  - Procedure using a needle for the percutaneous removal of a small amount of liver tissue
  - Histologic evaluation of liver tissue
- Nursing interventions before the procedure
  - Explain the procedure to the patient
  - Withhold food and fluids for 6 to 12 hours
  - Place an obtained written informed consent in the patient's chart
  - Assess baseline clotting studies and vital signs
  - Instruct the patient to exhale and hold his breath during insertion of the needle
- Nursing interventions after the procedure
  - Check the insertion site for bleeding
  - Monitor the patient's vital signs
  - Observe the patient for signs of shock and pneumothorax
  - Position the patient on the right lateral side for hemostasis

Colonoscopy
- Definition and purpose
  - Procedure using a flexible, lighted scope
  - Direct visualization of large intestine; biopsies can be obtained
- Nursing interventions before the procedure
  - Explain the procedure to the patient
  - Provide clear liquid diet 24 hours before test, if indicated
  - Administer bowel preparation
  - Explain that the patient will feel cramping and the sensation of needing to have a bowel movement
  - Explain the use of air to distend the bowel lumen
  - Obtain a signed informed consent per facility policy

Key facts about ERCP

- Radiographic examination of the hepatobiliary tree and pancreatic ducts using contrast medium and a lighted scope
- Used to evaluate the cause of obstructive jaundice
- Interventions:
- Check for signs of respiratory depression
- Withhold food until the gag reflex returns

Key facts about percutaneous transhepatic cholangiography

- Fluoroscopic examination of the biliary ducts through the use of contrast medium
- Used to evaluate the cause of severe jaundice and to diagnose obstruction
- Intervention: before the procedure, check for allergies; also check PT and PTT

- Nursing interventions after the procedure
  - Monitor for gross rectal bleeding
  - Withhold food and fluids for 2 hours
  - Check for blood in the stool if polyps are removed

● **Endoscopic retrograde cholangiopancreatography (ERCP)**
- Definition and purpose
  - Radiographic examination of the hepatobiliary tree and pancreatic ducts using contrast medium and a lighted scope
  - Used to evaluate the cause of obstructive jaundice
- Nursing interventions before the procedure
  - Explain the procedure to the patient
  - Withhold food and fluid after midnight
  - Check for allergies to iodine or seafood
  - Remove dentures
  - Explain that a local anesthetic will be used
  - Obtain a signed informed consent per facility policy
- Nursing interventions after the procedure
  - Check for signs of respiratory depression
  - Check for signs of urine retention
  - Provide comfort measures for throat irritation
  - Withhold food until the gag reflex returns

● **Percutaneous transhepatic cholangiography**
- Definition and purpose
  - Fluoroscopic examination of the biliary ducts through the use of contrast medium
  - Used to evaluate the cause of severe jaundice and to diagnose obstruction
- Nursing interventions before the procedure
  - Explain the procedure to the patient
  - Inform the patient that the X-ray table will be tilted and rotated during the procedure
  - Explain that transient pain will be felt with the injection of the anesthetic
  - Check for allergies to iodine or seafood
  - Check PT and PTT
  - Withhold food and fluid for 6 to 12 hours
  - Obtain a signed informed consent per facility policy
- Nursing interventions after the procedure
  - Instruct the patient to rest for at least 6 hours in the right side-lying position
  - Check for bleeding at the injection site
  - Monitor the patient's vital signs
  - Withhold food and fluids for 2 hours

PSYCHOSOCIAL IMPACT OF GI DISORDERS

- **Developmental impact**
  - Changes in body image
  - Feeling of lack of control over body function
  - Fear of rejection
  - Embarrassment from changes in body function and structure
  - Decreased self-esteem
- **Economic impact**
  - Disruption of employment
  - Cost of special diet
  - Cost of special diversion appliances
  - Cost of medications
- **Occupational impact**
  - Impact on occupation
  - Restrictions in physical activity
- **Social impact**
  - Changes in leisure activity
  - Changes in eating patterns and modes
  - Changes in elimination patterns and modes
  - Social withdrawal and isolation
  - Changes in sexual function

RISK FACTORS

- **Modifiable risk factors**
  - Diet
  - Smoking
  - Alcohol consumption
  - Inactivity
  - Stress
  - Contaminated water and food
  - Anger, fear, or anxiety
  - Culturally based reluctance to discuss personal hygiene and health habits
- **Nonmodifiable risk factors**
  - Family history of GI disorders
  - History of previous GI dysfunction

NURSING DIAGNOSES

- **Probable nursing diagnoses**
  - Constipation
  - Diarrhea
  - Acute pain
  - Imbalanced nutrition: Less than body requirements

Psychosocial impact of GI disorders

- Decreased self-esteem
- Disruption of employment
- Restrictions in physical activity
- Changes in eating patterns and modes
- Changes in elimination patterns and modes
- Social withdrawal and isolation
- Changes in sexual function

Modifiable risk factors for GI disorders

- Diet
- Smoking
- Inactivity
- Stress
- Alcohol

Nonmodifiable risk factors for GI disorders

- Family history
- History of GI dysfunction

TOP 4

Probable nursing diagnoses for a GI disorder

1. Constipation
2. Diarrhea
3. Acute pain
4. Imbalanced nutrition: Less than body requirements

Possible nursing diagnoses for GI disorders

- Disturbed body image
- Impaired skin integrity
- Toileting self-care deficit

- Imbalanced nutrition: More than body requirements
- Deficient fluid volume
- Anxiety
- Fear
- Deficient knowledge (specify)

● **Possible nursing diagnoses**
- Disturbed body image
- Situational low self-esteem
- Impaired skin integrity
- Noncompliance (specify)
- Sexual dysfunction
- Impaired swallowing
- Bowel incontinence
- Toileting self-care deficit
- Risk for infection

GALLBLADDER AND PANCREATIC SURGERIES

Types of gallbladder and pancreatic surgeries

- Cholecystostomy
- Choledochotomy
- Cholecystotomy
- Choledochostomy
- Cholecystectomy
- ESWL
- Laparoscopic cholecystectomy
- Pancreatectomy

● **Description**
- Cholecystostomy: surgical incision into the gallbladder to drain bile
- Choledochotomy: surgical incision into the common bile duct to remove stones
- Cholecystotomy: surgical incision into the gallbladder to remove gallstones
- Choledochostomy: surgical opening of the common bile duct to insert a T tube or catheter for drainage
- Cholecystectomy: surgical removal of the gallbladder
- Extracorporeal shock-wave lithotripsy (ESWL): use of shock waves to fragment gallstones into small pieces to be either removed by endoscopy or dissolved with solvents
- Laparoscopic cholecystectomy: removal of the gallbladder through a small incision in the abdomen and the use of a fiber-optic endoscope
- Pancreatectomy: surgical removal of part of or the entire pancreas

● **Preoperative nursing interventions**
- Complete patient and family preoperative teaching
  - Explain the procedure to the patient
  - Describe the operating room, postanesthesia care unit (PACU), and preoperative and postoperative routines
  - Demonstrate postoperative turning, coughing, deep breathing, splinting, and range-of-motion (ROM) exercises
  - Explain the postoperative need for drainage tubes, surgical dressings, oxygen therapy, I.V. therapy, and pain control
- Complete a preoperative checklist, and obtain a signed informed consent
- Administer preoperative medications, as prescribed
- Allay the patient's and his family's anxiety about surgery
- Document the patient's history and physical assessment database

Key nursing interventions before gallbladder and pancreatic surgeries

- Explain the procedure.
- Demonstrate turning, coughing, deep breathing, and splinting of the incision.
- Complete a preoperative checklist, and obtain an informed consent.

● **Postoperative nursing interventions**
- Check respiratory status and fluid balance
- Assess pain and administer postoperative analgesics, as prescribed
- Assess for nausea, vomiting, and abdominal distention
- Assess for return of peristalsis; give solid foods and liquids, as tolerated
- Administer I.V. fluids and transfusion therapy, as prescribed
- Allay the patient's anxiety
- Provide wound care and dressing changes, as directed
- Place the patient in semi-Fowler's position
- Encourage incentive spirometry, coughing, deep breathing, and splinting of the incision
- Encourage and assist with physical activity, as tolerated
- Monitor vital signs, intake and output (I/O), and laboratory studies
- Monitor and maintain the position and patency of drainage tubes: NG, wound drainage, T tube
- Administer antibiotics, as prescribed
- After pancreatic surgery
  – Monitor blood glucose levels
  – Monitor for signs of hyperglycemia
- Individualize home care instructions
  – Know about the disorder and its treatment
  – Follow instructions for medication use, and be aware of possible adverse effects
  – Avoid lifting for 6 weeks
  – Complete incision care daily, and observe for signs and symptoms of infection
  – Continue care of the T tube
  – Adhere to a low-fat diet for 6 weeks
  – Comply with medical follow-up

● **Possible surgical complications**
- Pneumonia
- Atelectasis
- Peritonitis
- Hemorrhage
- Infection

PORTOSYSTEMIC SHUNTS

● **Definition**
- Portacaval shunt: surgical anastomosis of the portal vein to the inferior vena cava that diverts blood from the portal system to decrease portal pressure
- Splenorenal shunt: surgical anastomosis of the splenic vein to the left renal vein that diverts blood from the portal system to decrease portal pressure

Key nursing interventions after gallbladder and pancreatic surgeries
- Check respiratory status and fluid balance.
- Provide wound care and dressing changes.
- Reinforce turning, coughing, deep breathing, and splinting of the incision.
- Monitor and maintain position and patency of drainage tubes: NG, wound drainage, T tube.

Types of portosystemic shunts
- Portocaval shunt
- Splenorenal shunt
- Mesocaval shunt
- TIPS

Key nursing interventions before portosystemic shunt surgery

- Demonstrate postoperative turning, coughing, deep breathing, incentive spirometry, splinting, and ROM exercises.
- Administer preoperative medications, as prescribed.
- Complete a preoperative checklist, and obtain an informed consent.

Key nursing interventions after portosystemic shunt surgery

- Assess cardiac, respiratory, and neurologic status and fluid balance.
- Assess pain and administer postoperative analgesics, as prescribed.
- Assess for return of peristalsis.
- Monitor vital signs, I/O, CVP, laboratory studies, ECG, neurovital signs, and pulse oximetry.
- Measure and record the patient's abdominal girth.
- Monitor stool and NG tube drainage for occult blood.
- Monitor for hemorrhage.

- Mesocaval shunt: surgical anastomosis of the inferior vena cava to the side of the superior mesenteric vein that diverts blood from the portal system to decrease portal pressure
- Transjugular intrahepatic portosystemic shunt (TIPS): shunt between the portal and systemic venous circulation using the right internal jugular vein and placement of a stent

● **Preoperative nursing interventions**
- Complete patient and family preoperative teaching
  - Explain the procedure to the patient
  - Describe the operating room, PACU, and preoperative and postoperative routines; demonstrate postoperative turning, coughing, deep breathing, incentive spirometry, splinting, and ROM exercises
  - Explain the postoperative need for drainage tubes, surgical dressings, oxygen therapy, I.V. therapy, and pain control
- Complete a preoperative checklist, and obtain a signed informed consent
- Administer preoperative medications, as prescribed
- Allay the patient's and his family's anxiety about surgery
- Document the patient's history and physical assessment database
- Monitor for bleeding and administer transfusion therapy, as prescribed
- Insert and maintain the patency of an NG tube, if ordered
- Monitor central venous pressure (CVP)
- Monitor laboratory values
- Provide fluids and electrolytes, as indicated
- Apply sequential compression devices

● **Postoperative nursing interventions**
- Assess cardiac, respiratory, and neurologic status and fluid balance
- Assess pain level, administer postoperative analgesics as prescribed, and evaluate effect
- Administer I.V. fluids, total parenteral nutrition (TPN), and transfusion therapy, as prescribed
- Provide emotional support and allay the patient's anxiety
- Provide wound care and dressing changes, as directed
- Encourage turning, coughing, deep breathing, incentive spirometry, and splinting of the incision
- Place the patient in semi-Fowler's position
- Maintain activity: bed rest, active and passive ROM and isometric exercises
- Administer oxygen, maintain the endotracheal tube to the ventilator, and provide suctioning, as needed
- Monitor vital signs, I/O, CVP, laboratory studies, electrocardiogram (ECG), neurovital signs, and pulse oximetry
- Monitor and maintain position and patency of drainage tubes: NG, indwelling urinary catheter, wound drainage
- Assess GI status, monitor the patient's abdominal girth, and observe for return of peristalsis
- Monitor stool and NG tube drainage for occult blood

- Monitor for signs and symptoms of bleeding
- Provide skin, nares, and mouth care
- Administer medications, as prescribed
- Elevate extremities and monitor for peripheral edema
- Apply sequential compression devices while in bed
- Individualize home care instructions
  - Know about the disorder and its treatment
  - Follow instructions for medication use, and be aware of possible adverse effects
  - Adhere to activity limitations
  - Complete incision care daily, and observe for signs and symptoms of infection
  - Avoid using alcohol
  - Adhere to a protein-restricted diet
  - Avoid using over-the-counter (OTC) medications unless directed by the physician
  - Observe for symptoms of bleeding
  - Comply with medical follow-up

● **Possible surgical complications**
- Acute hepatic failure
- Chronic portosystemic encephalopathy
- Coagulopathy
- Shunt malfunction
- Infection

GASTRIC SURGERY

● **Description**
- Vagotomy: surgical ligation of the vagus nerve to decrease the secretion of gastric acid
- Antrectomy: surgical removal of the antrum of the stomach
- Pyloroplasty: surgical dilatation of the pyloric sphincter to increase the rate of gastric emptying
- Gastroduodenostomy (Billroth I): surgical removal of the lower portion of the stomach with anastomosis of the remaining portion of the stomach to the duodenum
- Gastrojejunostomy (Billroth II): surgical removal of the antrum and distal portion of the stomach and duodenum with anastomosis of the stomach to the jejunum
- Subtotal gastrectomy: surgical removal of 60% to 80% of the stomach
- Esophagojejunostomy (total gastrectomy): surgical removal of the entire stomach with a loop of the jejunum anastomosed to the esophagus

● **Preoperative nursing interventions**
- Complete patient and family preoperative teaching
  - Explain the procedure to the patient

Types of gastric surgery

- Vagotomy
- Antrectomy
- Pyloroplasty
- Gastroduodenostomy
- Gastrojejunostomy
- Subtotal gastrectomy
- Esophagojejunostomy

Key nursing interventions before gastric surgery

- Complete patient and family teaching.
- Administer preoperative medications, as prescribed.
- Administer bowel preparation, as prescribed.

Key nursing interventions after gastric surgery

- Administer I.V. fluids, NG tube feedings, and transfusion therapy, as prescribed.
- Provide wound care and dressing changes.
- Assess for the return of peristalsis.
- Monitor and maintain the position and patency of drainage tubes: NG, indwelling urinary catheter, wound drainage.
- Apply sequential compression devices while in bed.

– Describe the operating room, PACU, and preoperative and postoperative routines
– Demonstrate postoperative turning, coughing, deep breathing, splinting, and leg and ROM exercises
– Explain the postoperative need for drainage tubes, surgical dressings, oxygen therapy, I.V. therapy, and pain control
- Complete a preoperative checklist, and obtain a signed informed consent
- Administer preoperative medications, as prescribed
- Allay the patient's and his family's anxiety about surgery
- Document the patient's history and physical assessment data
- Administer bowel preparation, as prescribed

● Postoperative nursing interventions
- Assess respiratory status and fluid balance
- Assess pain level, administer postoperative analgesics as prescribed, and evaluate effect
- Administer I.V. fluids, NG tube feedings, and transfusion therapy, as prescribed
- Allay the patient's anxiety and provide emotional support
- Provide wound care and dressing changes, as directed
- Encourage coughing, deep breathing, splinting of the incision, and use of incentive spirometry
- Place the patient in semi-Fowler's position
- Assess for the return of peristalsis
- Encourage activity, as tolerated
- Administer oxygen
- Monitor vital signs, I/O, laboratory studies, and pulse oximetry
- Monitor and maintain the position and patency of drainage tubes: NG, indwelling urinary catheter, wound drainage
- **Irrigate the NG tube only if ordered; don't reposition it; monitor drainage for signs of bleeding**
- Apply sequential compression devices while in bed
- Weigh the patient daily
- Individualize home care instructions
    – Know about the disorder and its treatment
    – Follow instructions for medication use, and be aware of possible adverse effects
    – Identify ways to reduce stress
    – Increase food intake gradually, and eat six small meals a day
    – Limit fluids with meals
    – Comply with medical follow-up

● Possible surgical complications
- Dumping syndrome after a partial gastrectomy
- Hemorrhage
- Dehydration
- Infection

- Dehiscence
- Evisceration

HEMORRHOIDECTOMY

- **Description**
  - Surgical removal of hemorrhoids by clamp, excision, or cautery
- **Preoperative nursing interventions**
  - Complete patient and family preoperative teaching
    - Explain the procedure to the patient
    - Describe the operating room, PACU, and preoperative and postoperative routines
    - Demonstrate postoperative turning, coughing, deep breathing, splinting, and ROM exercises
    - Explain the postoperative need for drainage tubes, surgical dressings, oxygen therapy, I.V. therapy, and pain control
  - Complete a preoperative checklist, and obtain a signed informed consent
  - Administer preoperative medications, as prescribed
  - Allay the patient's and his family's anxiety about surgery
  - Document the patient's history and physical assessment data
  - Administer bowel preparation, as prescribed
- **Postoperative nursing interventions**
  - Assess pain level, administer postoperative analgesics as prescribed, and evaluate effect
  - Assess for the return of peristalsis; give liquids, and advance diet as tolerated
  - Administer I.V. fluids
  - Allay the patient's anxiety and provide emotional support
  - Provide wound care and dressing changes, as directed
  - Encourage turning, coughing, deep breathing, and incentive spirometry
  - Keep the patient prone or on his side
  - Encourage activity, as tolerated
  - Monitor vital signs, I/O, and laboratory studies
  - Administer analgesics, stool softeners, or laxatives, as prescribed, before the first bowel movement
  - Provide sitz baths
  - Provide a flotation pad when sitting
  - Individualize home care instructions
    - Know about the disorder and its treatment
    - Follow instructions for medication use, and be aware of possible adverse effects
    - Avoid heavy lifting and prolonged standing or sitting
    - Perineal care
    - Anticipate a small amount of bleeding with bowel movements postoperatively

– Avoid Valsalva's maneuver
– Increase fluid and fiber intake
– Comply with medical follow-up

- **Possible surgical complications**
  - Rectal hemorrhage
  - Urine retention
  - Infection

BOWEL SURGERY

- **Description**
  - Abdominoperineal resection: removal of the distal sigmoid colon, rectum, and anus with the creation of a permanent colostomy (see *Reviewing types of ostomies*)
  - Colectomy: surgical excision of the right colon (right hemicolectomy) or left colon (left hemicolectomy)
  - Ileostomy: surgical opening of the ileum to the abdominal surface to form a stoma
  - Continent ileostomy: surgical creation of an intra-abdominal reservoir for stool
  - Bowel resection: surgical excision of a portion of the bowel
  - Permanent colostomy: surgical opening of the colon to the abdominal surface to form a single stoma after the distal portion of the bowel is removed
  - Loop colostomy: creation of proximal and distal stomas from a loop of intestine that has been pulled through an abdominal incision and supported with a plastic or glass rod
  - Double-barrel colostomy: surgical opening of the colon to the abdominal surface to form two stomas to prevent passage of stool into the distal bowel

- **Preoperative nursing interventions**
  - Complete patient and family preoperative teaching
    - Explain the procedure to the patient
    - Describe the operating room, PACU, and preoperative and postoperative routines
    - Demonstrate postoperative turning, coughing, deep breathing, splinting, and leg and ROM exercises; explain the need for early ambulation
    - Explain the postoperative need for drainage tubes, a gastrostomy feeding tube, surgical dressings, oxygen therapy, I.V. therapy, and pain control
  - Complete a preoperative checklist, and obtain a signed informed consent
  - Administer preoperative medications, as prescribed
  - Allay the patient's and his family's anxiety about surgery
  - Document the patient's history and physical assessment data
  - Administer bowel preparation, as prescribed
  - Arrange a preoperative visit with an enterostomal therapist

Types of bowel surgery

- Abdominoperineal resection
- Colectomy
- Ileostomy
- Continent ileostomy
- Bowel resection
- Permanent colostomy
- Loop colostomy
- Double-barrel colostomy

Key nursing interventions before bowel surgery

- Administer bowel preparation, as prescribed.
- Explain the postoperative need for drainage tubes, surgical dressings, and pain control.
- Arrange a preoperative visit with an enterostomal therapist.

Reviewing types of ostomies

The type of ostomy appropriate for a patient depends on the patient's condition. Temporary ones, such as a double-barrel or loop colostomy, help treat perforated sigmoid diverticulitis and other conditions in which intestinal healing is expected. Permanent colostomy or ileostomy accompanies extensive abdominal surgery such as the removal of a malignant tumor.

Types of ostomies

- Double-barrel colostomy: surgical opening of the colon to the abdominal surface to form two stomas to prevent passage of stool into the distal bowel
- Loop colostomy: creation of proximal and distal stomas from a loop of intestine that has been pulled through an abdominal incision and supported with a plastic or glass rod
- Permanent colostomy: surgical opening of the colon to the abdominal surface to form a single stoma after the distal portion of the bowel is removed
- Ileostomy: surgical opening of the ileum to the abdominal surface to form a stoma

DOUBLE-BARREL COLOSTOMY

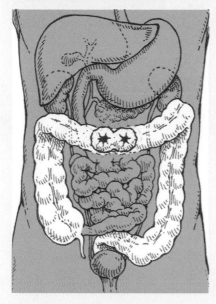

LOOP COLOSTOMY

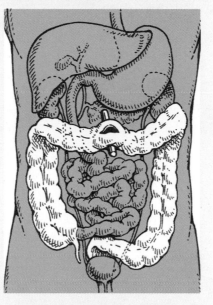

PERMANENT COLOSTOMY

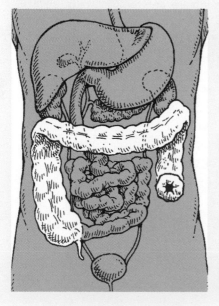

ILEOSTOMY

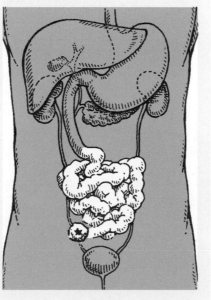

Key nursing interventions after bowel surgery

- Assess for the return of peristalsis; give solid foods and liquids, as tolerated.
- Monitor and maintain the position and patency of drainage tubes: NG, indwelling urinary catheter, wound drainage.
- Monitor and record the color, consistency, and amount of the patient's stool.
- Provide colostomy care.

- Encourage the patient to express his feelings about changes in his body image

● **Postoperative nursing interventions**
- Assess cardiac status and fluid balance
- Assess pain and administer postoperative analgesics, as prescribed
- Assess for the return of peristalsis before introducing clear liquids
- Administer I.V. fluids, TPN, and transfusion therapy, as prescribed
- Allay the patient's anxiety and provide emotional support
- Provide wound care and dressing changes, as directed
- Encourage coughing, deep breathing, incentive spirometry, and splinting of the incision
- Keep the patient in semi-Fowler's position
- Assist with ambulation, beginning in the first 24 hours
- Apply antiembolism or pneumatic stockings
- Monitor vital signs, I/O, laboratory studies, and pulse oximetry
- Monitor and maintain the position and patency of drainage tubes: NG, indwelling urinary catheter, wound drainage
- Encourage the patient to express his feelings about changes in his body function and image
- Monitor and record the color, consistency, and amount of the patient's stool
- Provide routine colostomy care
    - Prevent skin breakdown by thoroughly cleaning the skin around the stoma
    - Check the stoma for color and function
    - Change the ostomy bag as needed
- **Increase fluid intake to 3 qt (3 L)/day**
- Individualize home care instructions
    - Know about the disorder and its treatment
    - Follow instructions for medication use, and be aware of possible adverse effects
    - Recognize the signs and symptoms of intestinal obstruction
    - Check the condition of the stoma daily, and report bleeding and changes
    - Report changes in the consistency and color of stool
    - Perform colostomy and incision care daily
    - Avoid foods that cause flatus and irritability of the colon
    - Provide skin care around the stoma
    - Discuss concerns about sexual activities

● **Possible surgical complications**
- Infection
- Hemorrhage
- Dehiscence
- Evisceration
- Paralytic ileus
- Prolapsed stoma
- Abscess

HIATAL HERNIA

- **Definition**
  - Defect in the diaphragm that permits a portion of the stomach to pass through the diaphragmatic opening into the chest
  - Three types:
    - Sliding hernia
    - Paraesophageal hernia
    - Mixed hernia (see *Types of hiatal hernia,* page 240)
- **Causes**
  - Congenital weakness
  - Trauma
  - Increased abdominal pressure
- **Contributing factors**
  - Obesity
  - Pregnancy
  - Ascites
  - Aging
- **Pathophysiology**
  - The opening (hiatus) in the diaphragm where the esophagus enters the stomach becomes enlarged and weakened
  - The upper portion of the stomach enters the lower thorax
  - Sliding of the esophagus and stomach into the chest results in gastric acid reflux
- **Assessment findings**
  - Pyrosis
  - Dysphagia
  - Regurgitation
  - Sternal pain 1 to 4 hours after eating (heartburn), aggravated by reclining and belching
  - Vomiting
  - Feeling of fullness
  - Dyspnea
  - Cough
  - Tachycardia
  - Palpable bulge
- **Diagnostic test findings**
  - Esophagoscopy: incompetent cardiac sphincter
  - Barium swallow: protrusion of the hernia
  - Chest X-ray: protrusion of abdominal organs into the thorax
  - Gastric analysis: increased pH
  - Endoscopy: differentiates among hiatal hernia, varices, and other small gastroesophageal lesions

Key facts about hiatal hernia

- Protrusion of the stomach through the diaphragm into the thoracic cavity
- Sliding of the stomach into the chest results in gastric acid reflux

Common causes of hiatal hernia

- Congenital weakness
- Trauma
- Increased abdominal pressure

Key signs and symptoms of hiatal hernia

- Dysphagia
- Regurgitation
- Sternal pain after eating

Diagnosing hiatal hernia

- Esophagoscopy: incompetent cardiac sphincter
- Barium swallow: protrusion of the hernia

Types of hiatal hernia

- Sliding
- Paraesophageal (or rolling)

Types of hiatal hernia

These figures depict the normal stomach and the primary forms of hiatal hernia.

In a sliding hernia, both the stomach and the gastroesophageal junction slip up into the chest so that the gastroesophageal junction is above the diaphragmatic hiatus. This type of hernia causes symptoms if the lower esophageal sphincter (LES) is incompetent, which permits gastric reflux and heartburn.

In a paraesophageal (or rolling) hernia, a part of the greater curvature of the stomach rolls through the diaphragmatic defect. This type of hernia usually doesn't cause gastric reflux and heartburn because the closing mechanism of the LES is unaffected. However, it can cause displacement or stretching of the stomach or lead to strangulation of the herniated portion.

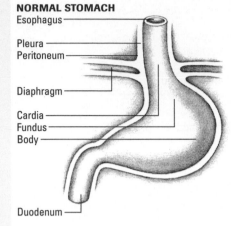

NORMAL STOMACH

Esophagus — Pleura — Peritoneum — Diaphragm — Cardia — Fundus — Body — Duodenum

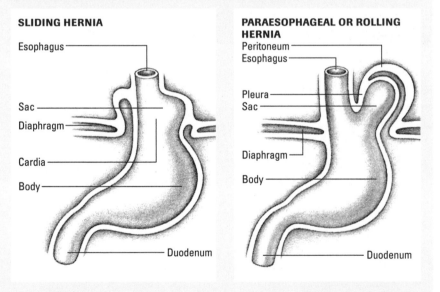

SLIDING HERNIA

Esophagus — Sac — Diaphragm — Cardia — Body — Duodenum

PARAESOPHAGEAL OR ROLLING HERNIA

Peritoneum — Esophagus — Pleura — Sac — Diaphragm — Body — Duodenum

Treating hiatal hernia

- Small, frequent meals
- Semi-Fowler's position
- H$_2$-receptor antagonists
- Proton pump inhibitor

Medical management

- Diet: small, frequent meals; avoidance of spicy or irritating foods
- Smoking cessation
- Position: semi-Fowler's during and after eating
- Activity: avoidance of activity that increases intra-abdominal pressure
- Monitoring: vital signs and I/O

TIME-OUT FOR TEACHING
Patients with GI disorders

Be sure to include these topics in your teaching plan for patients with GI disorders.

- Disorder and treatment plan
- Smoking cessation
- Stool monitoring, including color, amount, and consistency
- Glucose level monitoring
- Signs of hyperglycemia
- Weight maintenance program

- Medication therapy, including the action, adverse effects, and scheduling of medications
- Dietary recommendations and restrictions
- Rest and activity patterns
- Signs and symptoms of GI bleeding
- Self-monitoring for infection
- Relaxation techniques

- Cholinergic agent: bethanechol (Urecholine)
- Antacids: magnesium and aluminum hydroxide (Maalox), aluminum hydroxide gel (AlternaGEL)
- Histamine-2 (H$_2$) receptor antagonists: cimetidine (Tagamet), ranitidine (Zantac), famotidine (Pepcid), nizatidine (Axid)
- Proton pump inhibitor: omeprazole (Prilosec)
- Weight reduction, if indicated

● **Nursing interventions**
- Encourage small, frequent meals
- Assess respiratory status, and administer oxygen, if needed
- Keep the patient in semi-Fowler's position during and after meals
- Monitor and record vital signs, I/O, and daily weight
- Administer medications, as prescribed
- Allay the patient's anxiety through verbalization and medication
- Avoid flexion at the waist when positioning the patient
- Individualize home care instructions (for more information about teaching, see *Patients with GI disorders*)
  - Know about the disorder and its treatment
  - Eat small, frequent meals
  - Avoid spicy foods, alcohol, chocolate, peppermint, caffeine, and citrus foods
  - Remain upright for 2 hours after eating
  - Avoid wearing constrictive clothing
  - Avoid lifting, bending, straining, and coughing
  - Don't smoke
  - Lose weight (if indicated)

● **Complications**
- Hemorrhage
- Ulceration
- Aspiration

Key nursing interventions for a patient with hiatal hernia

- Assess respiratory status.
- Keep in semi-Fowler's position during and after meals.
- Administer medications.
- Provide home care instructions.

Key complications of hiatal hernia

- Esophagitis
- Ulceration

- Esophagitis
- Esophageal incarceration and strangulation
- Esophageal stricture
- **Surgical interventions**
  - Laparoscopy
  - Fundoplication

PEPTIC ULCER DISEASE

- **Definition**
  - Erosion of the mucosal or duodenal lining of the stomach
  - Peptic ulcer in the stomach is called a gastric ulcer; peptic ulcer in the duodenum is called a duodenal ulcer
- **Causes**
  - Severe physiologic stress
  - Drug-induced: salicylates, steroids, indomethacin, reserpine, nonsteroidal anti-inflammatory drugs (NSAIDs)
  - Gastritis
  - Zollinger-Ellison syndrome
  - Infection: *Helicobacter pylori*
  - Smoking and alcohol abuse (may be contributing factors)
- **Pathophysiology**
  - Increased emptying time of gastric acid from the gastric lumen into the small intestine causes an inflammatory reaction with tissue breakdown
  - Bile refluxes into the stomach if the pyloric valve is involved
  - Combination of hydrochloric acid and pepsin destroys gastric mucosa
  - Decreased resistance of gastric mucosa to action of hydrochloric acid
- **Assessment findings**
  - May be asymptomatic
  - Epigastric or upper abdominal pain that may worsen before or after eating or may occur in the early hours of the morning
  - Heartburn
  - Dyspepsia
  - Weight loss
  - Nausea and vomiting
  - Hematemesis
  - Melena
  - Anorexia
  - Relief from pain after administration of antacids
- **Diagnostic test findings**
  - Esophagogastroduodenoscopy (EGD): identifies ulcer
  - *H. pylori* test: positive
  - Hematology: decreased Hb, HCT, PT, and PTT
  - Gastric analysis: normal for gastric ulcer
  - Upper GI: location of the ulcer

- Barium swallow: ulceration of gastric mucosa
- Fecal occult blood: positive
- Serum gastrin: normal or increased (with Zollinger-Ellison syndrome)

● Medical management
- Diet: nothing by mouth if actively bleeding
- GI decompression: NG tube (with bleeding)
- Position: semi-Fowler's
- Monitoring: vital signs and I/O
- Smoking cessation
- Cessation of NSAIDs (if the cause)
- Triple therapy for *H. pylori* infection: amoxicillin, clarithromycin (Biaxin), and omeprazole (Prilosec)
- Laboratory studies: Hb and HCT
- Treatment: saline lavage by NG tube, if hemorrhaging
- Transfusion therapy: packed RBCs, if acute bleeding
- Anticholinergics (for duodenal ulcer): propantheline (Pro-Banthine), dicyclomine (Bentyl)
- For gastric and duodenal ulcers:
  - Antacids: magnesium and aluminum hydroxide (Maalox), aluminum hydroxide gel (AlternaGEL)
  - H_2-receptor antagonists: cimetidine (Tagamet), ranitidine (Zantac), nizatidine (Axid), famotidine (Pepcid)
  - Prostaglandin: misoprostol (Cytotec)
  - Mucosal barrier fortifier: sucralfate (Carafate)
- Endoscopic laser treatment or photocoagulation (for active bleeding)
- Hormone: vasopressin (Pitressin) for management of acute bleeding

● Nursing interventions
- Provide small, frequent meals, as tolerated
- Assess respiratory, GI, and cardiovascular status
- Maintain position, patency, and low suction of the NG tube if gastric decompression is ordered postoperatively
- Administer blood products as ordered
- Monitor and record vital signs, I/O, laboratory studies, and fecal occult blood
- Administer medications, as prescribed
- Allay the patient's anxiety and provide emotional support
- Minimize environmental stress and maintain a quiet environment
- Monitor the consistency, color, amount, and frequency of stools or emesis
- Apply sequential compression stockings while in bed
- Individualize home care instructions
  - Know about the disorder and its treatment
  - Follow instructions for medication use, and be aware of possible adverse effects
  - Identify ways to reduce stress
  - Avoid smoking
  - Comply with medical follow-up

Treating peptic ulcer disease
- Smoking cessation
- Endoscopic laser treatment or photocoagulation
- Triple therapy for *H. pylori* infection
- H_2-receptor antagonists
- Transfusion therapy, if acute bleeding

Key nursing interventions for a patient with peptic ulcer disease
- Assess respiratory, GI, and cardiovascular status.
- Maintain the position, patency, and low suction of the NG tube if gastric decompression is ordered.
- Monitor stools and emesis.
- Administer blood products as ordered.

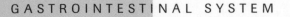

Key complications of peptic ulcer disease

- Hemorrhage
- Perforation

Key facts about gastric cancer

- Malignant stomach tumor
- May be primary or metastatic
- Usually develops in the distal third of the stomach
- Most common neoplasm is adenocarcinoma

Common causes of gastric cancer

- Unknown
- Risk factors: family history, smoking, gastritis

Key signs and symptoms of gastric cancer

- Nausea and vomiting
- Weight loss
- Epigastric fullness and pain
- Melena
- Anorexia

Diagnosing gastric cancer

- Gastroscopy: biopsy positive for cancer cells
- CEA: positive

- ● **Complications**
  - Hemorrhage
  - Perforation
  - Chemical peritonitis
  - Intestinal obstruction
- ● **Surgical interventions**
  - Vagotomy
  - Pyloroplasty
  - Gastrectomy

GASTRIC CANCER

- ● **Definition**
  - Malignant stomach tumor that's primary or metastatic
  - Most commonly affected areas are the pylores and the antrum
- ● **Cause**
  - Unknown
- ● **Risk factors**
  - High intake of salty and smoked foods
  - Family history
  - Smoking
  - High alcohol consumption
  - Type A blood
  - Gastritis with gastric atrophy
- ● **Pathophysiology**
  - Unregulated cell growth and uncontrolled cell division result in the development of a neoplasm
  - Tumor usually develops in the distal third of the stomach and metastasizes to the abdominal organs, lungs, and bones
  - Most common neoplasm is adenocarcinoma
- ● **Assessment findings**
  - Weakness and fatigue
  - Nausea and vomiting
  - Weight loss
  - Back, epigastric, or retrosternal pain not relieved with nonprescription medications
  - Vague feeling of fullness, heaviness, and moderate abdominal distention after meals
  - Dysphagia
  - Palpable mass
- ● **Diagnostic test findings**
  - CEA: positive
  - Hematology: decreased Hb and HCT; shortened or prolonged PT and PTT, depending on the location of the neoplasm

- Blood chemistry: increased AST, LD, and amylase
- GI series: gastric mass
- Gastroscopy: biopsy positive for cancer cells

Medical management
- Diet: based on condition; high-protein, high-calorie
- I.V. therapy for hydration
- GI decompression: NG tube postoperatively
- Activity: as tolerated
- Monitoring: vital signs and I/O
- Laboratory studies: Hb, HCT, and fecal occult blood
- Nutritional support: TPN and lipids
- Radiation therapy
- Antineoplastics: carmustine (BiCNU), 5-fluorouracil (Adrucil)
- Vitamin supplements: folic acid (Folvite), cyanocobalamin (vitamin B_{12})
- Analgesics: morphine (Roxanol), hydromorphone (Dilaudid)
- Antiemetic: ondansetron (Zofran)

Nursing interventions
- Monitor and record vital signs, I/O, laboratory studies, and daily weight
- Assess GI status
- Maintain position, patency, and low intermittent suction of the NG tube
- Keep the patient in semi-Fowler's position
- Administer medications, as prescribed
- Administer TPN and lipids until diet is resumed
- Encourage the patient to express his feelings about the diagnosis, and provide emotional support
- Monitor the color, consistency, amount, and frequency of stool and emesis
- Apply sequential compression stockings while in bed
- Assess pain level, administer analgesics as prescribed, and evaluate effect
- Provide postchemotherapeutic and postradiation nursing care
  - Provide prophylactic skin and mouth care
  - Administer antiemetics and antidiarrheals, as prescribed
  - Monitor for bleeding, infection, and electrolyte imbalance
  - Provide rest periods
- Provide information about the American Cancer Society
- Individualize home care instructions
  - Know about the disorder and its treatment
  - Follow instructions for medication use, and be aware of possible adverse effects
  - Avoid exposure to people with infections
  - Alternate rest periods with activity
  - Monitor self for signs and symptoms of infection
  - Recognize the signs and symptoms of ulceration
  - Complete skin care daily

Complications
- Intestinal obstruction

Treating gastric cancer
- Antineoplastics
- Gastric surgery
- Analgesics
- Radiation therapy

Key nursing interventions for a patient with gastric cancer
- Assess GI status.
- Assess pain level and administer analgesics
- Maintain the position, patency, and low intermittent suction of the NG tube.
- Monitor the consistency, amount, and frequency of stool.
- Provide postchemotherapeutic and postradiation nursing care.
- Provide home care instructions.

Key complications of gastric cancer
- Metastasis
- Intestinal obstruction
- Pneumonia

- Ulceration
- Metastasis
- Dumping syndrome
- Pneumonia
- Deep vein thrombosis (DVT)

● **Surgical interventions**
- Subtotal gastrectomy
- Total gastrectomy
- Gastroduodenostomy
- Gastrojejunostomy

ULCERATIVE COLITIS

● **Definition**
- Episodic inflammatory chronic disorder that causes ulceration of the mucosa of the colon

● **Causes**
- Unknown

● **Risk factors**
- Emotional stress
- Possible autoimmune disease
- Genetics
- Allergies

● **Pathophysiology**
- Inflammatory edema of the mucous membrane of the colon and rectum leads to bleeding and shallow ulcerations
- Abscess formation causes bowel-wall shortening, thinning, fragility, hypermotility, and decreased absorption
- Mucosal ulcerations begin in the distal end of the colon and ascend the large intestine

● **Assessment findings**
- Bloody, purulent, mucoid, watery stools (10 to 25/day)
- Abdominal tenderness and pain
- Weakness and fatigue
- Anorexia
- Nausea and vomiting
- Weight loss
- Abdominal cramping
- Tenesmus
- Abdominal distention
- Perianal irritation, hemorrhoids, and fissures
- Jaundice

Key facts about ulcerative colitis

- Inflammatory disorder of the large bowel
- Leads to bleeding and shallow ulcerations

Common causes of ulcerative colitis

- Unknown
- Risk factors: automimmune disease, genetics, allergies

Key signs and symptoms of ulcerative colitis

- Abdominal tenderness and pain
- Abdominal cramping
- Bloody, purulent, mucoid, watery stools (10 to 25/day)
- Hyperactive bowel sounds

Diagnostic test findings
- Sigmoidoscopy: increased mucosal friability, decreased mucosal detail, thick inflammatory exudate, edema, and erosion
- Blood chemistry: decreased potassium and magnesium
- Hematology: decreased Hb and HCT
- Stool specimen: positive for blood and mucus
- Biopsy: confirms diagnosis

Medical management
- Diet:
  - High-protein, high-calorie, low-residue; bland foods in small, frequent feedings with restricted intake of milk and gas-forming foods
  - No food and fluids, if severe
- I.V. therapy: hydration, electrolyte replacement
- Transfusion therapy: packed RBCs
- Position: semi-Fowler's
- Monitoring: vital signs, I/O, daily weight, calorie count, and stools for occult blood
- Laboratory studies: Hb, HCT, electrolytes, magnesium
- Nutritional support: TPN
- 5-Aminosalicylic agents: sulfasalazine (Azulfidine), mesalamine (Asacol)
- Tumor necrosis factor inhibitor: infliximab (Remicade)
- Corticosteroid: prednisone (Deltasone)
- Antiemetic: ondansetron (Zofran)
- Immunosuppressive agents: azathioprine (Imuran), cyclosporine (Sandimmune)
- Antimicrobials: ciprofloxacin (Cipro), metronidazole (Flagyl)
- Vitamin, mineral, and iron supplements
- Potassium supplements: potassium chloride (K-Lor), potassium gluconate (Kaon)

Nursing interventions
- Maintain the patient's diet; withhold food and fluids as needed
- Administer I.V. fluids, TPN, and transfusion therapy
- Assess GI status and fluid balance
- Keep the patient in semi-Fowler's position
- Monitor and record vital signs, I/O, laboratory studies, daily weight, calorie count, and fecal occult blood
- Administer medications, as prescribed
- Allay the patient's anxiety and provide emotional support
- Maintain bed rest and turn the patient every 2 hours (with severe episodes)
- Minimize environmental stress and maintain a quiet environment
- Provide rest periods
- Promote independence in activities of daily living (ADLs)
- Monitor the number, amount, and character of stools
- Assess perineal excoriation, and provide perianal care and sitz baths

Diagnosing ulcerative colitis
- Sigmoidoscopy: increased mucosal friability, decreased mucosal detail, thick inflammatory exudate, edema, and erosion
- Biopsy: confirms diagnosis

Treating ulcerative colitis
- Immunosuppressive agents
- 5-Aminosalicylic agents
- Tumor necrosis factor inhibitor
- Corticosteroids

Key nursing interventions for a patient with ulcerative colitis
- Assess GI status and fluid balance.
- Administer TPN.
- Monitor the number, amount, and character of stools.
- Provide information about the United Ostomy Association and the National Foundation of Ileitis and Colitis.

Key complications of ulcerative colitis

- Toxic megacolon
- GI obstruction
- Depression

- Provide information about the United Ostomy Association and the National Foundation of Ileitis and Colitis
- Individualize home care instructions
  - Know about the disorder and its treatment
  - Follow instructions for medication use, and be aware of possible adverse effects
  - Maintain a normal weight
  - Identify ways to reduce stress
  - Recognize the signs and symptoms of rectal hemorrhage and intestinal obstruction
  - Complete sitz baths and perianal care daily
  - Avoid highly seasoned foods, raw fruits and vegetables, and milk products

● **Complications**
- Anemia
- Malnutrition
- GI perforation
- Toxic megacolon
- GI obstruction
- Hemorrhage
- Depression

● **Surgical interventions**
- Ileostomy
- Total colectomy

CROHN'S DISEASE (REGIONAL ENTERITIS)

Key facts about Crohn's disease

- Chronic inflammatory bowel disease
- Usually affects the terminal ileum
- Extends through all layers of the intestinal wall

● **Definition**
- Chronic inflammatory bowel disease that may affect any part of the GI tract but commonly involves the terminal ileum
- Extends through all layers of the intestinal wall; may involve regional lymph nodes and mesentery

● **Cause**
- Unknown

● **Risk factors**
- Allergies
- Immune disorder
- Genetics

Common causes of Crohn's disease

- Unknown
- Risk factors: allergies, immune disorder, genetics

● **Pathophysiology**
- Ulcerations of intestinal mucosa are accompanied by congestion, thickening of the small bowel, and fissure formations (see *Bowel changes in Crohn's disease*)
- Enlarged regional mesenteric lymph nodes accompany fibrosis and narrowing of the intestinal wall

Bowel changes in Crohn's disease

As Crohn's disease progresses, fibrosis thickens the bowel wall and narrows the lumen. Narrowing—or stenosis—can occur in any part of the intestine and cause varying degrees of intestinal obstruction. At first, the mucosa may appear normal, but as the disease progresses, it takes on a "cobblestone" appearance, as shown.

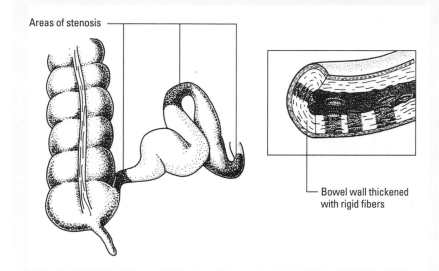

Areas of stenosis

Bowel wall thickened with rigid fibers

Assessment findings
- Fatigue and weakness
- Crampy, colicky pain in the right lower quadrant
- Mesenteric lymphadenitis
- Nausea
- Flatulence
- Weight loss
- Elevated temperature
- Chronic diarrhea; possible bloody stools
- Borborygmus

Diagnostic test findings
- Abdominal X-ray: congested, thickened, fibrosed, and narrowed intestinal wall
- Colonoscopy: patchy areas of inflammation and characteristic coarse irregularity ("cobblestone" appearance) of the mucosal surface
- Fecal occult blood: positive
- Fecal fat test: increased
- Barium enema: the classic "string sign" at the terminal ileum
- WBC count: elevated

Medical management
- Diet:

Bowel changes in Crohn's disease
- Thickening of the bowel wall and narrowing of the lumen can cause varying degrees of intestinal obstruction
- "Cobblestone" appearance of the intestinal mucosa

Key signs and symptoms of Crohn's disease
- Crampy, colicky pain in the right lower quadrant
- Chronic diarrhea
- Borborygmus

Diagnosing Crohn's disease
- Abdominal X-ray: congested, thickened, fibrosed, and narrowed intestinal wall
- Barium enema: classic "string sign" at the terminal ileum
- Colonoscopy: patchy areas of inflammation, characteristic coarse irregularity of the mucosal surface

Treating Crohn's disease

- Avoidance of dietary irritants
- 5-Aminosalicyclic acids
- Tumor necrosis factor inhibitor
- Anticholinergics
- Corticosteroids
- Antidiarrheal
- Anti-inflammatory agent
- Immunosuppressants

Key nursing interventions for a patient with Crohn's disease

- Assess GI status and fluid balance.
- Minimize stress and encourage expression of feelings.
- Monitor the number, amount, and character of stools.
- Provide home care instructions.

Key complications of Crohn's disease

- Intestinal obstruction
- Perianal abscess

    – Small, frequent feedings; avoidance of dietary irritants, such as raw fruits and vegetables, milk, and gas-forming foods

    – No food and fluids, if severe

- I.V. therapy: hydration, electrolyte replacement
- Activity: as tolerated
- Monitoring: vital signs, I/O, daily weight, and stools for occult blood
- Laboratory studies: electrolytes, Hb, HCT
- Nutritional support: TPN, if severe
- 5-Aminosalicylic acids: sulfasalazine (Azulfidine), mesalamine (Asacol)
- Tumor necrosis factor inhibitor: infliximab (Remicade)
- Anticholinergics: propantheline (Pro-Banthine), dicyclomine (Bentyl)
- Antidiarrheal: diphenoxylate (Lomotil)
- Vitamin, mineral, and iron supplements
- Potassium supplements: potassium chloride (K-Lor), potassium gluconate (Kaon)
- Anti-inflammatory: prednisone (Deltasone)
- Antimicrobial: metronidazole (Flagyl)
- Immunosuppressant: azathioprine (Imuran)

● **Nursing interventions**

- Maintain the patient's diet; withhold food and fluids as needed
- Assess GI status and fluid and electrolyte balance
- Monitor and record vital signs, I/O, laboratory studies, daily weight, urine specific gravity, and fecal occult blood
- **Monitor the number, amount, and character of stools**
- Administer TPN and lipids
- Administer medications, as prescribed
- Allay the patient's anxiety and provide emotional support
- Provide skin and perianal care
- Minimize the patient's stress, and encourage expression of his feelings
- Maintain a quiet environment
- Promote independence in ADLs
- Individualize home care instructions
  - Know about the disorder and its treatment
  - Follow instructions for medication use, and be aware of possible adverse effects
  - Avoid laxatives and aspirin
  - Complete perianal care daily
  - Identify ways to reduce stress
  - Recognize the signs and symptoms of rectal hemorrhage and intestinal obstruction
  - Comply with medical follow-up

● **Complications**

- Intestinal obstruction
- Anal fistulas
- Intestinal perforation
- Perianal abscess

- Malnutrition
- Malabsorption syndrome
- **Surgical interventions**
  - Bowel resection with anastomosis
  - Ileoanal reservoir
  - Colectomy with ileostomy

DIVERTICULAR DISEASE

- **Definition**
  - Diverticula: outpouching of intestinal mucosa through the muscular wall of the intestine
  - Diverticulosis: diverticula are present but asymptomatic
  - Diverticulitis: inflammation of diverticula
  - Typical sites: sigmoid colon, duodenum near the pancreatic border or the ampulla of Vater, jejunum
  - Diverticular disease of the ileum (Meckel's diverticulum) is the most common congenital anomaly of the GI tract (see *Meckel's diverticulum,* page 252)
- **Causes**
  - Diminished colonic motility and increased intralumenal pressure
  - Defects of the intestinal wall
- **Risk factors**
  - Low intake of roughage and fiber
  - Age
- **Pathophysiology**
  - Muscle tone is weakened in the intestinal wall, resulting in a saclike outpouching (diverticula)
  - Inflammation (diverticulitis) is caused by bacteria and fecal material trapped in the diverticula
  - Intestinal wall thickens and narrows
- **Assessment findings**
  - Diverticulosis
    - Asymptomatic
  - Diverticulitis
    - Left lower quadrant pain
    - Constipation and diarrhea
    - Severe abdominal cramping
    - Bloody stools
    - Low-grade fever
    - Rectal bleeding
    - Change in bowel pattern
    - Flatulence
    - Nausea

Key facts about diverticular disease

- Diverticula—outpouching of intestinal mucosa through the muscular wall of the intestine
- Diverticulosis—diverticula are present but asymptomatic
- Diverticulitis—inflammation of diverticula

Common causes of diverticular disease

- Diminished colonic motility and increased intralumenal pressure
- Congenital defects of the intestinal wall

Key signs and symptoms of diverticular disease

- Left lower quadrant pain
- Severe abdominal cramping
- Change in bowel pattern

Meckel's diverticulum

Meckel's diverticulum is a congenital abnormality that occurs when a blind tube like the appendix opens into the distal ileum near the ileocecal valve. This disorder results when the intra-abdominal portion of the yolk sac fails to close completely during fetal development. It occurs in about 2% of the population, mostly in males.

COMPLICATIONS

Uncomplicated Meckel's diverticulum produces no symptoms, but complications cause melena and abdominal pain, especially around the umbilicus. The lining of the diverticulum may be either gastric mucosa or pancreatic tissue. This disorder can lead to peptic ulceration, perforation, and peritonitis and may resemble acute appendicitis.

Meckel's diverticulum can also cause bowel obstruction when a fibrous band that connects the diverticulum to the abdominal wall, the mesentery, or other structures snares a loop of the intestine. This can cause intussusception into the diverticulum or volvulus near the diverticular attachment to the back of the umbilicus or another intra-abdominal structure.

Meckel's diverticulum should be considered in patients with GI obstruction or hemorrhage, especially when routine GI X-rays are negative.

TREATMENT

Treatment involves surgical resection of the inflamed bowel and antibiotic therapy, if infection occurs.

Key facts about Meckel's diverticulum

- Congenital abnormality
- Incomplete closure of the intra-abdominal portion of the yolk sac
- Complications: peptic ulceration, perforation, peritonitis
- Treatment: surgery

Diagnosing diverticular disease

- CT of the abdomen
- Sigmoidoscopy

Treating diverticular disease

- High-fiber, low-fat diet; avoid foods with seeds, kernels, or indigestible roughage
- Antibiotics
- Analgesic

- **Diagnostic test findings**
  - Computed tomography (CT) scan of the abdomen: diverticula, thickened wall, presence of abscess
  - Sigmoidoscopy (contraindicated during an acute episode): diverticula, thickened wall, inflamed mucosa
  - Barium enema (contraindicated in acute diverticulitis): inflammation, narrow lumen of the bowel, diverticula
  - Hematology: increased WBCs and erythrocyte sedimentation rate (ESR)
  - Stool for occult blood: positive

- **Medical management**
  - Diet:
    - High-fiber, low-fat; avoid foods with seeds, kernels or indigestible roughage
    - Liquid (with mild diverticulitis)
    - Withhold food and fluids (with acute diverticulitis)
  - I.V. therapy: fluids if dehydrated or not permitted oral intake
  - Position: semi-Fowler's
  - Activity: bed rest, active ROM and isometric exercises (during an acute episode)
  - Monitoring: vital signs and I/O
  - Laboratory studies: Hb, HCT, and WBCs
  - Nutritional support: TPN (if a prolonged episode)
  - Analgesic: morphine
  - Antibiotics: ciprofloxacin (Cipro), metronidazole (Flagyl), ampicillin/sulbactam (Unasyn)
  - Stool softener: docusate (Colace)

- **Nursing interventions**
  - Monitor and record vital signs, I/O, and laboratory studies
  - Assess GI status, abdominal distention, and pain
  - Administer medications, as prescribed
  - Maintain the patient's diet and encourage fluids, if not contraindicated
  - Keep the patient in semi-Fowler's position
  - Administer I.V. fluids or TPN
  - Assess pain level, administer analgesics as prescribed, and evaluate effect
  - Allay the patient's anxiety through verbalization and medication
  - Provide rest periods
  - Monitor the stool for occult blood
  - Provide preoperative and postoperative care as appropriate
  - Individualize home care instructions
    - Know about the disorder and its treatment
    - Follow instructions for medication use, and be aware of possible adverse effects
    - Identify ways to decrease constipation
    - Follow dietary recommendations and restrictions; avoid corn, nuts, and fruits and vegetables with seeds; increase fluid intake
    - Monitor stools for bleeding

- **Complications**
  - Bowel perforation
  - Peritonitis
  - Abscess
  - Fistula
  - Hemorrhage
  - Intestinal obstruction

- **Surgical intervention**
  - Bowel resection

INTESTINAL OBSTRUCTION

- **Definition**
  - Partial or complete blockage of the intestinal lumen
  - Three forms: simple, strangulated, close-looped
  - Medical emergency

- **Causes**
  - Adhesions
  - Strangulated hernias
  - Tumors
  - Fecal impaction
  - Mesenteric thrombosis
  - Paralytic ileus
  - Volvulus
  - Neurogenic abnormalities
  - Toxicity

Key nursing interventions for a patient with diverticular disease

- Assess abdominal distention.
- Monitor stools for occult blood.
- Assess bowel sounds.

Key complications of diverticular disease

- Intestinal obstruction
- Bowel perforation

Key facts about intestinal obstruction

- Partial or complete blockage of the intestinal lumen
- Medical emergency

Common causes of intestinal obstruction

- Strangulated hernias
- Tumors
- Fecal impaction

Key signs and symptoms of intestinal obstruction

- Abdominal cramping pain
- Abdominal distention
- Vomiting bile
- Absent bowel sounds below the obstruction

Diagnosing intestinal obstruction

- CT scan: identifies level and type of obstruction
- Barium enema: stops at the obstruction
- Abdominal X-rays: increased amount of gas in the bowel, "step ladder" pattern

Treating intestinal obstruction

- GI decompression
- Withhold food and fluids
- I.V. therapy and TPN

- Intussusception
- Foreign body

● Pathophysiology
- Gas, fluid, and digested substances accumulate proximal to the obstruction
- Fluids and gases cause bowel distention
- Peristalsis increases proximal to the obstruction
- Water and electrolytes are secreted into the blocked bowel
- Bowel inflammation increases, and absorption by bowel mucosa is inhibited
- Fluid loss results in dehydration

● Assessment findings
- Abdominal cramping pain
- Nausea
- Abdominal distention
- Vomiting green-colored bile
- Constipation
- Singultus
- Elevated temperature
- Absent bowel sounds below the obstruction; high-pitched bowel sounds above the obstruction
- Weight loss

● Diagnostic test findings
- CT scan of abdomen: identifies level and type of obstruction
- Blood chemistry: decreased sodium, potassium, and chloride
- Hematology: increased WBCs
- Barium enema: stops at obstruction
- Abdominal X-rays: increased amount of gas in the bowel; shows "step ladder" pattern (with small-bowel obstruction)

● Medical management
- Diet: withhold food and fluids until the obstruction is relieved; then high-fiber
- I.V. therapy: electrolyte replacement, hydration, TPN
- GI decompression: NG tube
- Position: semi-Fowler's
- Activity: bed rest
- Monitoring: vital signs and I/O
- Laboratory studies: electrolytes, complete blood count
- Antibiotics: cefazolin (Ancef), cefoxitin (Mefoxin)
- Analgesics: morphine
- Antiemetics: promethazine (Phenergan), ondansetron (Zofran)
- Anticoagulation: low-molecular-weight heparin
- Sequential compression stockings while in bed

● Nursing interventions
- Assess GI status; notify the physician of absent bowel sounds
- Measure and record the patient's abdominal girth

- Monitor and record the frequency, color, and amount of stools
- Monitor and record vital signs, I/O, and laboratory studies
- Administer medications, as prescribed
- Withhold food and fluids
- Administer I.V. fluids and TPN
- Maintain the position, patency, and low suction of the NG or Miller-Abbott tube
- Place the patient in semi-Fowler's position
- Use sequential compression stockings or administer low-molecular-weight heparin while on bed rest
- Encourage incentive spirometry
- Allay the patient's anxiety through verbalization and medication
- Provide nares and mouth care
- Provide preoperative and postoperative care as indicated
- Provide information about the American Ostomy Association
- Individualize home care instructions
  - Know about the disorder and its treatment
  - Follow instructions for medication use, and be aware of possible adverse effects
  - Avoid constipating foods
  - Monitor the frequency and color of stools
  - Recognize the signs and symptoms of obstruction

● **Complications**
  - Peritonitis
  - Strangulation or perforation of the bowel
  - Infection
  - Sepsis
  - Metabolic alkalosis or acidosis
  - Death

● **Surgical interventions**
  - Bowel resection
  - Colostomy

PERITONITIS

● **Definition**
  - Localized or generalized inflammation of the peritoneal cavity

● **Causes**
  - Bacterial infection
  - Chemical inflammation
  - Pancreatitis
  - Blunt or penetrating trauma
  - Inflammation of the colon or kidneys
  - Volvulus
  - Ruptured ectopic pregnancy

Key nursing interventions for a patient with an intestinal obstruction

- Administer I.V. fluids.
- Assess GI status.
- Measure and record the patient's abdominal girth.
- Maintain the position, patency, and low suction of the NG tube.

Key complications of intestinal obstruction

- Strangulation or perforation of the bowel
- Metabolic alkalosis or acidosis

Key facts about peritonitis

- Inflammation of the peritoneal cavity
- May be localized or generalized

Common causes of peritonitis

- Bacterial infection
- Pancreatitis
- Blunt or penetrating trauma
- Inflammation of the colon or kidneys
- Volvulus

Key signs and symptoms of peritonitis

- Constant, diffuse, and intense abdominal pain
- Rebound tenderness
- Elevated temperature
- Abdominal rigidity and distention
- Weak, rapid pulse
- Decreased or absent bowel sounds

Diagnosing peritonitis

- Abdominal X-ray: free air in the abdomen

Treating peritonitis

- Diet: withhold food and fluids
- I.V. therapy: hydration, electrolyte replacement
- GI decompression: NG tube
- Antibiotics

- Biliary tract disease with ascites
- Intestinal perforation
- Fistula
- Percutaneous endoscopic gastrotomy (PEG) tube displacement

● **Pathophysiology**
- Peritoneal irritants cause inflammatory edema, vascular congestion, and hypermotility of the bowel
- Movement of extracellular fluid into the peritoneal cavity leads to hypovolemia and decreased urine output

● **Assessment findings**
- Constant, diffuse, and intense abdominal pain
- Rebound tenderness
- Malaise
- Nausea
- Elevated temperature
- Abdominal rigidity and distention
- Anorexia
- Decreased urine output
- Shallow respirations
- Weak, rapid pulse
- Decreased or absent bowel sounds
- Abdominal resonance and tympany on percussion

● **Diagnostic test findings**
- Hematology: increased WBCs and HCT
- Peritoneal aspiration: positive for blood, pus, bile, bacteria, or amylase
- Abdominal X-ray: free air in the abdomen under the diaphragm

● **Medical management**
- Diet: withhold food and fluids
- Oxygen therapy, if distressed
- I.V. therapy: hydration, electrolyte replacement
- GI decompression: NG tube
- Position: semi-Fowler's
- Activity: bed rest until condition improves
- Monitoring: vital signs, I/O, CVP, and pulse oximetry
- Laboratory studies: Hb, HCT, potassium, sodium, calcium, osmolality, and WBCs
- Nutritional support: TPN
- Treatments: indwelling urinary catheter, incentive spirometry
- Antibiotics: gentamicin (Garamycin), clindamycin (Cleocin), cephalothin (Keflin), ampicillin or sulbactam (Unasyn)
- Analgesic: morphine
- Anticoagulant: low-molecular-weight heparin
- Sequential compression stockings while in bed

Nursing interventions
- Withhold food and fluids
- Administer I.V. fluids or TPN as ordered
- Encourage turning, coughing, deep breathing, and incentive spirometry
- Assess respiratory status and fluid balance
- Maintain the position, patency, and low suction of the NG tube
- Keep the patient in semi-Fowler's position
- Apply sequential compression stockings while in bed
- Monitor and record vital signs, I/O, laboratory studies, CVP, daily weight, and pulse oximetry
- Administer medications, as prescribed
- Allay the patient's anxiety and provide emotional support
- Provide nares and mouth care
- Reposition the patient every 2 hours, and encourage ambulation as soon as able
- Assess pain level, administer analgesics as prescribed, and evaluate effect
- Assess bowel sounds, and measure and record the patient's abdominal girth
- Avoid giving the patient laxatives
- Individualize home care instructions
    - Know about the disorder and its treatment
    - Follow instructions for medication use, and be aware of possible adverse effects
    - Recognize the signs and symptoms of infection
    - Monitor temperature daily
    - Recognize the signs and symptoms of GI obstruction
    - Comply with medical follow-up

Complications
- Adhesions
- Abscesses
- Intestinal obstruction
- Septic shock
- Respiratory failure

Surgical interventions
- Exploratory laparotomy
- Bowel resection
- Incision and drainage of abscess
- Closure of the perforation

HEMORRHOIDS

Definition
- Cluster of vascular tissue, smooth muscle, and connective tissue found in the superior or inferior hemorrhoidal venous plexus

- Classified as first, second, third, or fourth degree, based on severity
- May be internal or external

● **Causes**
- Chronic constipation
- Prolonged sitting or standing
- Straining at defecation
- Pregnancy
- Heavy lifting
- Portal hypertension
- Obesity

● **Pathophysiology**
- Increased abdominal pressure impairs blood flow through the hemorrhoidal venous plexus
- Decreased blood flow causes dilation and congestion of the vessels of the rectum and anus

● **Assessment findings**
- Anal pain with defecation, sitting, or walking
- Anal pruritus
- Prolapse of rectal mucosa
- Rectal mucus discharge
- Bleeding after defecation

● **Diagnostic test findings**
- Digital examination: hemorrhoids
- Anascopy: internal hemorrhoids

● **Medical management**
- Diet: high-fiber, low-roughage, with increased fluid intake
- Position: side-lying or prone
- Activity: avoidance of prolonged sitting
- Monitoring: vital signs, frequency of stools
- Laboratory studies: Hb and HCT
- Treatments: witch hazel compresses, sitz baths or tub baths
- Topical corticosteroid: hydrocortisone (Corticaine)
- Analgesic: acetaminophen (Tylenol)
- Stool softener: docusate (Colace)
- Anesthetic: lidocaine (Xylocaine)
- Laxative: magnesium hydroxide (milk of magnesia)
- Cryodestruction
- Injection sclerotherapy

● **Nursing interventions**
- Encourage increased fluids
- Assess bowel elimination and rectal bleeding
- Position the patient on his side or prone while in bed
- Encourage ambulation
- Monitor and record vital signs, I/O, and laboratory studies

- Administer medications, as prescribed
- Provide perineal care
- Administer sitz baths and witch hazel compresses for comfort
- Individualize home care instructions
  - Know about the disorder and its treatment
  - Follow instructions for medication use, and be aware of possible adverse effects
  - Use sitz baths and witch hazel compresses for comfort
  - Defecate when the urge is felt
  - Increase fluid and fiber intake to avoid constipation
  - Complete perineal care daily
  - Avoid prolonged sitting or standing
  - Avoid heavy lifting
  - Recognize the signs and symptoms of rectal bleeding
  - Comply with medical follow-up

Complications
- Infection
- Constipation
- Thrombosis of hemorrhoids

Surgical interventions
- Stapled hemorrhoid surgery
- Barron rubber-band ligation

COLORECTAL CANCER

Definition
- Malignant tumor of the colon or rectum that's primary or metastatic

Causes
- Unknown

Risk factors
- Digestive tract disorders
- Familial polyposis
- Aging (older than age 40)
- Low-fiber, high-protein diet
- Family history of colon cancer
- Excessive intake of saturated animal fat

Pathophysiology
- Unregulated cell growth and uncontrolled cell division result in the development of a neoplasm
- Metastasis commonly occurs in the liver
- Adenocarcinomas occur in the colon, rectum, jejunum, and duodenum
- Adenocarcinomas infiltrate and cause obstruction, ulcerations, and hemorrhage

Key signs and symptoms of colorectal cancer

- Rectal bleeding
- Change in bowel pattern

Diagnosing colorectal cancer

- Fecal occult blood: positive
- Sigmoidoscopy or colonoscopy: identification and location of the mass

Treating colorectal cancer

- Radiation therapy
- Antineoplastics
- Surgery
- Analgesics

Key nursing interventions for a patient with colorectal cancer

- Encourage the patient to express his feelings about his diagnosis; provide emotional support.
- Provide postchemotherapeutic and postradiation nursing care.
- Provide information about the United Ostomy Association and the American Cancer Society.

● **Assessment findings**
- Abdominal cramps and distention
- Change in bowel pattern
- Abnormal bowel sounds
- Abdominal tenderness
- Weakness
- Pallor
- Weight loss
- Anorexia
- Change in the shape of stool
- Rectal bleeding
- Fecal oozing
- Palpable mass
- Melena
- Vomiting

● **Diagnostic test findings**
- Fecal occult blood: positive
- Sigmoidoscopy or colonoscopy: identification and location of the mass
- Barium enema: location of the mass
- Biopsy: cytology positive for cancer cells
- CEA: positive

● **Medical management**
- Diet: high-fiber, low-fat, low–refined carbohydrate
- I.V. therapy: hydration
- Position: semi-Fowler's
- Activity: as tolerated
- Sequential compression stockings while in bed
- Monitoring: vital signs and I/O
- Laboratory studies: Hb and HCT
- Nutritional support: TPN
- Analgesics: morphine, hydromorphone (Dilaudid)
- Radiation therapy
- Cytotoxics: doxorubicin (Adriamycin), 5-fluorouracil (Adrucil), leucovorin (citrovorum factor)
- Monoclonal antibiotic therapy: bevacizumab (Avastin), cetuximab (Erbitux)
- Antiemetic: ondansetron (Zofran)
- Anticoagulant: low-molecular-weight heparin

● **Nursing interventions**
- Maintain the patient's diet, as tolerated
- Place the patient in semi-Fowler's position
- Apply sequential compression stockings while in bed
- Monitor and record vital signs, I/O, laboratory studies, and daily weight
- Administer I.V. fluids or TPN
- Administer medications, as prescribed

- Encourage the patient to express his feelings about his diagnosis; provide emotional support
- Monitor and record the color, consistency, amount, and frequency of stools
- Assess for signs and symptoms of intestinal obstruction and rectal bleeding
- Provide postchemotherapeutic and postradiation nursing care
  - Provide prophylactic skin and mouth care
  - Monitor dietary intake
  - Administer antiemetics and antidiarrheals, as prescribed
  - Monitor for bleeding, infection, and electrolyte imbalance
  - Provide rest periods
- Individualize home care instructions
  - Know about the disorder and its treatment
  - Follow instructions for medication use, and be aware of possible adverse effects
  - Monitor changes in bowel elimination
  - Monitor self for infection
  - Alternate rest periods with activity
  - Comply with medical follow-up
- Provide information about the United Ostomy Association and the American Cancer Society

● **Complications**
- Anemia
- Hemorrhage
- Intestinal obstruction
- Infection

● **Surgical interventions**
- Abdominoperincal resection with colostomy
- Bowel resection or right hemicolectomy
- Anterior or low anterior resection

CHOLECYSTITIS AND CHOLELITHIASIS

● **Definition**
- Cholecystitis: acute or chronic inflammation of the gallbladder
- Cholelithiasis: stones or calculi in the gallbladder

● **Causes**
- Infection of the gallbladder, estrogen therapy, trauma, reduced blood supply to the gallbladder, prolonged immobility, chronic dieting, prolonged anesthesia, opioid abuse (cholecystitis)
- Cholesterol, bile pigment, calcium stones (cholelithiasis)

● **Pathophysiology**
- Inflamed gallbladder can't contract in response to fatty foods entering the duodenum because of obstruction by calculi or edema (see *Common sites of calculi formation,* page 262)
- Inability to constrict causes pain

Key complications of colorectal cancer

- Infection
- Intestinal obstruction

Key facts about cholecystitis and cholelithiasis

- Inflammation of the gallbladder
- Stones or calculi in the gallbladder
- May be acute or chronic

Common causes of cholecystitis

- Infection of the gallbladder
- Reduced blood supply to the gallbladder
- Chronic dieting

Sites of calculi formation

- Liver
- Small bile duct
- Hepatic duct
- Cystic duct
- Pancreas
- Common bile duct
- Pancreatic ducts
- Greater duodenal papilla
- Gallbladder
- Duodenum

Key signs and symptoms of cholecystitis and cholelithiasis

- Indigestion or chest pain after eating fatty or fried foods
- Episodic colicky pain in epigastric area, which radiates to the back and right shoulder
- Jaundice
- Murphy's sign

Common sites of calculi formation

The illustration below shows sites where calculi typically collect. Stones vary in size; small stones may travel.

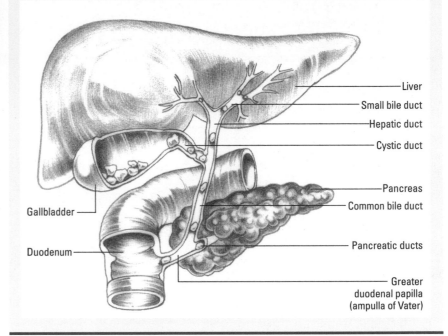

Liver

Small bile duct

Hepatic duct

Cystic duct

Pancreas

Common bile duct

Gallbladder

Pancreatic ducts

Duodenum

Greater duodenal papilla (ampulla of Vater)

- Accumulated bile is absorbed into the blood

● **Assessment findings**
- Severe right upper quadrant pain
- Indigestion or chest pain after eating fatty or fried foods or after fasting for an extended time
- Episodic colicky pain in the epigastric area, which radiates to the back and right shoulder
- Jaundice
- Nausea, vomiting, and chills
- Low-grade fever
- Flatulence
- Belching
- Clay-colored stools
- Dark amber urine
- Pruritus
- Steatorrhea
- Murphy's sign (with cholecystitis) (tenderness over the right upper quadrant that increases on inspiration)

● **Diagnostic test findings**
- Cholangiogram: stones in the biliary tree

- Gallbladder series: stones in the biliary tree
- Ultrasound: bile duct distention and calculi
- Percutaneous transhepatic cholangiography: calculi in the ducts
- Blood chemistry: increased alkaline phosphatase, bilirubin, direct bilirubin transaminase, amylase, lipase, AST, and LD (with common bile duct obstruction)
- Hematology: increased WBCs
- ERCP: narrowing of the bile ducts or identification of bile stones

● Medical management
- Diet:
  - Low-fat, in small, frequent feedings
  - No food and fluids if surgery is indicated
- I.V. therapy: hydration, electrolyte replacement
- Position: semi-Fowler's
- Activity: as tolerated
- Monitoring: vital signs, I/O, and wound and drainage after surgery
- Laboratory studies: amylase, lipase, bilirubin, alkaline phosphatase, and WBCs
- Treatments: incentive spirometry, tepid baths without soap
- Antibiotics: ampicillin/sulbactam (Unasyn), levofloxacin (Levaquin)
- Analgesics: meperidine (Demerol), morphine
- Antiemetics: prochlorperazine (Compazine), promethazine (Phenergan)
- Antipruritic: diphenhydramine (Benadryl)
- Bile salts: ursodiol (URSO)
- ESWL
- Endoscopic sphincterotomy

● Nursing interventions
- Maintain the patient's diet; withhold food and fluids as ordered
- Administer I.V. fluids
- Encourage turning, coughing, deep breathing, and incentive spirometry
- Assess pain level, administer analgesics as prescribed, and evaluate effect
- Maintain the position, patency, and low suction of the NG tube
- Place the patient in semi-Fowler's position
- Monitor and record vital signs, I/O, laboratory studies, and pulse oximetry
- Administer medications, as prescribed
- Provide preoperative and postoperative care
- Allay the patient's anxiety and provide emotional support
- Provide skin, nares, and mouth care
- Have the patient ambulate, as tolerated
- Maintain a quiet environment
- Individualize home care instructions
  - Know about the disorder and its treatment
  - Follow instructions for medication use, and be aware of possible adverse effects
  - Complete skin care daily
    Recognize the signs and symptoms of renal colic

Diagnosing cholecystitis and cholelithiasis
- Cholangiogram: stones in the biliary tree
- Ultrasound: bile duct distention and calculi

Treating cholecystitis and cholelithiasis
- Low-fat diet, in small, frequent feedings
- Analgesics
- Bile salts
- ESWL
- Cholecystectomy

Key nursing interventions for a patient with cholecystitis or cholelithiasis
- Withhold food and fluids.
- Assess pain and administer analgesics, as indicated.
- Maintain the position, patency, and low suction of the NG tube.
- Provide preoperative and postoperative care.

● **Complications**
- Gallbladder perforation
- Cholangitis
- Gallstone ileus

● **Surgical interventions**
- Cholecystectomy—open or laparoscopic
- Exploration of the common bile duct

PANCREATITIS

● **Definition**
- Acute or chronic inflammation of the pancreas with varying degrees of pancreatic edema, fat necrosis, and hemorrhage
- May lead to pancreatic function loss

● **Causes**
- Biliary tract disease
- Alcoholism
- Metabolic or endocrine disorders
- Trauma to the pancreas or abdomen
- Gallstones or common bile duct obstruction
- Pancreatic cyst or tumor
- Bacterial or viral infection
- Penetrating peptic ulcer

● **Risk factors**
- Medication induced: steroids, thiazide diuretics, hormonal contraceptives
- Renal failure and kidney transplantation
- Heredity
- ERCP

● **Pathophysiology**
- Acute: pancreatic enzymes are activated in the pancreas rather than the duodenum, resulting in tissue damage and autodigestion of the pancreas
- Chronic: chronic inflammation results in fibrosis and calcification of the pancreas, obstruction of the ducts, and destruction of the secreting acinar cells

● **Assessment findings**
- Nausea and vomiting
- Tachycardia
- Intense epigastric pain centered close to the umbilicus and radiating to the back between the 10th thoracic and 6th lumbar vertebrae
- Aching, burning, stabbing, pressing pain
- Abdominal tenderness and distention
- Elevated temperature
- Steatorrhea (chronic)
- Weight loss

- Jaundice
- Hypotension
- Pain after eating fatty food or consuming alcohol
- Dyspnea
- Dehydration
- Decreased or absent bowel sounds
- Positioning knee-chest, fetal, or leaning forward for comfort
- Cullen's sign (irregular, bluish hemorrhagic patches on the skin around the umbilicus)
- Turner's sign (a bruiselike discoloration of the skin of the flanks)

Diagnostic test findings
- CT scan: enlarged pancreas
- Blood chemistry: increased amylase, lipase levels
- Hematology: increased WBCs and RBCs
- Ultrasonography: cysts, bile duct inflammation and dilation
- Urine chemistry: increased amylase
- Fecal fat: positive (chronic)
- Arteriography: fibrous tissue and calcification of the pancreas
- Glucose tolerance test: increased
- ERCP: biliary obstruction

Medical management
- Respiratory support, if indicated
- Diet: withhold food and fluid until acute episode subsides; then gradual increase of low-fat, low-protein diet
- I.V. therapy: hydration, electrolyte replacement
- GI decompression: NG tube
- Position: semi-Fowler's
- Activity: bed rest during acute episode
- Alcohol and caffeine cessation
- Monitoring: vital signs, I/O, CVP, and urine glucose and ketones
- Laboratory studies: glucose, electrolytes, amylase, lipase, calcium, and lipids
- Nutritional support: TPN
- Transfusion therapy: packed RBCs
- Antibiotic: imipenem and cilastatin (Primaxin)
- Analgesics: meperidine (Demerol), tramadol (Ultram)
- Antiemetic: ondansetron (Zofran)
- Antianxiety agents: lorazepam (Ativan), alprazolam (Xanax)
- Digestant (with chronic form): pancrelipase (Viokase)
- Potassium supplements: potassium chloride (K-Lor), potassium gluconate (Kaon)
- Antidiabetic agent: insulin
- Mucosal barrier fortifier: sucralfate (Carafate)
- DVT prophylaxis: sequential compression stockings or low-molecular-weight heparin

Key signs and symptoms of pancreatitis
- Nausea and vomiting
- Tachycardia
- Intense epigastric pain centered close to the umbilicus and radiating to the back between the 10th thoracic and 6th lumbar vertebrae
- Turner's sign
- Cullen's sign
- Abdominal tenderness and distention

Diagnosing pancreatitis
- Blood chemistry: increased amylase and lipase levels
- Ultrasonography: cysts, bile duct inflammation and dilation
- CT scan: enlarged pancreas

Treating pancreatitis
- Respiratory support
- I.V. therapy: hydration, electrolyte replacement
- Bed rest
- Transfusion therapy
- Analgesics
- Corticosteroids
- Antidiabetic agents

Key nursing interventions for a patient with pancreatitis

- Assess GI, cardiac, and respiratory status.
- Assess fluid balance.
- Monitor and record vital signs, I/O, laboratory studies, CVP, daily weight, and blood glucose levels.

Key complications of pancreatitis

- Ileus
- Hypovolemic shock
- Diabetes mellitus
- Infection

Nursing interventions

- Withhold food and fluid during an acute episode
- Administer I.V. fluids, electrolyte replacements, or TPN, as ordered
- Assess fluid balance
- Assess GI, cardiac, and respiratory status
- Maintain the position, patency, and low suction of the NG tube
- Keep the patient in semi-Fowler's position
- Monitor and record vital signs, I/O, laboratory studies, CVP, daily weight, and blood glucose levels
- Administer medications, as prescribed
- Encourage incentive spirometry, coughing, and deep breathing
- Allay the patient's anxiety through verbalization and medication
- Provide skin, nares, and mouth care
- Encourage ambulation, if possible; reposition the patient every 2 hours while in bed
- Apply sequential compression stockings while in bed
- Provide a quiet, restful environment
- Monitor urine and stool for color, character, and amount
- Individualize home care instructions
  - Know about the disorder and its treatment
  - Follow instructions for medication use, and be aware of possible adverse effects
  - Monitor glucose levels with a blood glucose monitoring machine
  - Monitor the stool for steatorrhea
  - Monitor self for infection
  - Recognize the signs and symptoms of increased blood glucose
  - Avoid large meals and alcohol consumption
  - Adhere to activity limitations
  - Alternate rest periods with activity

Complications

- Disseminated intravascular coagulation
- GI bleeding
- Renal failure
- Pseudocysts
- Pancreatic cancer
- Multiorgan system failure
- Ileus
- Hypovolemic shock
- Diabetes mellitus
- Infection
- Pancreatic fistula
- Pancreatic abscess
- Septic shock
- Respiratory failure

● **Surgical intervention**
  • Pancreatectomy

CIRRHOSIS

● **Definition**
  • Chronic, progressive disease characterized by inflammation, fibrosis, and degeneration of liver parenchymal cells
  • Four types of cirrhosis
    – Laënnec's (micronodular)
    – Postnecrotic (macronodular)
    – Biliary
    – Idiopathic

● **Causes**
  • Unknown
  • Laënnec's
    – Alcohol use or abuse
    – Malnutrition
  • Postnecrotic
    – Viral hepatitis
    – Liver toxins
  • Biliary
    – Cholecystitis
    – Obstructions from neoplasms, strictures, or gallstones
  • Idiopathic
    – Chronic inflammatory bowel disease
    – Sarcoidosis

● **Pathophysiology**
  • Inflammation causes liver parenchymal cell destruction, with subsequent fibrosis
  • Fibrotic changes cause obstruction of hepatic blood flow and normal liver function
  • Obstruction causes portal hypertension
  • Decreased liver function results in changes in body chemistry
    – Decreased absorption and utilization of fat-soluble vitamins (A, D, E, and K)
    – Increased secretion of aldosterone
    – Ineffective detoxification of protein wastes
    – Prolonged clotting times

● **Assessment findings**
  • Nausea and vomiting
  • Weakness and fatigue
  • Anorexia and weight loss
  • Jaundice
  • Ecchymosis

Key facts about cirrhosis

• Chronic, progressive disease
• Characterized by inflammation, fibrosis, and degeneration of liver parenchymal cells
• Four types: Laënnec's, post-necrotic, biliary, and idiopathic

Common causes of cirrhosis

• Unknown
• Alcohol use
• Viral hepatitis
• Cholecystitis

Key signs and symptoms of cirrhosis

• Nausea and vomiting
• Anorexia
• Jaundice
• Pain in the right upper quadrant

- Palmar erythema
- Indigestion
- Pruritus
- Irregular bowel pattern
- Pain in the right upper quadrant
- Peripheral edema
- Petechiae
- Epistaxis
- Hematemesis
- Telangiectasis
- Gynecomastia and impotence
- Amenorrhea
- Hemorrhoids
- Hepatomegaly
- Melena
- Esophageal varices

Diagnostic test findings
- Blood chemistry: increased AST, ALT, LD, alkaline phosphatase, ammonia, bilirubin, and sulfobromophthalein test; decreased albumin and total protein
- Hematology: decreased Hb, HCT, and WBCs; increased PT, PTT, and International Normalized Ratio
- Abdominal X-ray: liver size, ascites
- Liver scan: fibrotic liver, increased blood flow
- Liver biopsy: destruction of parenchymal cells
- Esophagoscopy: esophageal varices
- Arterial blood gas (ABG) analysis: metabolic acidosis, respiratory acidosis, respiratory alkalosis
- Urine chemistry: proteinuria
- CT scan: ascites, liver size, liver masses

Medical management
- Oxygen therapy
- Monitoring: vital signs, I/O, neurovital signs, ECG, hemodynamic variables, and stools for occult blood
- I.V. therapy: hydration, electrolyte replacement
- Laboratory studies: AST, ALT, LD, PT, amylase, lipase, Hb, HCT, bilirubin, albumin, WBCs, and ABG analysis
- Diet: high-calorie, low-sodium, in small, frequent feedings with restricted intake of alcohol and fluids
- GI decompression: NG tube (with bleeding)
- Position: semi-Fowler's
- Activity: regular exercise unless actively bleeding
- Nutritional support: TPN, NG tube feedings
- Precautions: standard
- Transfusion therapy: platelets, packed RBCs, fresh frozen plasma (FFP)

Diagnosing cirrhosis
- Blood chemistry: increased AST, ALT, LD, alkaline phosphatase, ammonia, bilirubin, and sulfobromophthalein test; decreased albumin and total protein
- Liver biopsy: destruction of parenchymal cells
- CT scan: ascites

Treating cirrhosis
- Transfusion therapy: platelets, packed RBCs, FFP
- Diuretics
- Ammonia detoxicant
- Vitamins

- Diuretics: spironolactone (Aldactone), furosemide (Lasix)
- Sedative: phenobarbital (Luminal)
- Stool softener: docusate (Colace)
- Ammonia detoxicant: lactulose (Cephulac)
- Vitamin: zinc
- Analgesic: oxycodone (Tylox)
- Antihistamine: diphenhydramine (Benadryl)
- Endoscopy sclerotherapy: ethanolamine (Ethamolin)
- **Abdominal paracentesis (with ascites)**
- Balloon tamponade of varices: Sengstaken-Blakemore tube (with active bleeding)
- DVT prophylaxis: sequential compression stockings

● **Nursing interventions**
  - Administer oxygen
  - Assess respiratory, neurologic, and GI status, and fluid balance
  - Monitor and record vital signs, I/O, laboratory studies, hemodynamic variables, daily weight, and fecal occult blood
  - Maintain a low-sodium diet; withhold food and fluids as needed
  - Administer I.V. fluids or TPN, as ordered
  - Encourage turning, coughing, deep breathing, and incentive spirometry
  - Assess for bleeding
  - Maintain the position, patency, and low suction of the NG tube
  - Keep the patient in semi-Fowler's position
  - Monitor ammonia levels
  - Measure and record the patient's abdominal girth
  - Monitor for signs and symptoms of infection
  - Administer medications, as prescribed
  - Allay the patient's anxiety through verbalization and medication
  - Provide skin, nares, and mouth care
  - Maintain standard precautions
  - Maintain bed rest and a quiet environment
  - Monitor stool for color, consistency, and amount
  - Provide information on Alcoholics Anonymous (AA), or make a referral to a treatment program
  - Individualize home care instructions
    - Know about the disorder and its treatment
    - Follow instructions for medication use, and be aware of possible adverse effects
    - Avoid using OTC medications
    - Avoid alcohol use
    - Avoid exposure to people with infections
    - Complete skin care daily
    - Avoid straining while defecating, vigorously blowing the nose, coughing, and using a hard toothbrush
    - Comply with medical follow-up

Key nursing interventions for a patient with cirrhosis

- Assess respiratory status, GI bleeding, and fluid balance.
- Assess for bleeding.
- Monitor and record vital signs, I/O, laboratory studies, hemodynamic variables, daily weight, and fecal occult blood.
- Observe for signs of behavioral or personality changes.
- Monitor ammonia levels.
- Provide information on AA, or make a referral to a treatment program.

- **Complications**
  - Ascites
  - Esophageal varices
  - Hemorrhoids
  - Hemorrhage
  - Estrogen and androgen imbalance
  - Portal hypertension
  - Hepatic coma
  - Pancytopenia
  - Liver cancer
- **Surgical interventions**
  - Portacaval shunt
  - LeVeen peritoneovenous shunt
  - TIPS
  - Liver transplant

VIRAL HEPATITIS

- **Definition**
  - Infection and inflammation of the liver caused by a virus
  - Six types of hepatitis
    - Hepatitis A
    - Hepatitis B
    - Hepatitis C
    - Hepatitis D
    - Hepatitis E
    - Hepatitis G
- **Causes, transmission**
  - Hepatitis A: contaminated food (usually by preparers with poor hand washing), milk, water, feces (food-borne most common)
  - Hepatitis B: parenteral, sexual, oral, transmitted through contact with any infected body fluid
  - Hepatitis C: blood or serum (blood transfusions, exposure to contaminated blood), transmitted through contact with any infected body fluid
  - Hepatitis D: similar to type B virus (HBV); can become active only in the presence of HBV
  - Hepatitis E: fecal (usually from contact with sewage-contaminated water), oral route
  - Hepatitis G: thought to be blood-borne, with transmission similar to hepatitis B and C
- **Pathophysiology**
  - Inflammation of liver tissue leads to diffuse injury and necrosis of hepatocytes
  - Hypertrophy and proliferation of Kupffer's cells and bile stasis occur

● **Assessment findings**
  • Prodromal stage
    – Anorexia
    – Nausea and vomiting
    – Fatigue
    – Weight loss
    – Malaise
    – Elevated temperature
    – Changes in senses of taste and smell
    – Clay-colored stools
    – Dark urine
    – Headache, photophobia
    – Arthralgia, myalgia (hepatitis B)
  • Clinical jaundice stage
    – Anorexia
    – Abdominal pain or tenderness in the right upper quadrant
    – Indigestion
    – Rashes, erythematous patches or hives
    – Cervical adenopathy
    – Hepatomegaly
    – Jaundice
    – Splenomegaly
    – Pruritus
  • Posticteric stage
    – Decreasing hepatomegaly
    – Decreasing jaundice
    – Improved appetite

● **Diagnostic test findings**
  • Blood chemistry: increased ALT, AST, alkaline phosphatase, LD, bilirubin, ESR
  • Hepatitis profile: identifies antibodies specific to the causative virus, establishing the type of hepatitis
  • Hematology: increased PT
  • Sulfobromophthalein: increased
  • Urine chemistry: increased urobilinogen
  • Liver biopsy: shows chronic hepatitis

● **Medical management**
  • Diet: high-calorie, moderate-protein, with avoidance of alcohol
  • Activity: frequent rest periods
  • Monitoring: vital signs and I/O
  • Laboratory studies: ALT, AST, LD, bilirubin, PT, PTT
  • Precautions: standard
  • Alpha interferons: interferon alfa-2b (Intron A), interferon alfa-2b and ribavirin (Rebetron)
  • Antivirals: lamivudine (Epivir), entecavir (Baraclude), adefovir (Hepsera)

Key signs and symptoms of hepatitis

● Fatigue
● Anorexia
● Clay-colored stools
● Dark urine
● Hepatomegaly
● Jaundice

Diagnosing hepatitis

● Increased ALT, AST, alkaline phosphatase, LD, bilirubin, ESR
● Hepatitis profile: identifies type of hepatitis
● Liver biopsy: shows chronic hepatitis

Treating hepatitis

● Alpha interferons
● Antivirals

Key nursing interventions for a patient with hepatitis

- Provide rest periods.
- Provide skin care.
- Assess for signs and symptoms of bleeding.

Key complications of hepatitis

- Fulminant hepatitis
- Esophageal varices
- Liver failure

Key facts about esophageal varices

- Dilation of esophageal veins in the lower part of the esophagus
- After the esophageal veins dilate, they protrude into the esophageal lumen

- Antiemetic: prochlorperazine (Compazine)

● **Nursing interventions**
- Maintain the patient's diet and monitor nutritional status
- Monitor and record vital signs, I/O, and laboratory studies
- Administer medications, as prescribed
- Allay the patient's anxiety and provide emotional support
- Maintain standard precautions
- Provide frequent rest periods
- Provide skin care
- Assess for signs and symptoms of bleeding
- Individualize home care instructions
    - Know about the disorder and its treatment
    - Follow instructions for medication use, and be aware of possible adverse effects
    - Avoid exposure to people with infections
    - Avoid alcohol use
    - Increase fluid intake to 3 qt (3 L)/day
    - Use safe sex practices

● **Complications**
- Fulminant hepatitis
- Primary liver cancer
- Esophageal varices
- Liver failure
- Cirrhosis

● **Surgical intervention**
- Liver transplant (with hepatitis C)

ESOPHAGEAL VARICES

● **Definition**
- Dilated, torturous veins in the submucosa of the lower part of the esophagus, resulting from portal hypertension

● **Causes**
- Portal hypertension
- Increased intra-abdominal pressure
- Alcohol abuse
- Cirrhosis
- Mechanical obstruction and occlusion of the hepatic veins

● **Pathophysiology**
- Venous drainage from the liver into the portal vein is decreased
- Drainage obstruction results in portal hypertension
- Return of venous blood from the intestinal tract and spleen to the right atrium via the collateral circulation is obstructed

- The increased pressure dilates the esophageal veins, which then protrude into the esophageal lumen

● **Assessment findings**
- Anorexia
- Nausea and vomiting
- Hematemesis
- Fatigue and weakness
- Tachycardia
- Tachypnea
- Hypotension
- Splenomegaly
- Ascites
- Peripheral edema
- Melena
- Dysphagia
- Pallor
- Jaundice

● **Diagnostic test findings**
- Hematology: increased PT; decreased RBCs, Hb, and HCT
- Blood chemistry: increased BUN, sodium, total bilirubin, and ammonia levels; decreased albumin
- Coagulation studies: prolonged PT
- Endoscopy: ruptured varix

● **Medical management**
- Oxygen therapy, if in respiratory distress
- Diet: soft; withhold food and fluids with active bleeding
- I.V. therapy: hydration
- GI decompression: NG tube
- Position: semi-Fowler's
- Activity: bed rest while actively bleeding
- Monitoring: vital signs and I/O
- Laboratory studies: Hb, HCT, PT, and PTT
- Transfusion therapy: packed RBCs and FFP
- Esophageal balloon tamponade: Sengstaken-Blakemore or Minnesota tube
- Paracentesis
- Endoscopy sclerotherapy: ethanolamine (Ethamolin)
- Vasoconstrictor: vasopressin (Pitressin)
- Vasodilator: nitroglycerin (Nitro-Bid)
- Nonselective beta-adrenergic blocker: propranolol (Inderal)
- Antisecretory agents: somatostatin (Zecnil), octreotide (Sandostatin)
- Vitamins: vitamin K (AquaMEPHYTON)
- Iced saline lavage by NG tube during active bleeding
- Stool softener: docusate (Colace)
- Mucosal barrier fortifier: sucralfate (Carafate)

Key nursing interventions for a patient with esophageal varices

- Maintain the position, patency, and low suction of the NG tube.
- Assess for signs of bleeding.
- Avoid activities that increase intra-abdominal pressure.
- Assess neurologic status.
- Administer I.V. fluids and blood products.

Key complications of esophageal varices

- Hemorrhage
- Hepatic failure
- Shock

● Nursing interventions
- Assess cardiovascular and respiratory status
- Monitor and record vital signs, I/O, laboratory studies, CVP, and daily weight
- Administer oxygen
- Withhold food and fluids
- Administer I.V. fluids and blood products
- Assess skin turgor
- Maintain the position, patency, and low suction of the NG tube or Sengstaken-Blakemore tube
  - Maintain emergency measures for gastric balloon rupture
  - Have suction and scissors to cut the tube available
- Place the patient in semi-Fowler's position
- Administer medications, as prescribed
- Allay the patient's anxiety and provide emotional support
- Provide nares and mouth care
- Minimize environmental stress
- Assess for signs of bleeding
- Avoid activities that increase intra-abdominal pressure
- Monitor and record the amount, color, frequency, and consistency of stools and NG drainage
- Assess neurologic status
- Individualize home care instructions
  - Know about the disorder and its treatment
  - Follow instructions for medication use, and be aware of possible adverse effects
  - Monitor stools for occult blood
  - Avoid lifting and straining
  - Avoid alcohol use
- Provide information about AA, or refer the patient to a treatment program

● Complications
- Hepatic failure
- Hemorrhage
- Shock
- Metabolic imbalance
- Sudden death

● Surgical interventions
- Ligation of varices
- Portacaval shunt
- Splenorenal shunt
- Mesocaval shunt
- TIPS

GASTROESOPHAGEAL REFLUX DISEASE (GERD)

- **Definition**
  - Backflow of gastric or duodenal contents into the esophagus and past the lower esophageal sphincter (LES) without associated belching or vomiting
- **Causes**
  - Impaired LES functioning
  - Increased intra-abdominal pressure —for example, obesity, pregnancy, constricting waistline, and bending over
- **Risk factors**
  - Hiatal hernia
  - Alcohol ingestion
  - Smoking
  - Gastric distention such as from large meals or ascites
  - Prolonged NG intubation
  - Ingestion of peppermint or spearmint
  - Medications, such as morphine, calcium channel blockers, anticholinergics, and nitrates
- **Pathophysiology**
  - Reflux occurs when LES pressure is deficient or when pressure within the stomach exceeds LES pressure (see *How heartburn occurs,* page 276)
  - Acidic contents cause injury and inflammation to the esophageal mucosa
- **Assessment findings**
  - Dyspepsia (pyrosis or heartburn) in the epigastric region
  - Pain worsens with lying down or bending over
  - Hypersalivation (water brash)
  - Regurgitation of warm, sour, or bitter fluid in the throat
  - Chronic pain radiating to the neck, jaws, and arms that may mimic angina pectoris
  - Laryngitis and morning hoarseness
  - Chronic cough
- **Diagnostic test findings**
  - Esophageal acidity tests: reveals the degree of reflux
  - Gastroesophageal scintillation: reveals reflux
  - Endoscopy: allows visualization and confirmation of pathologic changes in the mucosa
  - Barium swallow: identifies evidence of recurrent reflux
  - Esophageal manometry: abnormal LES pressure and sphincter incompetence
- **Medical management**
  - Lifestyle modifications
  - Diet: small, frequent meals, with increased fluid intake; avoid meals before bedtime
  - Position: upright during and after meals; sleep with the head of the bed elevated

Key facts about GERD

- Backflow of gastric or duodenal contents into the esophagus and past the LES
- Acidic contents cause injury and inflammation to the esophageal mucosa

Common causes of GERD

- Impaired LES functioning
- Increased intra-abdominal pressure
- Risk factors: hiatal hernia, alcohol ingestion

Common signs and symptoms of GERD

- Dyspepsia (pyrosis or heartburn) in the epigastric region; may radiate to the jaw or arms, occurs after meals
- Pain worsens with lying down or bending over
- Regurgitation of warm, sour, or bitter fluid in the throat
- Laryngitis
- Chronic cough

Diagnosing GERD

- Endoscopy
- Barium swallow
- Esophageal manometry

Treating GERD

- Position: upright during and after meals; sleep with the head of the bed elevated
- Antacids
- H_2-receptor antagonists
- Proton pump inhibitors
- Cholinergic agent

What happens in heartburn

- Hormonal fluctuations, mechanical stress, and the effects of certain foods and drugs can lower LES pressure.
- When LES pressure falls and intra-abdominal or intragastric pressure rises, the normally contracted LES relaxes inappropriately and allows the reflux of gastric acid or bile secretions in the lower esophagus.
- The reflux irritates and inflames the esophageal mucosa, causing pyrosis.

Nursing interventions for a patient with GERD

- Advise the patient to maintain an upright position during and after meals.
- Provide information on alcohol and smoking cessation.
- Individualize home care instructions such as instructing the patient to eat small, frequent meals.

How heartburn occurs

Hormonal fluctuations, mechanical stress, and the effects of certain foods and drugs can decrease lower esophageal sphincter (LES) pressure. When LES pressure falls and intra-abdominal or intragastric pressure rises, the normally contracted LES relaxes inappropriately and allows the reflux of gastric acid or bile secretions into the lower esophagus. There, the reflux irritates and inflames the esophageal mucosa, causing pyrosis.

Persistent inflammation can cause LES pressure to decrease even more and may trigger a recurrent cycle of reflux and pyrosis.

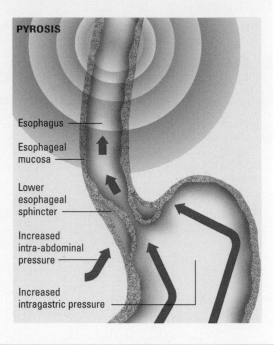

- Antacids: magnesium and aluminum hydroxide (Maalox), aluminum hydroxide gel (AlternaGEL)
- H$_2$-receptor antagonists: cimetidine (Tagamet), ranitidine (Zantac), famotidine (Pepcid), nizatidine (Axid)
- Proton pump inhibitors: omeprazole (Prilosec), lansoprazole (Prevacid), esomeprazole (Nexium)
- Cholinergic agent: bethanechol (Urecholine)
- Smoking cessation

● Nursing interventions

- Maintain the patient's diet with small, frequent feedings
- Advise the patient to maintain an upright position during and after meals
- Monitor and record vital signs, I/O, and laboratory studies
- Monitor respiratory status
- Encourage increased fluid intake
- Administer medications, as prescribed
- Individualize home care instructions
  - Know about the disorder and its treatment
  - Follow instructions for medication use, and be aware of possible adverse effects
  - Adjust the diet by consuming small, frequent meals (see *Factors affecting LES pressure*)

Factors affecting LES pressure

Various dietary and lifestyle elements can increase or decrease lower esophageal sphincter (LES) pressure. Take these into account as you plan the patient's treatment program.

WHAT INCREASES LES PRESSURE
- Protein
- Carbohydrates
- Nonfat milk
- Low-dose ethanol

WHAT DECREASES LES PRESSURE
- Fat
- Whole milk
- Orange juice
- Tomatoes
- Antiflatulents (simethicone)
- Chocolate
- Coffee
- Carbonated soft drinks
- High-dose ethanol
- Cigarette smoking
- Lying on the right or left side
- Sitting

Key factors affecting LES pressure
- Smoking
- Coffee
- Alcohol
- Lying on the right or left side

– Maintain the prescribed position during and after meals and during sleep
– Recognize signs and symptoms of reflux
– Avoid alcohol use and smoking
– Identify and practice ways to avoid increasing intra-abdominal pressure
– Comply with medical follow-up

● **Complications**
- Barrett's epithelium
- Esophagitis with possible ulceration
- Esophageal stricture
- Esophageal bleeding
- Aspiration pneumonia
- Tracheoesophageal fistula

● **Surgical interventions**
- Belsey Mark IV operation (invaginates the esophagus into the stomach)
- Hill or Nissen procedures (creates a gastric wraparound with or without fixation)
- Vagotomy
- Pyloroplasty

Key complications of GERD
- Barrett's epithelium
- Esophageal bleeding
- Aspiration pneumonia

APPENDICITIS

● **Definition**
- Inflammation of the vermiform appendix
- Most common major abdominal disease requiring surgery

● **Causes**
- Mucosal ulceration

Key facts about appendicitis
- Inflammation of the appendix
- Blood flow is restricted, and infection occurs

**Common causes
of appendicitis**

- Mucosal ulceration
- Fecal mass
- Stricture

**Key signs and symptoms
of appendicitis**

- Abdominal rigidity
- Rebound tenderness
- Generalized abdominal pain that becomes localized in the right lower abdomen
- Anorexia
- Rovsing sign
- Obturator sign
- Psoas sign

Treating appendicitis

- GI decompression: NG tube
- Antibiotic
- Analgesic
- Surgery

**Key nursing
interventions for
a patient with
appendicitis**

- Withhold food and fluids.
- Provide preoperative and postoperative care.
- Monitor vital signs and laboratory studies.

- Fecal mass
- Stricture
- Barium ingestion
- Viral infection
- Foreign body
- Neoplasm

● **Pathophysiology**
- Lumen of the appendix becomes obstructed, and inflammation occurs
- Mucosa continues to secrete fluid, and pressure in the lumen of the appendix increases
- Blood flow is restricted, and infection occurs
- Gangrene from hypoxia or perforation may occur

● **Assessment findings**
- Generalized abdominal pain that becomes localized in the right lower abdomen and intensifies when moving
- Anorexia
- Nausea
- Vomiting
- Abdominal rigidity (boardlike)
- Rebound tenderness
- Low-grade fever (late sign)
- Sudden cessation of pain (indicates rupture)
- Rovsing sign
- Obturator sign
- Positive psoas sign

● **Diagnostic test findings**
- Hematology: elevated WBCs
- Ultrasound: inflammation of the appendix
- CT scan: enlarged appendix; perforation or abscess

● **Medical management**
- Diet: nothing by mouth until after surgery
- I.V. therapy: fluid and electrolyte replacement
- Activity: bed rest until after surgery
- Monitoring: vital signs, I/O, and laboratory values
- Antibiotic: ampicillin (Principen)
- Analgesic: morphine

● **Nursing interventions**
- Withhold food and fluids until after surgery
- Administer I.V. fluids
- Assess GI status and fluid balance
- Monitor and record vital signs, I/O, and laboratory studies
- Administer medications, as prescribed
- Maintain bed rest until after surgery; then encourage ambulation
- Provide preoperative and postoperative care, as appropriate

- Individualize home care instructions
  - Know about the disorder and its treatment
  - Follow instructions for medication use, and be aware of possible adverse effects
  - Recognize the signs and symptoms of infection

● **Complications**
  - Peritonitis
  - Wound infection
  - Intra-abdominal abscess
  - Intestinal obstruction
  - Fecal fistula
  - Death (from rupture)

● **Surgical intervention**
  - Appendectomy: open or laparoscopic

GASTROENTERITIS

● **Definition**
  - Self-limiting inflammation of the stomach and small intestine

● **Causes**
  - Amoebae, especially *Entamoeba histolytica*
  - Bacteria (responsible for acute food poisoning): *Staphylococcus aureus, Salmonella, Shigella, Clostridium botulinum, Escherichia coli, Clostridium perfringens*
  - Drug reactions (especially antibiotics)
  - Enzyme deficiencies
  - Food allergens
  - Ingestion of toxins: plants or toadstools
  - Parasites: *Ascaris, Enterobius, Trichinella spiralis*
  - Viruses (may be responsible for traveler's diarrhea): adenovirus, echovirus, or coxsackievirus

● **Pathophysiology**
  - Infecting organism may attack the intestinal mucosa through the release of an enterotoxin
  - The organism may attach to the mucosal epithelium, destroying the intestinal villi
  - The organism may overwork the absorptive capacity of the small bowel
  - The result is hypermotility of the GI tract, leading to altered secretions of fluids and electrolytes

● **Assessment findings**
  - Watery, frequent diarrhea
  - Increased or hyperactive bowel sounds
  - Nausea and vomiting
  - Abdominal tenderness
  - Malaise and fatigue
  - Signs and symptoms of dehydration, if prolonged

Key complications of appendicitis

- Peritonitis
- Wound infection
- Death

Key facts about gastroenteritis

- Inflammation of the digestive tract
- Infecting organism causes hypermotility of the GI tract

Key signs and symptoms of gastroenteritis

- Watery, frequent diarrhea
- Vomiting
- Nausea
- Abdominal tenderness

Diagnosing gastroenteritis

- Stool culture: identifies the organism
- Blood culture: identifies the organism

Treating gastroenteritis

- I.V. therapy: fluid and electrolyte replacement
- Bismuth-containing compound
- Antiemetics

Key nursing interventions for a patient with gastroenteritis

- Assess GI status and fluid balance.
- Provide perianal care.
- Monitor and record vital signs, I/O, daily weight, and laboratory studies.

Key facts about IBS

- Functional GI disorder
- Characterized by chronic diarrhea, abdominal pain, and bloating

Common causes of IBS

- Ingestion of irritants
- Lactose intolerance
- Food allergies

● **Diagnostic test findings**
- Stool culture: identifies the organism
- Blood culture: identifies the organism

● **Medical management**
- Diet: advance the diet from clear liquid to soft foods, as tolerated
- I.V. therapy: fluid and electrolyte replacement
- Activity: as tolerated, bed rest with acute episodes
- Monitoring: vital signs, I/O, and laboratory tests
- Bismuth-containing compound: bismuth subsalicylate (Pepto-Bismol)
- Antiemetics: prochlorperazine (Compazine), trimethobenzamide (Tigan)

● **Nursing interventions**
- Maintain the patient's diet: advance diet as tolerated; avoid milk products
- Assess GI status and fluid balance
- Monitor and record vital signs, I/O, daily weight, and laboratory studies
- Administer medications as ordered
- Provide skin and perianal care
- Maintain bed rest with acute episodes
- Report the infection to the local health department, depending on the cause of the gastroenteritis
- Individualize home care instructions
  - Know about the disorder and its treatment
  - Follow dietary recommendations
  - Use proper hand-washing technique

● **Complications**
- Dehydration
- Electrolyte imbalance

● **Surgical interventions**
- None

IRRITABLE BOWEL SYNDROME (IBS)

● **Definition**
- A functional GI disorder characterized by chronic or periodic diarrhea alternating with constipation, abdominal pain, and bloating

● **Causes**
- Stress
- Ingestion of irritants
- Lactose intolerance
- Hormonal changes
- Food allergies
- Laxative abuse

● **Pathophysiology**
- Impaired motor function of the GI tract, resulting in changes in normal bowel elimination patterns
- Follows a pattern of remissions and exacerbations

Assessment findings
- Diarrhea, constipation, or both
- Abdominal pain or cramps relieved by defecation
- Abdominal distention
- Mucus with stool passage
- Flatus
- Pasty, pencil-like stools

Diagnostic test findings
- Barium enema: may reveal colonic spasm or a tubular appearance of the descending colon
- Sigmoidoscopy or colonoscopy: normal bowel mucosa, spastic contractions
- Stool culture: to rule out ova, parasites, and bacteria
- Lactose intolerance testing: to rule out lactose intolerance

Medical management
- Diet: small, frequent meals; avoiding food irritants
- Activity: as tolerated, regular exercise
- Monitoring: vital signs, I/O, and laboratory values
- Antidiarrheals: diphenoxylate with atropine (Lomotil), loperamide (Imodium)
- Anticholinergic: dicyclomine (Bentyl)
- Bulk-forming laxative: methylcellulose (Citrucel)
- Tricyclic antidepressants: imipramine (Tofranil), amitriptyline (Elavil)
- Prokinetic: tegaserod (Zelnorm)
- Serotonin receptor antagonist: alosetron (Lotronex)
- Chloride-channel activator: lubiprostone (Amitiza)
- Stress management and behavior modification

Nursing interventions
- Assist with the identification of dietary habits and food irritants
- Assess GI status and fluid balance
- Administer medications, as prescribed
- Teach stress-management techniques
- Individualize home care instructions
  - Know about the disorder and its treatment
  - Take medications, as directed
  - Exercise regularly
  - Practice stress-management techniques
  - Avoid food irritants; eat small, frequent meals
  - Drink 6 to 8 glasses of water daily
  - Obtain adequate sleep

Complications
- Diverticulitis
- Colon cancer
- Chronic inflammatory bowel disease

Surgical intervention
- None

NCLEX CHECKS

It's never too soon to begin your NCLEX preparation. Now that you've reviewed this chapter, carefully read each of the following questions and choose the best answer. Then compare your responses to the correct answers.

1. A nurse is providing discharge teaching for a client with GERD. Which statement by the client indicates that he understands the instructions?

- ☐ **1.** "I will lie down after meals."
- ☐ **2.** "I will restrict fluids."
- ☒ **3.** "I will sleep with the head of the bed elevated."
- ☐ **4.** "I will no longer use a pillow."

2. Which finding in a client with appendicitis alerts the nurse to a ruptured appendix?

- ☐ **1.** Pain in the right lower abdomen
- ☒ **2.** Sudden cessation of abdominal pain
- ☐ **3.** Rebound tenderness
- ☐ **4.** Psoas sign

3. While preparing a client for an endoscopy, the nurse should implement which of the following? Select all that apply.

- ☐ **1.** Administer a preparation to clean the GI tract, such as GoLYTELY or Fleet Phospho-soda.
- ☒ **2.** Tell the client that he shouldn't eat or drink for 6 to 12 hours before the procedure.
- ☐ **3.** Tell the client that he must be on a clear-liquid diet for 24 hours before the procedure.
- ☒ **4.** Inform the client that he'll receive a sedative before the procedure.
- ☐ **5.** Tell the client that he may eat and drink immediately after the procedure.

4. A nurse is evaluating the effectiveness of dietary instructions in a client with diverticulitis. Regular consumption of which food would indicate that the client hasn't understood the instructions?

- ☐ **1.** Fiber
- ☐ **2.** Bananas
- ☐ **3.** Milk products
- ☒ **4.** Cucumbers

5. A client with a history of peptic ulcer disease develops a fever of 101° F (38.3° C). Which accompanying sign most strongly indicates that the client has peritonitis?

- ☐ **1.** Leukopenia
- ☐ **2.** Hyperactive bowel sounds
- ☒ **3.** Abdominal rigidity
- ☐ **4.** Polyuria

6. A nurse is planning care for a female client with acute hepatitis A. What's the primary mode of transmission for hepatitis A?

- ☒ **1.** Fecal contamination and oral ingestion
- ☐ **2.** Exposure to contaminated blood
- ☐ **3.** Sexual activity with an infected partner
- ☐ **4.** Sharing a contaminated needle or syringe

7. Peritonitis is a complication of a ruptured appendix. Another possible cause of peritonitis may be:

- ☒ **1.** PEG tube displacement.
- ☐ **2.** indwelling urinary catheter displacement.
- ☐ **3.** GERD.
- ☐ **4.** gastroenteritis.

8. A nurse is caring for a client who's experiencing abdominal cramping pain, vomiting green bile, and exhibiting absent bowel sounds. The physician should be notified immediately because the client may have which life-threatening disorder?

- ☐ **1.** Colorectal cancer
- ☐ **2.** Esophageal varices
- ☐ **3.** Hepatitis
- ☒ **4.** Intestinal obstruction

9. A modifiable risk factor for gastric cancer is:

- ☐ **1.** family history of gastric cancer.
- ☐ **2.** work environment.
- ☒ **3.** high intake of salty and smoked foods.
- ☐ **4.** aging.

10. A self-limiting GI disorder is:

- ☐ **1.** pancreatitis.
- ☐ **2.** diverticulitis.
- ☐ **3.** cholecystitis.
- ☒ **4.** gastroenteritis.

ANSWERS AND RATIONALES

1. CORRECT ANSWER: 3

The client with GERD should sleep with the head of the bed elevated to reduce intra-abdominal pressure. The head of the bed should remain elevated during and after meals to reduce reflux. Fluid intake should be increased to wash gastric contents out of the esophagus. Lying flat in bed increases intra-abdominal pressure and the risk of reflux.

2. CORRECT ANSWER: 2

Sudden cessation of abdominal pain indicates perforation or infarction of the appendix. Pain in the right lower abdomen, rebound tenderness, and psoas are all signs and symptoms of appendicitis.

3. CORRECT ANSWER: 2, 4

The client shouldn't eat or drink for 6 to 12 hours before the procedure to ensure that his upper GI tract is clear for viewing. The client will receive a sedative before the endoscope is inserted that will help him relax but allow him to remain conscious. GI tract cleaning and a clear-liquid diet are interventions for a client having a lower GI tract procedure such as colonoscopy. Food and fluids must be withheld until the gag reflex returns.

4. CORRECT ANSWER: 4

With diverticulitis, vegetables with seeds are prohibited in the diet because the seeds can lodge in diverticula and cause flare-ups of diverticulitis. Fiber and residue are recommended in the diet. Bananas and milk products aren't contra-indicated.

5. CORRECT ANSWER: 3

Abdominal rigidity is a classic sign of peritonitis. The client would typically have leukocytosis, hypoactive bowel sounds, and decreased urine output.

6. CORRECT ANSWER: 1

Hepatitis A is predominantly transmitted by the ingestion of fecally contaminated food. Transmission is more likely to occur with poor hygiene, crowded conditions, and poor sanitation. Hepatitis B and C may be transmitted through exposure to contaminated blood and blood products. Sexual activity with an infected partner and sharing contaminated needles or syringes may transmit hepatitis B.

7. CORRECT ANSWER: 1

PEG tube displacement may result in peritonitis. Other causes include ruptured ectopic pregnancy, pancreatitis, intestinal perforation, biliary tract disease, fistula, and bacterial infection.

8. CORRECT ANSWER: 4

Abdominal cramping pain, green bile emesis, and absent bowel sounds may indicate an intestinal obstruction, which may be life-threatening if left untreated.

9. CORRECT ANSWER: 3

Modifiable risk factors for gastric cancer include high intake of salty and smoked foods, smoking, and high alcohol consumption.

10. CORRECT ANSWER: 4

Gastroenteritis is a self-limiting inflammation of the stomach and small intestines that causes nausea, vomiting, and diarrhea.

6

Endocrine system

1. A modifiable risk factor for diabetes mellitus (type 2) is:

☐ 1. blood pressure.

☐ 2. age.

☐ 3. family history.

☐ 4. weight.

CORRECT ANSWER: 4

2. Which laboratory finding may indicate diabetes insipidus?

☐ 1. Serum glucose level greater than 126 mg/dl

☐ 2. Urine specific gravity less than 1.004

☐ 3. Serum glucose level greater than 200 mg/dl

☐ 4. Urine specific gravity greater than 1.004

CORRECT ANSWER: 2

3. Symptoms of hyperpituitarism may include:

☐ 1. skeletal abnormalities with a protruding jaw.

☐ 2. short stature with an enlarged tongue.

☐ 3. absent postpartum lactation and amenorrhea.

☐ 4. hypothermia and depigmentation of the nipples.

CORRECT ANSWER: 1

4. An important nursing intervention for the care of a client after a thyroidectomy is:

☐ 1. monitoring blood glucose levels.

☐ 2. keeping a tracheostomy tray at the bedside.

☐ 3. providing nutritional supplements.

☐ 4. restricting fluid intake.

CORRECT ANSWER: 2

5. A possible sign or complication of hyperparathyroidism is:

☐ 1. hyperglycemia.

☐ 2. hypoglycemia.

☐ 3. renal calculi.

☐ 4. hypovolemia.

CORRECT ANSWER: 3

LEARNING OBJECTIVES

After studying this chapter, you should be able to:

● Describe the psychosocial impact of endocrine disorders.

● Differentiate between modifiable and nonmodifiable risk factors in the development of an endocrine disorder.

● List three probable and three possible nursing diagnoses for a patient with an endocrine disorder.

● Identify the nursing interventions for a patient with an endocrine disorder.

● Identify three teaching topics for a patient with an endocrine disorder.

CHAPTER OVERVIEW

Caring for the patient with an endocrine disorder requires a sound understanding of endocrine anatomy and physiology and fluid and electrolyte balance. A thorough assessment is essential to planning and implementing appropriate patient care. The assessment includes a complete history, a physical examination, diagnostic testing, identification of modifiable and nonmodifiable risk factors, and information related to the psychosocial impact of the disorder on the patient.

Nursing diagnoses focus primarily on altered nutrition, fluid volume excess or deficit, and body image disturbance. Nursing interventions are designed to assess patient hydration and nutritional status, teach the patient and his family about long-term use of medications, and assist the patient in adjusting to changes in body image and the effects of chronic illness. Patient teaching—a crucial nursing activity—involves providing information about the disorder and its implications, medication regimens, signs and symptoms of possible complications, reducing modifiable risk factors through adherence to dietary and medication recommendations and restrictions, and medical follow-up.

ANATOMY AND PHYSIOLOGY

- **Hypothalamus**
  - Controls temperature, respiration, and blood pressure
  - Affects the emotional states of fear, anxiety, anger, rage, pleasure, and pain
  - Produces hypothalamic-stimulating hormones, which affect the inhibition and release of pituitary hormones
- **Pituitary gland**
  - Considered the "master gland"
  - Composed of anterior and posterior lobes
    - Posterior lobe (neurohypophysis) secretes vasopressin (antidiuretic hormone [ADH]) and oxytocin
    - Anterior lobe (adenohypophysis) secretes follicle-stimulating hormone (FSH), luteinizing hormone (LH), prolactin, corticotropin, thyroid-stimulating hormone (TSH), and growth hormone (GH)
  - Affects all hormonal activity; factors altering pituitary gland function affect all hormonal activity
- **Thyroid gland**
  - Accelerates cellular reactions, including basal metabolic rate and growth
  - Controlled by secretion of TSH
  - Produces thyroxine (T_4), triiodothyronine (T_3), and thyrocalcitonin
- **Parathyroid glands**
  - Secrete parathyroid hormone (parathormone [PTH]), which regulates calcium and phosphorus metabolism
  - Require the active form of vitamin D for PTH function
- **Adrenal glands**
  - Adrenal cortex secretes three major hormones

What the hypothalamus controls

- Temperature
- Respiration
- Blood pressure

Key facts about the pituitary gland

- Considered the "master gland"
- Affects all hormone activity

The role of the thyroid gland

- Accelerates cellular reactions
- Produces T_4, T_3, and thyrocalcitonin

Key facts about the parathyroid glands

- Secrete PTH
- Require the active form of vitamin D

Key facts about the adrenal glands

- Adrenal cortex: secretes hormones such as glucocorticoids
- Adrenal medulla: secretes hormones such as norepinephrine

The role of the pancreas

- Aids in digestion
- Secretes digestive enzymes
- Secretes hormones such as insulin

- – Glucocorticoids (cortisol)
- – Mineralocorticoids (aldosterone)
- – Sex hormones (androgens, estrogens, and progesterone)
- Adrenal medulla secretes two hormones
  - – Norepinephrine
  - – Epinephrine

- **Pancreas**
  - Accessory gland of digestion
    - – Exocrine function: secretion of digestive enzymes
      - · Amylase
      - · Lipase
      - · Trypsin
    - – Endocrine function: secretion of hormones from the islets of Langerhans
      - · Insulin
      - · Glucagon
      - · Somatostatin
  - Main pancreatic duct joins the common bile duct and empties into the duodenum at the ampulla of Vater

ASSESSMENT FINDINGS

Key signs and symptoms of endocrine disorders

- Changes in weight; hair quality and distribution; and body proportions, muscle mass, and fat distribution
- Change in mood or behavior
- Changes in menses and libido
- Intolerance of heat or cold

- **History**
  - Changes in weight; hair quality and distribution; and body proportions, muscle mass, and fat distribution (see *Assessing endocrine dysfunction: Some common signs and symptoms*)
  - Fatigue and weakness
  - Change in mood or behavior
  - Anorexia
  - Constipation, diarrhea, urinary frequency
  - Change in menses and libido
  - History of infections
  - Intolerance of heat or cold

Key physical examination findings in endocrine disorders

- Skin color and temperature changes
- Change in skin texture
- Change in LOC
- Change in urinary patterns
- Change in thirst

- **Physical examination**
  - Vital sign changes
  - Skin color and temperature changes
  - Change in skin texture
  - Change in level of consciousness (LOC) or altered mental status
  - Pattern and character of respirations
  - Change in urinary patterns
  - Change in thirst
  - Abnormalities of nails
  - Change in visual acuity

Assessing endocrine dysfunction: Some common signs and symptoms

SIGN OR SYMPTOM	POSSIBLE CAUSES
Abdominal pain	Diabetic ketoacidosis (DKA), myxedema, addisonian crisis, thyroid storm
Anemia	Hypothyroidism, panhypopituitarism, adrenal insufficiency, Cushing's disease, hyperparathyroidism
Anorexia	Hyperparathyroidism, Addison's disease, DKA, hypothyroidism
Body temperature changes	*Increase:* Thyrotoxicosis, thyroid storm, primary hypothalamic disease (after pituitary surgery) *Decrease:* Addison's disease, hypoglycemia, myxedema coma, DKA
Hypertension	Primary aldosteronism, pheochromocytoma, Cushing's syndrome
Libido changes, sexual dysfunction	Thyroid or adrenocortical hypofunction or hyperfunction, diabetes mellitus, hypopituitarism, gonadal failure
Skin changes	*Hyperpigmentation:* Addison's disease (after bilateral adrenalectomy for Cushing's syndrome), corticotropin-secreting pituitary tumor *Hirsutism:* Cushing's syndrome, adrenal hyperplasia, adrenal tumor, acromegaly *Coarse, dry skin:* Myxedema, hypoparathyroidism, acromegaly *Excessive sweating:* Thyrotoxicosis, acromegaly, pheochromocytoma, hypoglycemia
Tachycardia	Hyperthyroidism, pheochromocytoma, hypoglycemia, DKA
Weakness, fatigue	Addison's disease, Cushing's syndrome, hypothyroidism, hyperparathyroidism, hyperglycemia or hypoglycemia, pheochromocytoma
Weight gain	Cushing's syndrome, hypothyroidism, pituitary tumor
Weight loss	Hyperthyroidism, pheochromocytoma, Addison's disease, hyperparathyroidism, diabetes mellitus, diabetes insipidus

Common signs and symptoms of endocrine dysfunction

- Abdominal pain
- Anemia
- Anorexia
- Body temperature changes
- Hypertension
- Libido changes, sexual dysfunction
- Skin changes
- Tachycardia
- Weakness, fatigue
- Weight gain
- Weight loss

DIAGNOSTIC TESTS AND PROCEDURES

- **Hematologic studies**
  - Definition and purpose
    - Laboratory test of a blood sample
    - Analysis for white blood cells, red blood cells, erythrocyte sedimentation rate, platelets, prothrombin time, partial thromboplastin time, hemoglobin (Hb), and hematocrit (HCT)
  - Nursing interventions
    - Explain the procedure to the patient
    - Note current drug therapy that might alter test results

Key facts about hematologic studies

- Laboratory test of blood
- Analyze blood cells
- Intervention: note current drug therapy that might alter test results

Key facts about blood chemistry studies

- Laboratory test of blood
- Analyzes chemical components of blood
- Intervention: check the venipuncture site for bleeding

Key facts about fasting serum glucose and 2-hour postprandial glucose test

- Laboratory test of a blood sample
- Measures the body's use and disposal of glucose
- Intervention: assess the patient for hypoglycemia or hyperglycemia

Key facts about glucose tolerance test

- Laboratory test of blood and urine
- Measures absorption of carbohydrates
- Intervention: list any medications that might interfere with the test

Key facts about adrenocorticotropic hormone stimulation test

- Laboratory test of a blood sample
- Analyzes cortisol
- Intervention: monitor 24-hour I.V. infusion of corticotropin after the sample is drawn

– Check the venipuncture site for bleeding after the procedure

● **Blood chemistry**
- Definition and purpose
  – Laboratory test of a blood sample
  – Analysis for potassium, sodium, calcium, phosphorus, ketones, glucose, osmolality, chloride, blood urea nitrogen (BUN), creatinine, T_3, T_4, protein-bound iodine, cortisol
- Nursing interventions
  – Explain the procedure to the patient
  – Check the venipuncture site for bleeding after the procedure

● **Fasting serum glucose and 2-hour postprandial glucose test**
- Definition and purpose
  – Laboratory test of a blood sample
  – Analysis to measure the body's use and disposal of glucose
- Nursing interventions
  – Explain the procedure to the patient
  – Withhold food and fluids for 12 hours before the fasting sample is drawn
  – Withhold insulin until the test is completed
  – Administer the ordered amount of glucose orally, and schedule the laboratory to draw blood 2 hours later
  – Check the venipuncture site for bleeding after the procedure
  – Assess the patient for hypoglycemia or hyperglycemia

● **Glucose tolerance test (GTT)**
- Definition and purpose
  – Laboratory test of blood and urine
  – Analysis to measure absorption of carbohydrates
- Nursing interventions
  – Explain the procedure to the patient
  – List any medications that might interfere with the test
  – Note pregnancy, trauma, or infectious disease
  – Provide the patient with a high-carbohydrate diet 2 days before the test; then have the patient fast for 12 hours before the test
  – Instruct the patient to avoid smoking, caffeine, alcohol, and exercise for 12 hours before the procedure
  – Withhold all medications after midnight
  – Obtain fasting serum glucose and urine specimen
  – Administer test load oral glucose, and record the time
  – Schedule laboratory collection of serum glucose and urine specimens at 30, 60, 120, and 180 minutes
  – Check the venipuncture site for bleeding after the procedure
  – Assess the patient for hyperglycemia or hypoglycemia

● **Adrenocorticotropic hormone stimulation test**
- Definition and purpose
  – Laboratory test of a blood sample
  – Analysis for cortisol level

- Nursing interventions
  - Explain the procedure to the patient
  - List any medications that might interfere with the test
  - Monitor 24-hour I.V. infusion of corticotropin after the baseline serum sample is drawn
  - Check the venipuncture site for bleeding after the procedure

Dexamethasone suppression test
- Definition and purpose
  - Laboratory test of urine samples
  - Analysis of serum cortisol and urinary 17-hydroxycorticosteroids (17-OHCS) after the administration of dexamethasone
- Nursing interventions
  - Explain the procedure to the patient
  - Administer dexamethasone and an antacid, as prescribed
  - Obtain single urine and 24-hour urine samples, as directed
  - Place a 24-hour urine sample on ice until the entire specimen is obtained
  - List any medications that might interfere with the test

24-hour urine test for 17-ketosteroids (17-KS) and 17-OHCS
- Definition and purpose
  - Laboratory test of urine samples
  - Quantitative laboratory analysis of urine collected over 24 hours to determine hormone precursors
- Nursing interventions
  - Explain the procedure to the patient
  - Withhold all medications for 48 hours before the test
  - Instruct the patient to void, and note the time (collection of urine starts with the next voiding)
  - Place the urine container on ice until the entire specimen is collected
  - Measure each voided urine
  - Instruct the patient to void at the end of the 24-hour period
  - List any medications that might interfere with the test

Urine vanillylmandelic acid (VMA) test
- Definition and purpose
  - Laboratory test of urine samples
  - Quantitative analysis of urine collected over 24 hours to determine the end products of catecholamine metabolism (epinephrine and norepinephrine)
- Nursing interventions
  - Explain the procedure to the patient
  - List any medications, previous tests, and medical conditions that might interfere with the test
  - Restrict foods that contain vanilla, coffee, tea, citrus fruits, bananas, nuts, and chocolate for 3 days before the 24-hour urine collection

Key facts about dexamethasone suppression test
- Laboratory test of urine
- Analyzes serum cortisol and 17-OHCS after dexamethasone administration
- Intervention: obtain single urine and 24-hour urine samples, as directed

Key facts about 24-hour urine test
- Laboratory test of urine samples
- Analyzes urine collected over 24 hours
- Intervention: withhold all medications for 48 hours before the test

Key facts about VMA test
- Laboratory test of urine
- Analyzes urine collected over 24 hours to determine the end products of epinephrine and norepinephrine metabolism
- Intervention: restrict foods that contain vanilla, coffee, tea, citrus fruits, bananas, nuts, and chocolate for 3 days before the 24-hour urine collection

Key facts about basal metabolic rate test

- Noninvasive test
- Indirect measurement of oxygen consumed by the body during a given time
- Intervention: list medications taken before the procedure

Key facts about computed tomography

- Noninvasive scan
- Visualizes the sella turcica and abdomen
- Intervention: note the patient's allergies before the procedure

Key facts about ultrasonography

- Noninvasive procedure
- Uses echoes from sound waves to visualize the thyroid, pelvis, and abdomen
- Intervention: determine the patient's ability to lie still

Key facts about closed percutaneous thyroid biopsy

- Involves aspiration of thyroid tissue
- Histologic evaluation
- Intervention: assess the patient for esophageal or tracheal puncture

– Instruct the patient to void, and note the time (collection of urine starts with the next voiding)
– Place the urine container on ice until the entire specimen is collected
– Measure each voided urine
– Instruct the patient to void at the end of the 24-hour period

● **Basal metabolic rate test**
  • Definition and purpose
    – Noninvasive test
    – Indirect measurement of oxygen consumed by the body during a given time
  • Nursing interventions
    – Explain the procedure to the patient
    – List medications taken before the procedure
    – Note environmental and emotional stressors

● **Computed tomography (CT)**
  • Definition and purpose
    – Noninvasive scan that may use I.V. injection of contrast dye
    – Visualization of the sella turcica and abdomen
  • Nursing interventions
    – Explain the procedure to the patient
    – Note the patient's allergies to iodine, seafood, and radiopaque dyes
    – Complete paperwork per facility policy
    – Inform the patient about possible throat irritation and flushing of the face, if contrast dye is used

● **Ultrasonography**
  • Definition and purpose
    – Noninvasive procedure using echoes from sound waves
    – Visualization of the thyroid, pelvis, and abdomen
  • Nursing interventions
    – Explain the procedure to the patient
    – Determine the patient's ability to lie still

● **Closed percutaneous thyroid biopsy**
  • Definition and purpose
    – Sterile aspiration of a small amount of thyroid tissue for histologic evaluation
  • Nursing interventions before the procedure
    – Explain the procedure to the patient
    – Withhold food and fluids from midnight before the procedure
    – Place an obtained written informed consent in the patient's chart
  • Nursing interventions after the procedure
    – Maintain bed rest for 24 hours
    – Monitor vital signs

– Check the biopsy site for bleeding

– Assess the patient for esophageal or tracheal puncture

● **Thyroid uptake (radioactive iodine uptake [RAIU])**
  • Definition and purpose
    – Administration of oral or I.V. radioactive iodine to measure the amount of radioactive iodine (^{131}I) taken up by the thyroid gland in 24 hours
  • Nursing interventions before the procedure
    – Explain the procedure to the patient
    – Advise the patient not to eat iodine-rich foods, such as iodized salt or shellfish, for 24 hours before the test
    – Discontinue all thyroid and cough medications 7 to 10 days before the test
    – Schedule a thyroid scan before tests using iodine-based dyes

● **Thyroid scan**
  • Definition and purpose
    – Administration of an oral or I.V. radioactive isotope to visualize radioactivity distribution in the thyroid gland through imaging
  • Nursing interventions before the procedure
    – Explain the procedure to the patient
    – Advise the patient not to eat iodine-rich foods, such as iodized salt or shellfish, for 24 hours before the test
    – Discontinue all thyroid and cough medications 7 to 10 days before the test
    – Schedule the scan before other tests using iodine-based dyes or radioactive iodine

● **Arteriography**
  • Definition and purpose
    – Injection of a radiopaque dye through a catheter to examine the arterial blood supply to the parathyroid, adrenal, or pancreatic glands through fluoroscopy
  • Nursing interventions before the procedure
    – Explain the procedure to the patient
    – Place an obtained written informed consent in the patient's chart
    – Note the patient's allergies to iodine, seafood, and radiopaque dyes
    – Inform the patient about possible throat irritation and flushing of the face after the dye injection
    – Withhold food and fluids from midnight before the procedure
  • Nursing interventions after the procedure
    – Monitor vital signs
    – Check the insertion site for bleeding
    – Ensure that the patient keeps the affected extremity straight for the prescribed time

---

Key facts about thyroid uptake test

● Uses oral or I.V. radioactive iodine
● Measures the amount of radioactive iodine taken up by the thyroid gland
● Intervention: advise the patient not to eat iodine-rich foods for 24 hours before the test

Key facts about thyroid scan

● Uses an oral or I.V. radioactive isotope
● Provides visual imaging of radioactivity distribution in the thyroid gland
● Intervention: advise the patient not to eat iodine-rich foods for 24 hours before the procedure

Key facts about arteriography

● Uses an injection of radiopaque dye through a catheter
● Examines the arterial blood supply
● Intervention: note the patient's allergies before the procedure; ensure that the patient keeps the affected extremity straight for the prescribed time

Key facts about Sulkowitch's test

- Laboratory test of urine
- Measures the amount of calcium being excreted
- Intervention: collect a urine sample before or after a meal, depending on what disorder is indicated

Psychosocial impact of endocrine disorders

- Decreased self-esteem
- Disruption of employment
- Cost of medications
- Adjustment to change in occupation
- Changes in eating patterns

Modifiable risk factors for endocrine disorders

- Medication
- Diet

Nonmodifiable risk factors for endocrine disorders

- Family history
- Aging

● **Sulkowitch's test**
  - Definition and purpose
    - Laboratory test of urine
    - Analysis to measure the amount of calcium being excreted
  - Nursing interventions
    - Explain the procedure to the patient
    - If hypercalcemia is suspected, collect a single urine sample before a meal
    - If hypocalcemia is suspected, collect a single urine sample after a meal

PSYCHOSOCIAL IMPACT OF ENDOCRINE DISORDERS

● **Developmental impact**
  - Decreased self-esteem
  - Changes in body image
  - Embarrassment or anxiety from the changes in body function and structure, such as changes in secondary sex characteristics and sexual functioning

● **Economic impact**
  - Disruption of employment
  - Cost of vocational retraining
  - Cost of medications
  - Cost of special diet
  - Cost of hospitalizations and follow-up care

● **Occupational and recreational impact**
  - Physical activity restrictions
  - Adjustment to change in occupation

● **Social impact**
  - Social withdrawal and isolation
  - Changes in eating patterns
  - Changes in role performance
  - Changes in sexual function

RISK FACTORS

● **Modifiable risk factors**
  - Medication
  - Stress
  - Diet
  - Obesity

● **Nonmodifiable risk factors**
  - Family history of endocrine illness
  - History of trauma
  - Aging

NURSING DIAGNOSES

● **Probable nursing diagnoses**
- Excess fluid volume
- Risk for imbalanced fluid volume
- Risk for imbalanced nutrition: More than body requirements
- Disturbed body image
- Impaired urinary elimination
- Imbalanced nutrition: Less than body requirements
- Anxiety
- Fear
- Deficient knowledge (disorder and treatment)

● **Possible nursing diagnoses**
- Risk for injury
- Social isolation
- Noncompliance
- Disturbed sensory perception: visual
- Disturbed sensory perception: tactile
- Risk for impaired skin integrity
- Disturbed thought processes

ADRENALECTOMY

● **Description**
- Surgical removal of one or both adrenal glands

● **Preoperative nursing interventions**
- Complete patient and family preoperative teaching
  - Explain the procedure to the patient
  - Describe the operating room, postanesthesia care unit (PACU), and preoperative and postoperative routines
  - Demonstrate postoperative turning, coughing, deep breathing, splinting, and range-of-motion (ROM) exercises
  - Explain the postoperative need for drainage tubes, surgical dressings, oxygen therapy, I.V. therapy, and pain control
- Complete a preoperative checklist; check that a signed informed consent has been placed in the patient's chart
- Administer preoperative medications, as prescribed
- Allay the patient's and his family's anxiety about surgery
- Document the patient's history and physical assessment data
- Administer steroids, as prescribed
- Administer vasopressors, as prescribed

● **Postoperative nursing interventions**
- Assess cardiac, respiratory, and neurologic status
  - Monitor fluid intake and output (I/O) and serum electrolyte levels

---

Probable nursing diagnoses in endocrine disorders

- Excess fluid volume
- Risk for imbalanced fluid volume
- Disturbed body image
- Impaired urinary elimination
- Imbalanced nutrition: Less than body requirements

Possible nursing diagnoses in endocrine disorders

- Noncompliance
- Risk for impaired skin integrity

Key facts about adrenalectomy

- Surgical removal of one or both adrenal glands

Key nursing interventions before adrenalectomy

- Administer steroids, as prescribed.
- Administer vasopressors, as prescribed.

Key nursing interventions after adrenalectomy

- Assess cardiac, respiratory, and neurologic status.
- Monitor vital signs, I/O, CVP, laboratory studies, cardiac rhythm, daily weight, and pulse oximetry.
- Administer hormone replacements and vasopressors.

– Keep in mind that adrenalectomy disturbs mineralocorticoid and glucocorticoid secretion, resulting in altered fluid and electrolyte balance
- Assess pain level, administer analgesics as prescribed, and evaluate effect
- Assess for the return of peristalsis; provide liquids, as tolerated
- Administer I.V. fluids
- Allay the patient's anxiety and provide emotional support
- Inspect the surgical dressing and change, as directed
- Encourage turning, coughing, deep breathing, the use of an incentive spirometer, and splinting of the incision
- Keep the patient in semi-Fowler's position
- Maintain activity, as tolerated
- Monitor vital signs, I/O, central venous pressure (CVP), laboratory studies, cardiac rhythm, daily weight, and pulse oximetry
- Monitor and maintain the position and patency of drainage tubes (nasogastric, indwelling urinary catheter, and wound drainage) as appropriate
- Encourage the patient to express his feelings about changes in his body image and the need for lifelong medication replacement
- Administer medications, as prescribed
- Maintain a quiet environment
- Individualize home care instructions
  - Know about the disorder and its treatment
  - Follow instructions for medication use, and be aware of possible adverse effects
  - Recognize the signs and symptoms of infection, hypovolemia, and hypoglycemia
  - Avoid exposure to people with infections
  - Complete incision care daily, as directed
  - Monitor blood pressure daily
  - Avoid extreme temperatures
  - Comply with medical follow-up

● **Possible surgical complications**
- Shock
- Hypoglycemia
- Hemorrhage
- Peptic ulcers
- Adrenal crisis
- Pneumothorax
- Acute renal failure
- Infection

HYPOPHYSECTOMY

Key facts about hypophysectomy

- Surgical removal of part or all of the pituitary gland

● **Description**
- Surgical removal of part or all of the pituitary gland

● **Preoperative nursing interventions**
  • Complete patient and family preoperative teaching
    – Explain the procedure to the patient
    – Describe the operating room, PACU, and preoperative and postoperative routines
    – Demonstrate postoperative turning, coughing, deep breathing, splinting, and ROM exercises
    – Explain the postoperative need for drainage tubes, surgical dressings, oxygen therapy, I.V. therapy, and pain control
  • Complete a preoperative checklist; check that a signed informed consent has been placed in the patient's chart
  • Administer preoperative medications, as prescribed
  • Allay the patient's and his family's anxiety about surgery
  • Document the patient's history and physical assessment data

● **Postoperative nursing interventions**
  • Assess cardiac, respiratory, and neurologic status and fluid balance
  • Assess pain level, administer analgesics as prescribed, and evaluate effect
  • Assess for the return of peristalsis; provide liquids, as tolerated
  • Administer I.V. fluids
  • Allay the patient's anxiety and provide emotional support
  • Inspect the surgical dressing or nasal drip pad and change, as directed
  • Test nasal drainage for glucose
  • Encourage turning, coughing, deep breathing, and the use of an incentive spirometer
  • Keep the patient in semi-Fowler's position
  • Maintain activity, as tolerated
  • Monitor vital signs, I/O, CVP, laboratory studies, neurovital signs, daily weight, and pulse oximetry
  • Monitor and maintain the position and patency of the indwelling urinary catheter
  • Institute seizure precautions
  • Administer medications, as prescribed
  • **Observe the patient for signs of increased intracranial pressure (ICP)**
  • Check for rhinorrhea
  • Provide mouth and eye care but avoid brushing the patient's teeth
  • Individualize home care instructions
    – Know about the disorder and its treatment
    – Follow instructions for medication use, and be aware of possible adverse effects
    – Recognize the signs and symptoms of infection, seizure activity, and hormone deficiencies
    – Avoid coughing, blowing the nose, lifting, straining while defecating, and sneezing
    – Comply with lifelong hormone replacement

Key nursing interventions before hypophysectomy
● Administer steroids, as prescribed.
● Administer antibiotics, as prescribed.

Key nursing interventions after hypophysectomy
● Assess cardiac, respiratory, and neurologic status and fluid balance.
● Inspect the surgical dressing or nasal drip pad and change, as directed.
● Test nasal drainage for glucose.
● Monitor vital signs, I/O, CVP, laboratory studies, neurovital signs, daily weight, and pulse oximetry.
● Institute seizure precautions.
● Administer medications.
● Check for rhinorrhea.
● Avoid brushing the patient's teeth.

Key facts about thyroidectomy and parathyroidectomy

- Surgical removal of part or all of the thyroid gland (thyroidectomy)
- Surgical removal of one or more parathyroid glands (parathyroidectomy)

Key nursing interventions before thyroid and parathyroid surgery

- Administer iodine preparations.
- Administer antithyroid medications.

Key nursing interventions after thyroid or parathyroid surgery

- Assess respiratory status.
- Monitor vital signs, I/O, CVP, laboratory studies (especially calcium and phosphorus), and pulse oximetry.
- Keep calcium gluconate or calcium chloride and a tracheostomy tray available.
- Keep the patient in semi-Fowler's position.

● **Possible surgical complications**
- Diabetes insipidus
- Increased ICP
- Hemorrhage
- Adrenal crisis
- Thyroid storm
- Meningitis
- Diplopia

THYROID AND PARATHYROID SURGERIES

● **Description**
- Thyroidectomy: surgical removal of part or all of the thyroid gland
- Parathyroidectomy: surgical removal of one or more parathyroid glands

● **Preoperative nursing interventions**
- Complete patient and family preoperative teaching
  - Explain the procedure to the patient
  - Describe the operating room, PACU, and preoperative and postoperative routines
  - Demonstrate postoperative turning, coughing, deep breathing, splinting, and ROM exercises
  - Explain the postoperative need for drainage tubes, surgical dressings, oxygen therapy, I.V. therapy, and pain control
- Complete a preoperative checklist; check that a signed informed consent has been placed in the patient's chart
- Administer preoperative medications, as prescribed
- Allay the patient's and his family's anxiety about surgery
- Document the patient's history and physical assessment data

● **Postoperative nursing interventions**
- Assess respiratory status
- Assess pain level, administer analgesics as prescribed, and evaluate effect
- Assess for the return of peristalsis; provide liquids, as tolerated
- Administer I.V. fluids
- Allay the patient's anxiety and provide emotional support
- Inspect the surgical dressing for bleeding, especially at the back of the neck, and change the dressing, as directed
- Encourage turning, coughing, deep breathing, the use of an incentive spirometer, and splinting of the incision
- Keep the patient in semi-Fowler's position, with neutral alignment and support to his neck
- Maintain activity, as tolerated
- Monitor vital signs, I/O, CVP, laboratory studies (especially calcium and phosphorus), and pulse oximetry
- Monitor and maintain the position and patency of wound drainage tubes
- Maintain seizure precautions

- Encourage the patient to express his feelings about a fear of choking or the loss of his voice
- Assess for tetany
- Assess for hoarseness and aphasia
- Assess for thyroid storm
- Keep calcium gluconate or calcium chloride and a tracheostomy tray available
- Discourage talking
- Provide specific parathyroidectomy care
  - Provide a high-calcium diet with vitamin D
  - Administer calcium and vitamin D supplements, as prescribed
- Individualize home care instructions
  - Know about the disorder and its treatment
  - Follow instructions for medication use, and be aware of possible adverse effects
  - Recognize the signs and symptoms of infection, seizure activity, and hypothyroidism
  - Alternate periods of talking with voice rest
  - Complete incision care daily, as directed
  - Complete ROM exercises of the neck daily
  - Comply with medical follow-up

- ● **Possible surgical complications**
  - Hypocalcemia
  - Laryngeal nerve damage
  - Hypothyroidism
  - Respiratory failure
  - Vocal cord paralysis
  - Laryngeal obstruction
  - Hemorrhage
  - Arrhythmias

HYPERTHYROIDISM

- ● **Definition**
  - Increased synthesis of thyroid hormone from overactivity (Graves' disease) or a change in the thyroid gland (toxic nodular goiter) function

- ● **Causes**
  - Autoimmune and genetic factors
  - Graves' disease
  - Increased TSH secretion
  - Thyroid adenomas
  - Pituitary tumors
  - Precipitating factors
    - Psychological or physiologic stress
    - Infection

     – Diabetic ketoacidosis
     – Excessive iodine intake
     – Surgery
     – Toxemia of pregnancy

● **Pathophysiology**
  - Thyroid-stimulating antibodies have a slow, sustained, stimulating effect on thyroid metabolism
  - Accelerated metabolism causes increased synthesis of thyroid hormone and signs and symptoms of sympathetic nervous system stimulation

● **Assessment findings**
  - Anxiety
  - Flushed, smooth skin
  - Heat intolerance
  - Mood swings
  - Diaphoresis
  - Tachycardia
  - Palpitations
  - Dyspnea
  - Weakness
  - Increased systolic blood pressure
  - Tachypnea
  - Fine hand tremors
  - Exophthalmos
  - Weight loss despite increased appetite
  - Diarrhea
  - Hyperhidrosis
  - Bruit or thrill over the thyroid
  - Fertility problems
  - Oligomenorrhea or amenorrhea

● **Diagnostic test findings**
  - Thyroid scan: nodules
  - Blood chemistry: increased T_3, T_4, protein-bound iodine, and ^{131}I; decreased TSH and cholesterol
  - Electrocardiogram (ECG): atrial fibrillation
  - RAIU: increased

● **Medical management**
  - Diet: restrict stimulants such as caffeine
  - I.V. therapy as needed
  - Activity: bed rest
  - Monitoring: vital signs and I/O
  - Laboratory studies: T_3, T_4
  - Sedative: lorazepam (Ativan)
  - Radiation therapy
  - Thyroid hormone antagonists: propylthiouracil

Key signs and symptoms of hyperthyroidism

- Heat intolerance
- Diaphoresis
- Tachycardia
- Palpitations
- Exophthalmos
- Bruit or thrill over the thyroid

Diagnosing hyperthyroidism

- Thyroid scan: nodules
- Blood chemistry: increased T_3, T_4, protein-bound iodine, and ^{131}I; decreased TSH and cholesterol

Treating hyperthyroidism

- I.V. therapy
- Radiation therapy
- Thyroid hormone antagonists
- [131]I
- Beta-adrenergic blocking agents
- Glucocorticoids

TIME-OUT FOR TEACHING

Patients with endocrine disorders

Be sure to include the following topics in your teaching plan when caring for patients with endocrine disorders.

- Optimal body weight maintenance
- Medication therapy, including the action, adverse effects, and scheduling of medications
- Dietary recommendations and restrictions
- Fluid intake recommendations and restrictions
- Rest and activity patterns, including any limitations or restrictions
- Safe, quiet environment
- Ways to reduce stress
- Medical identification jewelry
- Community agencies and resources for supportive services
- Follow-up care

- Radioactive iodine: single dose of ^{131}I
- Beta-adrenergic blocking agent: propranolol (Inderal)
- Glucocorticoids: prednisone (Deltasone); I.V. hydrocortisone (Solu-Cortef) for thyroid storm

● **Nursing interventions**
- Assess cardiovascular status
- Monitor vital signs, I/O, daily weight, and laboratory studies
- Avoid giving the patient stimulants, such as drugs and foods that contain caffeine
- Administer I.V. fluids
- Administer medications, as prescribed
- Provide rest periods in a quiet, cool environment
- Allay the patient's anxiety and provide emotional support
- Provide postradiation nursing care
  - Provide prophylactic skin, mouth, and perineal care
  - Monitor dietary intake
  - Provide rest periods
- Individualize home care instructions (for teaching tips, see *Patients with endocrine disorders*)
  - Know about the disorder and its treatment
  - Follow instructions for medication use, and be aware of possible adverse effects
  - Stop smoking
  - Recognize the signs and symptoms of thyroid storm
  - Adhere to activity limitations
  - Avoid exposure to people with infections
  - Monitor self for infection
  - Comply with medical follow-up

Key teaching topics for a patient with an endocrine disorder
- Medication therapy
- Optimal weight maintenance
- Diet and fluid recommendations
- Follow-up care

Key nursing interventions for a patient with hyperthyroidism
- Assess cardiovascular status.
- Avoid giving the patient stimulants.
- Monitor vital signs, I/O, daily weight, and laboratory studies.
- Provide postradiation care.

Key facts about thyroid storm

- Overproduction of T_3 and T_4 hormones causes an increase in systemic adrenergic activity that results in severe hypermetabolism
- Leads to cardiac, GI, and sympathetic nervous system decompensation
- Initial symptoms include tachycardia, vomiting, and stupor
- Onset is usually abrupt

Key complications of hyperthyroidism

- Thyroid storm
- Arrhythmias
- Diabetes mellitus

Key facts about hypothyroidism

- Underactive state of the thyroid gland
- Results in the absence or decreased secretion of thyroid hormone

Common causes of hypothyroidism

- Autoimmune disease: Hashimoto's thyroiditis
- Thyroidectomy
- Overuse of antithyroid drug

Understanding thyroid storm

Thyrotoxic crisis—also known as thyroid storm—usually occurs in patients with preexisting, though commonly unrecognized, thyrotoxicosis. Left untreated, it's usually fatal.

PATHOPHYSIOLOGY

The thyroid gland secretes the thyroid hormones triiodothyronine (T_3) and thyroxine (T_4). When T_3 and T_4 are overproduced, systemic adrenergic activity increases. The result is epinephrine overproduction and severe hypermetabolism, leading rapidly to cardiac, GI, and sympathetic nervous system decompensation.

ASSESSMENT FINDINGS

Initially, the patient may have marked tachycardia, vomiting, and stupor. If left untreated, he may experience vascular collapse, hypotension, coma, and death. Other findings may include a combination of irritability and restlessness; visual disturbances such as diplopia; tremor and weakness; angina; shortness of breath; cough; and swollen extremities. Palpation may disclose warm, moist, flushed skin, and a high fever that begins insidiously and rises rapidly to a lethal level.

PRECIPITATING FACTORS

Onset is usually abrupt and evoked by a stressful event, such as trauma, surgery, or infection. Other less common precipitating factors include:
- insulin-induced ketoacidosis
- hypoglycemia or diabetic ketoacidosis
- stroke
- myocardial infarction
- pulmonary embolism
- sudden discontinuation of antithyroid drug therapy
- initiation of radioactive iodine therapy
- preeclampsia
- subtotal thyroidectomy with accompanying excessive intake of synthetic thyroid hormone.

⬤ **Complications**
- Thyroid storm (thyroid crisis): tachycardia, delirium, agitation, coma, death, hyperpyrexia, dehydration, arrhythmias, diarrhea (see *Understanding thyroid storm*)
- Arrhythmias (especially atrial fibrillation)
- Diabetes mellitus
- Osteoporosis

⬤ **Surgical intervention**
- Subtotal thyroidectomy when euthyroid state is established

HYPOTHYROIDISM

⬤ **Definition**
- Underactive state of the thyroid gland, resulting in the absence or decreased secretion of thyroid hormone

⬤ **Causes**
- Autoimmune disease: Hashimoto's thyroiditis
- Thyroidectomy
- Overuse of antithyroid drugs

- Malfunction of the pituitary gland
- Use of radioactive iodine
- Inflammatory conditions
- Toxemia of pregnancy

● **Pathophysiology**
- Thyroid gland fails to secrete a satisfactory quantity of thyroid hormone
- Hyposecretion of thyroid hormone results in overall decrease in metabolism

● **Assessment findings**
- Fatigue
- Weight gain
- Dry, flaky, "doughy" skin
- Edema
- Cold intolerance
- Coarse hair
- Alopecia
- Thick tongue, swollen lips
- Mental sluggishness
- Menstrual disorders
- Constipation
- Hypersensitivity to opioids, barbiturates, and anesthetics
- Anorexia
- Decreased diaphoresis
- Hypothermia

● **Diagnostic test findings**
- Blood chemistry: decreased T_3, T_4, protein-bound iodine, sodium; increased TSH, cholesterol
- RAIU: decreased
- ECG: sinus bradycardia

● **Medical management**
- Thyroid hormone replacements: levothyroxine (Synthroid), liothyronine (Cytomel), thyroglobulin, liotrix (Thyrolar)
- Activity: caution with contact sports or heavy physical labor
- Monitoring: vital signs, I/O, and laboratory studies (T_3, T_4, and sodium)

● **Nursing interventions**
- Encourage fluids
- Monitor and record vital signs, I/O, and laboratory studies
- Observe for signs and symptoms of myxedema coma (see *Managing myxedema coma,* page 304)
- Administer medications, as prescribed
- Encourage physical activity and mental stimulation, as tolerated
- Provide a warm environment
- **Avoid sedation: administer one-third to one-half the normal dose of sedatives or opioids**
- Assess for constipation and edema
- Provide frequent rest periods

Key signs and symptoms of hypothyroidism

- Fatigue
- Weight gain
- Dry, flaky, "doughy" skin
- Cold intolerance
- Mental sluggishness
- Menstrual disorders
- Hypothermia

Diagnosing hypothyroidism

- T_3, T_4, protein-bound iodine, sodium: decreased
- TSH, cholesterol: increased

Treating hypothyroidism

- Thyroid hormone replacement: levothyroxine, liothyronine, thyroglobulin, liotrix
- Monitoring vital signs, I/O, and laboratory studies (T_3, T_4, and sodium)

Key nursing interventions for a patient with hypothyroidism

- Observe for signs and symptoms of myxedema coma.
- Encourage physical activity and mental stimulation, as tolerated.
- Avoid sedation: Administer one-third to one-half the normal dose of sedatives or opioids.

Key facts about myxedema coma

- Medical emergency
- May develop abruptly
- Nursing interventions include:
- maintaining a patent airway
- providing fluid replacement
- warming the patient
- monitoring laboratory values
- administering thyroid hormone and corticosteroids

Managing myxedema coma

Myxedema coma is a medical emergency that's commonly fatal. Progression is usually gradual, but when stress aggravates severe or prolonged hypothyroidism, coma may develop abruptly. Examples of severe stress are infection, exposure to cold, and trauma. Other precipitating factors include thyroid medication withdrawal and the use of a sedative, an opioid, or an anesthetic.

Patients in myxedema coma have significantly depressed respirations, so their partial pressure of carbon dioxide in arterial blood may increase. Decreased cardiac output and worsening cerebral hypoxia may also occur. The patient is stuporous and hypothermic, and her vital signs reflect bradycardia and hypotension.

NURSING INTERVENTIONS

If your patient becomes comatose, begin these interventions as soon as possible:
- Maintain airway patency with ventilatory support, if necessary.
- Maintain circulation through I.V. fluid replacement.
- Provide continuous electrocardiogram monitoring.

- Monitor arterial blood gas levels to detect hypoxia and metabolic acidosis.
- Warm the patient by wrapping her in blankets. Don't use a warming blanket because it might increase peripheral vasodilation, causing shock.
- Monitor body temperature until stable with a low-reading thermometer.
- Replace thyroid hormone by administering large doses of I.V. levothyroxine as ordered. Monitor vital signs because rapid correction of hypothyroidism can cause adverse cardiac reactions.
- Monitor intake and output and daily weight. With treatment, urine output should increase and body weight should decrease; if not, report this to the physician.
- Replace fluids and other substances such as glucose. Monitor serum electrolyte levels.
- Administer a corticosteroid as ordered.
- Check for possible sources of infection, such as blood, sputum, or urine, which may have precipitated coma. Treat infections or any other underlying illness.

- Individualize home care instructions
  - Know about the disorder and its treatment
  - Follow instructions for medication use, and be aware of possible adverse effects
  - Exercise regularly
  - Recognize the signs and symptoms of myxedema coma
  - Comply with medical follow-up

● Complications
- Myxedema coma: hypoventilation, hypothermia, respiratory acidosis, syncope, bradycardia, hypotension, seizures, and cerebral hypoxia
- Coronary artery disease (CAD)
- Heart failure
- Acute organic psychosis
- Angina
- Myocardial infarction

Key complications of hypothyroidism

- Myxedema coma
- CAD
- Heart failure

● **Surgical intervention**
  • None

THYROID CANCER

● **Definition**
  • Malignant, primary tumor of the thyroid that doesn't affect thyroid hormone secretion

● **Causes**
  • Chronic overstimulation of the pituitary gland
  • Chronic overstimulation of the thymus gland
  • Neck radiation

● **Pathophysiology**
  • Unregulated cell growth and uncontrolled cell division result in the development of a neoplasm
  • Papillary carcinoma: well-differentiated columnar cells form a solitary nodule in the thyroid gland that spreads to the cervical lymph nodes
  • Follicular carcinoma: encapsulated, well-differentiated cells that invade blood vessels and lymphatics
  • Anaplastic carcinoma: either squamous, spindle, or small round cells
  • Medullary carcinoma: solid, differentiated tumor arising from calcitonin-producing C cells

● **Assessment findings**
  • Enlarged thyroid gland
  • Painless, firm, irregular, and enlarged thyroid nodule or mass
  • Palpable cervical lymph nodes
  • Dysphagia
  • Hoarseness
  • Dyspnea

● **Diagnostic test findings**
  • RAIU: "cold" or nonfunctioning nodule
  • Ultrasound: thyroid nodules or mass
  • Thyroid biopsy: cytology positive for cancer cells
  • Thyroid function tests: normal
  • Blood chemistry: increased calcitonin, serotonin, and prostaglandins

● **Medical management**
  • Radiation therapy
  • Chemotherapy: chlorambucil (Leukeran), doxorubicin (Adriamycin), vincristine (Oncovin)
  • Thyroid hormone replacements (after surgery): levothyroxine (Synthroid), liothyronine (Cytomel), thyroglobulin
  • Pulse oximetry
  • Antiemetics: prochlorperazine (Compazine), ondansetron (Zofran)

Key facts about thyroid cancer

• Malignant, primary tumor of the thyroid
• Doesn't affect thyroid hormone secretion
• Types of thyroid carcinomas: papillary, follicular, anaplastic, and medullary

Common causes of thyroid cancer

• Chronic overstimulation of the pituitary gland
• Chronic overstimulation of the thymus gland

Key signs and symptoms of thyroid cancer

• Enlarged thyroid gland
• Painless, firm, irregular, and enlarged thyroid nodule or mass

Diagnosing thyroid cancer

• RAIU: "cold" or nonfunctioning nodule
• Ultrasound: thyroid nodules or mass
• Thyroid biopsy: cytology positive for cancer cells

Treating thyroid cancer

• Radiation therapy
• Chemotherapy
• Thyroidectomy
• Thyroid hormone replacements (after surgery)

- Diet: high-protein, high-carbohydrate, high-calorie, with supplemental feedings
- I.V. therapy as needed
- Activity: as tolerated
- Monitoring: vital signs and I/O
- Laboratory studies: calcitonin, serotonin

● **Nursing interventions**
- Assess respiratory status
- Assess the patient's ability to swallow
- Monitor and record vital signs, I/O, and laboratory studies
- Administer medications, as prescribed
- Encourage the patient to express his feelings about fear of dying
- Provide postchemotherapeutic and postradiation nursing care
  - Provide prophylactic skin, mouth, and perineal care
  - Monitor dietary intake
  - Administer antiemetics and antidiarrheals, as prescribed
  - Monitor for bleeding, infection, and electrolyte imbalance
  - Provide rest periods
- Provide postoperative care, as appropriate
  - Monitor the wound and dressing
  - Monitor calcium levels
  - Assess pain level, administer analgesics as prescribed, and evaluate effect
- Individualize home care instructions
  - Know about the disorder and its treatment
  - Follow instructions for medication use, and be aware of possible adverse effects
  - Know the signs and symptoms of complications
  - Perform wound care, if appropriate
  - Provide information about the American Cancer Society
  - Recognize the signs and symptoms of respiratory distress and difficulty swallowing
  - Comply with medical follow-up

● **Complications**
- Laryngotracheal obstruction
- Respiratory failure
- Esophageal obstruction

● **Surgical interventions**
- Thyroidectomy
- Modified neck dissection

SIMPLE GOITER

● **Definition**
- Enlarged thyroid gland that manifests as swelling in the anterior portion of the neck

- Classified as endemic (colloid) or sporadic (nontoxic)

● **Causes**
- Endemic
  - Living in an area with iodine-depleted soil
  - Decreased iodine intake
- Sporadic
  - Unknown
  - Possibly due to the use of certain drugs, such as lithium or amino-glutethimide

● **Pathophysiology**
- Low levels of thyroid hormone stimulate increased secretion of TSH by the pituitary gland
- TSH stimulation causes the thyroid to increase in size to compensate for the low levels of thyroid hormone

● **Assessment findings**
- Swelling in the neck
- Dysphagia
- Dyspnea, cough, wheezing

● **Diagnostic test findings**
- Blood chemistry: normal or decreased T_4
- RAIU: normal or increased
- TSH: increased
- Ultrasound: thyroid nodules
- Thyroid biopsy: rules out cancer

● **Medical management**
- Radioactive iodine to shrink the goiter
- Diet: avoid goitrogenic foods; use iodized salt
- Monitoring: vital signs, I/O, and laboratory studies (T_4)
- Thyroid hormone replacements: levothyroxine (Synthroid), liothyronine (Cytomel), thyroglobulin
- Avoid goitrogenic drugs, such as sulfonamides, salicylates, and lithium

● **Nursing interventions**
- Assess respiratory status and the patient's ability to swallow
- Monitor and record vital signs, I/O, and laboratory studies
- Administer medications, as prescribed
- Encourage the patient to express his feelings about changes in his body image
- Provide postoperative care, as indicated
  - Monitor the wound and dressings
  - Monitor calcium levels
  - Assess pain level, administer analgesics as prescribed, and evaluate effect
- Individualize home care instructions
  - Know about the disorder and its treatment

– Follow instructions for medication use, and be aware of possible adverse effects
– Know the signs and symptoms of complications
– Perform wound care, if appropriate
– Comply with medical follow-up

Key complications of simple goiter

- Respiratory failure
- Laryngotracheal obstruction

● **Complications**
  • Respiratory failure
  • Laryngotracheal obstruction

● **Surgical intervention**
  • Subtotal thyroidectomy

HYPERPARATHYROIDISM

Key facts about hyperparathyroidism

- Overactivity of one or more parathyroid glands, resulting in increased PTH secretion
- Classified as primary or secondary

● **Definition**
  • Overactivity of one or more parathyroid glands, resulting in increased PTH secretion
  • Classified as primary or secondary

● **Causes**
  • Chronic renal failure
  • Bone disease
  • Benign adenomas
  • Hypertrophy of the parathyroid gland
  • Malignant tumors of the parathyroid gland
  • Vitamin D deficiency
  • Malabsorption

Common causes of hyperparathyroidism

- Chronic renal failure
- Bone disease
- Malignant tumors of the parathyroid gland

● **Pathophysiology**
  • Primary
      – One or more of the parathyroid glands enlarge
      – PTH secretion increases; serum calcium level elevates
  • Secondary: excessive compensatory production of PTH stems from a hypocalcemia-producing abnormality outside the parathyroid gland that isn't responsive to PTH

● **Assessment findings**
  • Recurring nephrolithiasis
  • Arrhythmias
  • Constant epigastric pain that radiates to the back
  • Constipation
  • Anorexia
  • Nausea and vomiting
  • Depression
  • Lethargy
  • Fatigue
  • Muscle weakness, particularly in the legs
  • Personality disturbances

- Chronic low back pain
- Psychomotor disturbances
- Skin necrosis
- Cataracts
- Subcutaneous calcifications
- Polydipsia
- Polyuria
- Hematuria
- Pathologic fractures

● **Diagnostic test findings**
- Primary
  - Blood chemistry: increased calcium, PTH, creatinine, chloride, and alkaline phosphatase; decreased phosphorus
  - Osteocalcin: increased
  - Tartrate-resistant acid phosphatase: increased
  - Basal acid secretion: may increase
  - Urine chemistry: increased calcium and chloride
  - X-ray: may show diffuse bone demineralization, bone cysts, outer cortical bone absorption, and subperiosteal erosion of the phalanges and distal clavicles
- Secondary
  - Serum calcium: normal or slightly decreased
  - Serum phosphorus: variable
  - Serum PTH: increased

● **Medical management**
- Diet: increase fluid intake to 3,000 ml/day
- I.V. therapy: fluids as needed
- Monitoring: vital signs, I/O, and laboratory studies (calcium, phosphorus, BUN, creatinine, potassium, and sodium)
- Bisphosphonate: alendronate (Fosamax)
- Calcitonin (Miacalcin)
- Analgesic (after surgery): oxycodone (Vicodin)
- Antacid (secondary): aluminum hydroxide gel (AlternaGEL)
- Antineoplastic (primary, if disease is metastatic): plicamycin (Mithracin)
- Phosphate salts (primary): K-Phos, Neutra-Phos
- Dialysis using calcium-free dialysate
- Vitamin D (secondary)
- Glucocorticoid: prednisone (secondary)

● **Nursing interventions**
- Administer I.V. fluids; encourage increased oral fluids
- Assess renal status
- Monitor and record vital signs, I/O, and laboratory studies
- Administer medications, as prescribed
- Encourage the patient to express his feelings about his illness
- Encourage ambulation after surgery

Key signs and symptoms of hyperparathyroidism
- Recurring nephrolithiasis
- Arrhythmias
- Nausea and vomiting
- Muscle weakness, particularly in the legs
- Personality disturbances
- Polydipsia
- Polyuria

Diagnosing hyperparathyroidism
- Primary: increased osteocalcin and tartrate-resistant acid phosphatase
- Secondary: normal or slightly decreased serum calcium; increased urine calcium and chloride

Treating hyperparathyroidism
- Monitoring vital signs, I/O, and laboratory studies
- Bisphosphonate
- Calcitonin
- Antineoplastic
- Phosphate salts

Key nursing interventions for a patient with hyperparathyroidism

- Administer I.V. fluids; encourage increased oral fluids.
- Assess bone and flank pain.
- Move the patient carefully to prevent pathologic fractures.

Key complications of hyperparathyroidism

- Renal colic and calculi
- Arrhythmias
- Pathologic fractures

Key facts about hypoparathyroidism

- Decrease in PTH secretion
- Classified as idiopathic, acquired, or reversible

Common causes of hypoparathyroidism

- Abnormalities of the calcium sensor receptor
- Autoimmune disease
- Parathyroidectomy
- Massive thyroid irradiation

- Assess bone and flank pain
- Move the patient carefully to prevent pathologic fractures
- Limit strenuous activity
- Monitor serum electrolytes and calcium, phosphate, and magnesium levels
- Provide postoperative care, as appropriate
    - Keep a tracheostomy tray at the bedside
    - Maintain seizure precautions
    - Support the patient's head and neck with sandbags
    - Monitor for signs of tetany; administer calcium chloride as ordered
- Individualize home care instructions
    - Know about the disorder and its treatment
    - Follow instructions for medication use, and be aware of possible adverse effects
    - Recognize the signs and symptoms of complications
    - Comply with medical follow-up

● **Complications**
- Peptic ulcer
- Depression
- Arrhythmias
- Renal colic and calculi
- Renal failure
- Osteoporosis
- Pathologic fractures
- Muscle atrophy

● **Surgical intervention**
- Parathyroidectomy

HYPOPARATHYROIDISM

● **Definition**
- Decrease in PTH secretion
- Classified as idiopathic, acquired, or reversible

● **Causes**
- Abnormalities of the calcium sensor receptor
- Congenital absence or malformation of the parathyroid glands
- Hypomagnesemia
- Hypercalcemia
- Trauma
- Autoimmune disease
- Parathyroidectomy
- Massive thyroid irradiation
- Use of radioactive iodine
- Parathyroid tumor

GO WITH THE FLOW

What happens in acute hypoparathyroidism

Causes of acute hypoparathyroidism include injury to the glands, accidental removal of the parathyroid glands during thyroidectomy or other neck surgery, autoimmune disease, tumor, tuberculosis, sarcoidosis, hemochromatosis, and severe magnesium deficiency associated with alcoholism and intestinal malabsorption. These disorders and conditions cause a cascade of effects that result in severe hypocalcemia and hyperphosphatemia, which can lead to seizures, tetany, laryngospasm, and central nervous system (CNS) abnormalities, as shown in the flowchart below.

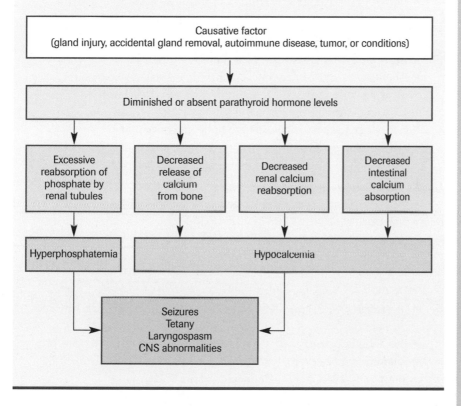

Pathophysiology

- Decreased PTH decreases stimulation to osteoclasts, resulting in decreased release of calcium and phosphorus from bone (see *What happens in acute hypoparathyroidism*)
- Decreased circulating PTH reduces GI absorption of calcium and increases absorption of phosphorus
- Decreased blood calcium causes a rise in serum phosphates and decreased phosphate excretion by the kidney

Assessment findings

- Anxiety

Key signs and symptoms of hypoparathyroidism

- Tingling in the fingers, around the mouth and, occasionally, in the feet
- Increased deep tendon reflexes
- Nausea, vomiting, abdominal pain
- Transverse and longitudinal ridges in the fingernails
- Trousseau's and Chvostek's signs: positive

Diagnosing hypoparathyroidism

- Blood chemistry: decreased PTH, calcium; increased phosphorus
- Urine chemistry: decreased calcium
- CT scan: frontal lobe and basal ganglia calcifications

Treating hypoparathyroidism

- I.V. calcium salts
- Oral calcium salts
- Monitoring vital signs, I/O, and laboratory studies

Key nursing interventions for a patient with hypoparathyroidism

- Assess neurologic status.
- Maintain seizure precautions.
- Keep a tracheostomy tray and I.V. calcium gluconate available.

- Depression
- Muscle and abdominal spasms
- Trousseau's sign: positive
- Chvostek's sign: positive
- Tingling in the fingers, around the mouth and, occasionally, in the feet
- Arrhythmias
- Seizures
- Nausea, vomiting, abdominal pain
- Dyspnea
- Laryngeal stridor
- Personality changes
- Brittle nails
- Transverse and longitudinal ridges in the fingernails
- Alopecia
- Deep tendon reflexes: increased

● **Diagnostic test findings**
- Blood chemistry: decreased PTH, calcium; increased phosphorus
- Urine chemistry: increased creatinine; decreased calcium
- CT scan of frontal lobe and basal ganglia: calcifications
- X-ray: increased bone density and bone malformation
- ECG: prolonged QT interval
- Sulkowitch's test: decreased

● **Medical management**
- I.V. calcium salts: calcium chloride or calcium gluconate
- Oral calcium salts: calcium gluconate (Kalcinate), calcium carbonate (Os-Cal)
- Diet: high-calcium, low-phosphorus
- Activity: as tolerated
- I.V. therapy: fluids as needed
- Monitoring: vital signs, I/O, and laboratory studies (PTH, calcium, and phosphorus)
- Precautions: seizure
- Vitamins: ergocalciferol (vitamin D), dihydrotachysterol (Hytakerol)
- Hormone replacement: parathyroid extract (PTH)

● **Nursing interventions**
- Assess neurologic status
- Maintain seizure precautions
- Monitor and record vital signs, I/O, and laboratory studies
- Administer medications, as prescribed
- Allay the patient's anxiety and provide emotional support
- Keep a tracheostomy tray and I.V. calcium gluconate available
- Maintain a calm environment
- Individualize home care instructions
    - Recognize the signs and symptoms of seizure activity
    - Follow dietary recommendations

- **Complications**
  - Heart failure
  - Nephrolithiasis
- **Surgical intervention**
  - None

CUSHING'S SYNDROME (HYPERCORTISOLISM)

- **Definition**
  - Hyperactivity of the adrenal cortex that results in excessive secretion of glucocorticoids, particularly cortisol
  - Possible increase in mineralocorticoids and sex hormones
- **Causes**
  - Hyperplasia of the adrenal glands
  - Hypothalamic stimulation of the pituitary gland
  - Adenoma or carcinoma of the pituitary gland
  - Exogenous secretion of corticotropin by malignant neoplasms in the lungs or gallbladder
  - Excessive or prolonged administration of glucocorticoids or corticotropin
  - Adenoma or carcinoma of the adrenal cortex
- **Pathophysiology**
  - Hypothalamic stimulation of the pituitary gland causes excessive secretion of corticotropin
  - Excessive secretion of corticotropin causes increased plasma cortisol (see *Understanding corticosteroid excess,* pages 314 and 315)
  - Elevated blood cortisol levels don't diminish secretion of hypothalamic corticotropin-releasing hormone
- **Assessment findings**
  - Weight gain
  - Hirsutism
  - Amenorrhea
  - Weakness and fatigue
  - Ecchymosis, petechiae, and purple striae
  - Edema
  - Hypertension
  - Mood swings
  - Fragile skin
  - Poor wound healing
  - Truncal obesity with thin extremities
  - Buffalo hump
  - Moon face
  - Gynecomastia
  - Enlarged clitoris
  - Decreased libido
  - Muscle weakness

Key results of corticosteroid excess

- Loss of muscle mass
- Obesity and abnormal fat distribution
- Hepatic gluconeogenesis and glycolysis stimulation
- Mineral corticoid activity
- Decreased lymphocytes, especially T lymphocytes
- Varied mood states and alterations in mental abilities
- Blood component changes
- Decreased androgen production leading to virilizing effects in females

Understanding corticosteroid excess

The following are possible results of corticosteroid excess in Cushing's syndrome.

ALTERED PROTEIN METABOLISM

Excessive catabolism of proteins leads to loss of muscle mass with various consequences, including:
- muscle wasting of the extremities—arms and legs become thin
- difficulty pulling up from low chairs and climbing stairs
- generalized weakness and fatigue
- loss of protein bone matrix leading to osteoporosis; compression fractures of the spine; complaints of backache, bone pain, and pathological fractures
- loss of collagen support to the skin, causing thin, fragile skin; purple striae seen after rapid weight gain; skin bruising easily
- delayed wound healing.

ALTERED FAT METABOLISM

Alterations in fat metabolism lead to obesity and abnormal fat distribution.
- Moon face is seen from fatty deposits in the cheeks and face.
- Buffalo hump occurs as a result of intracapsular fat deposits in the upper back.
- Truncal obesity is seen from mesenteric fat deposits.
- Weight gain is usually experienced.

ALTERED CARBOHYDRATE METABOLISM

Increased cortisol level stimulates hepatic gluconeogenesis and glycolysis.
- Postprandial hyperglycemia is a result of impaired insulin metabolism.
- Serum blood glucose level is elevated.
- Steroid-induced diabetes mellitus may develop.

ALTERED WATER AND MINERAL METABOLISM

Increased cortisol produces mineral corticoid activity.

- Sodium and water are retained, contributing to weight gain and edema.
- Hypertension may develop.
- Hypokalemia, hypochloremia, and alkalosis may be present.
- Increased calcium resorption from bone contributes to osteoporosis and can contribute to the formation of renal calculi.

ALTERED IMMUNE RESPONSE

Increased cortisol causes a decrease in lymphocytes, especially T lymphocytes.
- Cell-mediated immunity is decreased.
- Neutrophil count increases.
- Antibody activity is altered.
- Vulnerability to viral and fungal infections, especially opportunistic infections, increases.
- Early signs of infection, particularly fever, are masked.
- Wound healing is delayed.

ALTERED EMOTIONAL STABILITY

Elevated cortisol level contributes to varied mood states and affects mental abilities.
- Mood swings, euphoria, and depression may occur.
- Anxiety, irritability, and psychosis may occur.
- Difficulty concentrating and poor memory may occur.
- Sleep patterns may be altered, and difficulty falling asleep may occur.

ALTERED HEMATOLOGIC ACTIVITY

Excessive cortisol results in changes of many blood components.
- Red blood cell count, hemoglobin level, and hematocrit may be high. This may contribute to a facial

---

Understanding corticosteroid excess *(continued)*

plethora commonly seen in Cushing's disease.
- Leukocytosis, lymphopenia, and eosinopenia may occur.
- Increased platelet count and clotting factors may contribute to thrombus formation.

ALTERED ANDROGEN ACTIVITY
Excessive cortisol results in increased androgen production, leading to viril-

izing effects in females, including:
- hirsutism—a downy covering of hair on face and body
- facial acne
- loss of scalp hair
- menstrual irregularities, including amenorrhea
- altered libido.

- Recurrent infections
- Acne

● **Diagnostic test findings**
- Dexamethasone suppression test: no decrease in plasma cortisol levels
- CT scan, magnetic resonance imaging (MRI), ultrasonography: pituitary or adrenal tumors
- Urine chemistry: elevated free cortisol; decreased specific gravity; glycosuria
- Blood chemistry: increased cortisol, aldosterone, sodium, corticotropin, and glucose; decreased potassium and calcium

● **Medical management**
- Diet: low-sodium, low-calorie, high-potassium, high-protein
- Activity: as tolerated
- Monitoring: vital signs, I/O, and laboratory studies (sodium, potassium, cortisol, BUN, and glucose)
- Radiation therapy
- Glucocorticoids (after surgery and with the use of adrenal suppressants): prednisone (Deltasone)
- Potassium supplements: potassium chloride (K-Lor), potassium gluconate (Kaon)
- Adrenal suppressants: metyrapone (Metopirone), aminoglutethimide (Cytadren), ketoconazole (Nizoral)
- Hypoglycemics: rapid-acting; short-acting (regular); intermediate-acting (NPH); long-acting (Lente, Lantus); glyburide (DiaBeta, Micronase, Amaryl); glipizide (Glucotrol, Glucotrol XL)

● **Nursing interventions**
- Maintain the patient's diet
- Monitor and record vital signs, I/O, daily weight, blood glucose levels, and laboratory studies
- Assess edema and fluid balance
- Check for infections of the skin and the respiratory and urinary tracts
- Protect the patient from falls and bruising

Diagnosing Cushing's syndrome
- Dexamethasone suppression test: no decrease in plasma cortisol levels
- CT scan: pituitary or adrenal tumors
- Blood chemistry: increased cortisol, aldosterone, sodium, corticotropin, and glucose; decreased potassium and calcium

Treating Cushing's syndrome
- Radiation therapy
- Glucocorticoids (after surgery and with the use of adrenal suppressants)
- Adrenal suppressants
- Hypoglycemics

Key nursing interventions for a patient with Cushing's syndrome
- Assess edema and fluid balance.
- Protect the patient from infection.
- Provide postradiation care.
- Provide postoperative care.

- Protect from infection
- Administer medications, as prescribed
- Encourage the patient to express his feelings about changes in his body image and sexual function
- Provide rest periods and minimize environmental stress
- Provide postradiation nursing care
  - Provide prophylactic skin care
  - Monitor dietary intake
  - Provide rest periods
  - Assess for hypoglycemia
- Provide posttransphenoidal hypophysectomy care, as appropriate
  - Keep the head of the bed elevated at least 30 degrees
  - Maintain nasal packing
  - Provide frequent mouth care
  - Avoid activities that increase intracerebral pressure
  - Monitor neurologic status
  - Assess for signs and symptoms of diabetes insipidus
- Individualize home care instructions
  - Know about the disorder, and be aware of possible adverse effects
  - Recognize the signs and symptoms of infection and fluid retention
  - Avoid exposure to people with infections
  - Monitor self for infection

Complications
- Adrenal insufficiency
- Infection
- Peptic ulcers
- Hypertension
- Osteoporosis
- Fractures
- Heart failure
- Psychosis
- Diabetes insipidus
- Diabetes mellitus
- Arteriosclerosis

Surgical interventions
- Adrenalectomy
- Transphenoidal hypophysectomy

ADDISON'S DISEASE

Definition
- Chronic hypoactivity of the adrenal cortex, resulting in insufficient secretion of glucocorticoids (cortisol) and mineralocorticoids (aldosterone)
- Classified as primary or secondary

Causes
- Idiopathic atrophy of adrenal glands
- Surgical removal of adrenal glands
- Autoimmune disease
- Tuberculosis
- Metastatic lesions from lung cancer
- Pituitary hypofunction
- Infection
- Trauma

Pathophysiology
- Autoimmune theory: body produces adrenocortical antibodies, resulting in adrenal hypofunction
- Decreased aldosterone causes disturbances in sodium, water, and potassium metabolism
- Decreased cortisol causes abnormal metabolism of fat, protein, and carbohydrate

Assessment findings
- Hypoglycemia
- Weakness and lethargy
- Bronzed skin pigmentation of nipples and scars (primary)
- Increased pigmentation of buccal mucosa (primary)
- Vitiligo
- Anorexia, nausea, vomiting
- Decreased pubic and axillary hair in females
- Orthostatic hypotension
- Irregular pulse
- Poor coordination
- Craving for salty foods
- Decreased libido
- Chronic diarrhea
- Weight loss
- Depression

Diagnostic test findings
- Blood chemistry: decreased HCT, Hb, cortisol, glucose, sodium, chloride and aldosterone; increased BUN and potassium
- Urine chemistry: decreased 17-KS and 17-OHCS
- Basal metabolic rate (BMR): decreased
- Fasting serum glucose: hypoglycemia
- Metyrapone test: no rise in plasma cortisol precursor level (secondary)
- Corticotropin-stimulating test: no rise in plasma and urine cortisol levels
- X-ray: small heart and adrenal calcification

Medical management
- Mineralocorticoid (aldosterone): fludrocortisone (Florinef)
- Glucocorticoids: cortisone (Cortone), hydrocortisone (Solu-Cortef)

Common causes of Addison's disease
- Idiopathic atrophy of adrenal glands
- Surgical removal of adrenal glands
- Autoimmune disease
- Tuberculosis

Key signs and symptoms of Addison's disease
- Hypoglycemia
- Weakness and lethargy
- Orthostatic hypotension
- Weight loss
- Bronzed pigmentation of nipples and scars

Diagnosing Addison's disease
- Metryrapone test: plasma levels of cortisol precursor don't rise
- Corticotropin-stimulating test: plasma and urine cortisol levels don't rise

Treating Addison's disease

- I.V. therapy
- Glucocorticoids
- Mineralocorticoids
- Monitoring vital signs, I/O, daily weight, and laboratory studies

Key nursing interventions for a patient with Addison's disease

- Administer medications.
- Protect the patient from falls.
- Encourage fluid intake.

Key complications of Addison's disease

- Addisonian crisis
- Hyperpyrexia
- Hypoglycemia

Key facts about pheochromocytoma

- Catecholamine-secreting neo-plasm associated with hyper-functioning adrenal medulla
- Increased catecholamines cause hypertension, increased BMR, and hyperglycemia

- Diet: high-carbohydrate, high-protein, high-sodium, low-potassium, in small, frequent feedings before steroid therapy; high-potassium and low-sodium when on steroid therapy
- I.V. therapy: hydration, electrolyte replacement
- Activity: bed rest (with adrenal crisis)
- Monitoring: vital signs, I/O, daily weight, and laboratory studies
- Vasopressors: phenylephrine (Neo-Synephrine), norepinephrine (Levophed), dopamine (Intropin) (with adrenal crisis)

● **Nursing interventions**
- Monitor and record vital signs, I/O, daily weight, and laboratory studies
- Administer I.V. fluids
- Administer medications, as prescribed
- Allay the patient's anxiety and provide emotional support
- Protect the patient from falls
- Encourage fluid intake
- Assist with activities of daily living
- Maintain a quiet environment
- Individualize home care instructions
  – Know about the disorder and its treatment
  – Follow instructions for medication use, and be aware of possible adverse effects
  – Avoid strenuous exercise, particularly in hot weather
  – Recognize the signs and symptoms of adrenal crisis
  – Increase fluid intake in hot weather
  – Carry medical identification regarding steroid use
  – Carry injectable dexamethasone (Decadron)
  – Avoid using over-the-counter (OTC) drugs
  – Comply with medical follow-up

● **Complications**
- Addisonian crisis (adrenal crisis)
- Hyperpyrexia
- Hypoglycemia
- Hypovolemic shock
- Renal failure

● **Surgical interventions**
- None

PHEOCHROMOCYTOMA

● **Definition**
- Catecholamine-secreting neoplasm associated with hyperfunctioning adrenal medulla

● **Causes**
- May be inherited as an autosomal dominant trait

- Risk factors
  - Anesthesia
  - Medication
  - Radiation contrast dye
  - Childbirth
- **Pathophysiology**
  - Tumor in the adrenal medulla secretes large amounts of catecholamines (epinephrine and norepinephrine)
  - Increased catecholamines cause hypertension, increased BMR, and hyperglycemia
- **Assessment findings (during paroxysms or crisis)**
  - Labile malignant hypertension
  - Throbbing headaches
  - Diaphoresis
  - Palpitations
  - Tachycardia
  - Excessive anxiety
  - Vertigo
  - Tachypnea
  - Angina
  - Nausea and vomiting
  - Visual disturbances
  - Seizures
  - Tremors
- **Diagnostic test findings**
  - CT scan: adrenal tumor
  - Angiography: adrenal tumor
  - MRI: adrenal tumor
  - VMA: increased
  - Blood chemistries: increased BUN, creatinine, glucose, and catecholamines
  - Urine chemistries: increased glucose and catecholamines
  - Iodine-131-meta-iodobenzyl-guanidine scan: confirms pheochromocytoma
- **Medical management**
  - Diet: high-protein with adequate calories
  - Activity: rest during acute attacks
  - Monitoring: vital signs, I/O, and daily weight
  - Laboratory studies: BUN, creatinine, and glucose
  - Alpha-adrenergic blockers: phenoxybenzamine (Dibenzyline), labetalol (Normodyne)
  - Beta-adrenergic blocker: propranolol (Inderal)
  - Vasodilator (during crisis): nitroprusside (Nipride)
  - Catecholamine synthesis antagonist: metyrosine (Demser)

Common causes of pheochromocytoma

- Autosomal dominant trait
- Risk factors: anesthesia, medication, radiation contrast dye, childbirth

Key signs and symptoms of pheochromocytoma

During paroxysms or crisis:
- Labile malignant hypertension
- Throbbing headaches
- Diaphoresis
- Tachycardia
- Tachypnea

Diagnosing pheochromocytoma

- CT scan: adrenal tumor
- Iodine-131-meta-iodobenzyl-guanidine scan: confirms neoplasm

Treating pheochromocytoma

- Alpha-adrenergic blockers
- Beta-adrenergic blocker
- Catecholamine synthesis antagonist

● **Nursing interventions**
- Assess cardiovascular status
- Keep the patient in semi-Fowler's position
- Monitor vital signs, I/O, orthostatic blood pressure, daily weight, and laboratory studies
- Administer medications, as prescribed
- Allay the patient's anxiety and provide emotional support
- Protect the patient from falls
- Provide rest periods and minimize environmental stress
- Provide postradiation nursing care
  - Provide skin and mouth care
  - Monitor dietary intake
  - Provide rest periods
- Provide postoperative care, as appropriate
  - Monitor vital signs
  - Assess the wound and dressings for signs of hemorrhage
  - Assess pain level, administer analgesics as prescribed, and evaluate effect
- Individualize home care instructions
  - Know about the disorder and its treatment
  - Follow instructions for medication use, and be aware of possible adverse effects
  - Stop smoking
  - Recognize the signs and symptoms of renal failure
  - Monitor blood pressure

● **Complications**
- Cardiac arrest or arrhythmia
- Stroke
- Retinopathy
- Renal failure
- Acute pulmonary edema
- Heart failure

● **Surgical intervention**
- Removal of pheochromocytoma

HYPERALDOSTERONISM (PRIMARY ALDOSTERONISM, CONN'S SYNDROME)

● **Definition**
- Hypersecretion of aldosterone (mineralocorticoids) from the adrenal cortex
- Classified as primary or secondary

● **Causes**
- Adenoma of the adrenal cortex
- Adrenal hyperplasia
- Adrenal carcinoma

Effects of excessive aldosterone secretion

Excessive aldosterone secretion fosters serious electrolyte imbalances. The chart below shows what happens.

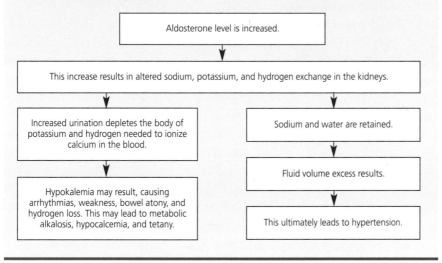

- Bartter syndrome
- Nephrotic syndrome
- Hepatic cirrhosis with ascites

● **Pathophysiology**
- Aldosterone's primary effect on the renal tubules causes the kidneys to retain sodium and water and excrete potassium and hydrogen (see *Effects of excessive aldosterone secretion*)

● **Assessment findings**
- Vision disturbances
- Muscle weakness
- Polyuria
- Polydipsia
- Hypertension
- Postural hypotension
- Headache
- Abdominal distention
- Paresthesia
- Intermittent flaccid paralysis
- Fatigue
- Nocturia

● **Diagnostic test findings**
- Blood chemistry: decreased potassium; increased sodium, bicarbonate
- Arterial blood gas (ABG) analysis: metabolic alkalosis
- Urine chemistry: increased aldosterone, protein, pH; decreased specific gravity

Key signs and symptoms of hyperaldosteronism

- Vision disturbances
- Muscle weakness
- Headache
- Paresthesia
- Intermittent flaccid paralysis

Diagnosing hyperaldosteronism

- Plasma aldosterone: increased
- Plasma renin: increased
- Adrenal angiography or CT scan: localizes the tumor

- Plasma aldosterone: increased
- Plasma renin: increased (secondary)
- Suppression test: distinguishes between primary and secondary
- Adrenal angiography or CT scan: localizes the tumor

● **Medical management**
- Treatment of the underlying cause (secondary)
- Diet: high-potassium, low-sodium
- Monitoring: vital signs, I/O, cardiac rhythm, and laboratory studies (serum electrolytes, calcium, and ABG analysis)
- Potassium supplements: potassium chloride (KCl), potassium gluconate (Kaon)
- Potassium-sparing diuretics: spironolactone (Aldactone), acetazolamide (Diamox)

● **Nursing interventions**
- Assess for signs and symptoms of tetany
- Maintain the patient's diet, as tolerated
- Monitor and record vital signs, I/O, orthostatic blood pressure, daily weight, and laboratory studies
- Administer medications, as prescribed
- Allay the patient's anxiety and provide emotional support
- Provide a quiet environment
- Provide postoperative care, as appropriate
    - Assess for signs and symptoms of adrenal hypofunction
    - Monitor the wound and dressings
    - Assess pain level, administer analgesics as prescribed, and evaluate effect
- Individualize home care instructions
    - Know about the disorder and its treatment
    - Follow instructions for medication use, and be aware of possible adverse effects
    - Recognize the signs and symptoms of fluid overload and muscle irritability
    - Comply with medical follow-up

● **Complications**
- Seizures
- Arrhythmias
- Heart failure

● **Surgical intervention**
- Adrenalectomy

DIABETES MELLITUS

● **Definition**
- Chronic disorder of absolute or relative insulin deficiency or resistance
- Characterized by disturbances in carbohydrate, protein, and fat metabolism

---

Treating hyperaldosteronism

- Treatment of the underlying cause
- Potassium supplements
- Potassium-sparing diuretics

Key nursing interventions for a patient with hyperaldosteronism

- Assess fluid balance.
- Monitor vital signs, I/O, orthostatic blood pressure, daily weight, and laboratory studies.
- Provide postoperative care.

Key complications of hyperaldosteronism

- Seizures
- Arrhythmias
- Heart failure

Key facts about diabetes mellitus

- Chronic disorder of absolute or relative insulin deficiency or resistance
- Two types: type 1, type 2

- Two primary forms
  - Type 1, characterized by absolute insulin insufficiency
  - Type 2, characterized by insulin resistance with varying degrees of insulin secretory defects

Causes
- Autoimmune disease (type 1)
- Genetic factors

Risk factors
- Viral infections (type 1)
- Obesity (type 2)
- Physiologic or emotional stress
- Sedentary lifestyle (type 2)
- Pregnancy
- Medications such as adrenal corticosteroids

Pathophysiology
- Type 1 results from an inability to produce endogenous insulin by the beta cells in the islets of Langerhans in the pancreas
- Type 2 is a deficit in insulin release or an insulin-receptor defect in peripheral tissues
- Insulin deprivation of insulin-dependent cells leads to a marked decrease in the cellular rate of glucose uptake
- Glucogenesis increases because of decreased stimulation of glucose metabolism with resulting hyperglycemia and glycosuria
- Decreased insulin triggers release of free fatty acids that can't be metabolized and are released as ketone bodies in blood and urine
- Decreased insulin depresses protein synthesis, causing a release of amino acids that the liver converts into glucose and ketones
- The formation of urea results in overall nitrogen loss

Assessment findings
- Weight loss
- Anorexia
- Polyphagia
- Acetone breath
- Weakness
- Fatigue
- Dehydration
- Paresthesia
- Polyuria
- Polydipsia
- Kussmaul's respirations
- Frequent infections
- Muscle wasting
- Poor wound healing
- Peripheral and visceral neuropathies
- Retinopathy
- Sexual dysfunction

Common causes of diabetes mellitus
- Autoimmune disease
- Genetic factors
- Risk factors: viral infection, obesity, pregnancy, medications

Key signs and symptoms of diabetes mellitus
- Polyphagia
- Polyuria
- Polydipsia
- Weight loss
- Frequent infections

Diagnosing diabetes mellitus

- Fasting serum glucose: increased on at least two occasions
- Postprandial blood glucose: hyperglycemia

Treating diabetes mellitus

- Diet: individually prescribed diet based on ideal weight, metabolic activity, and personal activity levels
- Hypoglycemics
- Monitoring vital signs, I/O, blood glucose levels, and laboratory studies
- Regular exercise program

Key nursing interventions for a patient with diabetes mellitus

- Monitor and record vital signs, I/O, blood glucose levels, and laboratory studies.
- Provide meticulous skin and foot care.
- Monitor the patient for infection.
- Monitor wound healing.

● **Diagnostic test findings**
- Random blood glucose level: 200 mg/dl or more
- Fasting serum glucose: 126 mg/dl or more on at least two occasions
- Glycosylated Hb assay: increased
- Blood chemistry: increased potassium, chloride, ketones, cholesterol, and triglycerides; decreased carbon dioxide; pH less than 7.4
- Urine chemistry: increased glucose, ketones
- GTT: hyperglycemia
- Postprandial blood glucose: hyperglycemia

● **Medical management**
- Diet: individually prescribed diet based on ideal weight, metabolic activity, and personal activity levels
- Activity: regular exercise program
- Monitoring: vital signs, I/O, and laboratory studies
- Hypoglycemics: rapid-acting, short-acting (regular), intermediate-acting (NPH), long-acting (Ultralente, Lantus); glyburide (DiaBeta, Micronase, Amaryl); glipizide (Glucotrol, Glucotrol XL); metformin (Glucophage); pioglitazone (Actos); rosiglitazone (Avandia); repaglinide (Prandin)
- Vitamin and mineral supplements

● **Nursing interventions**
- Evaluate the patient's diet, and formulate an appropriate diet with a dietician's help
- Monitor and record vital signs, I/O, blood glucose levels, and laboratory studies
- Administer medications, as prescribed
- Encourage the patient to express his feelings about the diagnosis
- Provide meticulous skin and foot care
- Monitor the patient for infection
- Maintain a warm and quiet environment
- Monitor wound healing
- Observe for Somogyi phenomena and Sjögren's syndrome
- Provide information about the American Diabetes Association
- Determine the patient's knowledge of his diet, exercise, and medication regimens, and develop a teaching plan
- Individualize home care instructions
  - Know about the disorder and its treatment
  - Follow instructions for medication use, and be aware of possible adverse effects
  - Monitor blood glucose levels
  - Follow nutritional recommendations
  - Administer insulin, if appropriate
  - Exercise regularly
  - Smoking cessation
  - Recognize the signs and symptoms of hyperglycemia and hypoglycemia

- Monitor self for infection, skin breakdown, changes in peripheral circulation, poor wound healing, and numbness in extremities
- Adjust diet and insulin for changes in work, exercise, trauma, infection, fever, and stress
- Complete daily skin and foot care
- Carry an emergency supply of glucose and know when to use it
- Seek counseling for sexual dysfunction
- Avoid the use of OTC medication without the physician's approval
- Avoid alcohol
- Know the location of available resource and support groups
- Comply with medical follow-up

Complications
- Ketoacidosis (diabetic coma) (see *Understanding DKA and HHNS,* page 326)
- Hyperosmolar hyperglycemic nonketotic syndrome (HHNS)
- Hypoglycemia
- Infections
- Peripheral neuropathies
- Glaucoma
- Impotence
- CAD
- Stroke
- Chronic renal failure
- Diabetic retinopathy
- Peripheral vascular disease

Surgical intervention
- Pancreas transplant

DIABETES INSIPIDUS

Definition
- Disorder of water balance regulation
- Characterized by a deficiency of ADH (vasopressin) that's secreted by the posterior lobe of the pituitary gland (neurohypophysis)
- Also known as DI

Causes
- Trauma to the pituitary gland or hypothalamus
- Tumor of the posterior lobe of the pituitary gland
- Neurosurgery
- Head injury
- Failure of a kidney to respond to vasopressin (nephrogenic DI)
- Congenital malformation of the central nervous system
- Medications such as lithium
- Idiopathic
- Infection

Key facts about DKA and HHNS

- Acute complications of hyperglycemic crisis
- DKA occurs more commonly in patients with type 1 diabetes
- HHNS occurs more commonly in patients with type 2 diabetes
- Insulin-deprived cells can't utilize glucose, and the response is rapid metabolism of protein
- A loss of intracellular potassium and phosphorus occurs, along with excessive liberation of amino acids
- Amino acids are converted into urea and glucose by the liver
- Blood glucose levels become grossly elevated
- Increased serum osmotic diuresis occurs, creating a massive fluid loss and dehydration
- Dehydration is perpetuated, decreasing the glomerular filtration rate and reducing the amount of glucose excreted in the urine
- Diminished glucose excretion raises blood glucose levels, producing hyperosmolarity and dehydration, which cause shock, coma, and death

Understanding DKA and HHNS

Diabetic ketoacidosis (DKA) and hyperosmolar hyperglycemic nonketotic syndrome (HHNS) are acute complications of hyperglycemic crisis that may occur with diabetes. If not treated properly, either may result in coma or death.

DKA occurs more commonly in patients with type 1 diabetes and may be the first evidence of the disease. HHNS occurs more commonly in patients with type 2 diabetes, but it also occurs in anyone whose insulin tolerance is stressed and in patients who have undergone certain therapeutic procedures, such as peritoneal dialysis, hemodialysis, tube feedings, or total parenteral nutrition.

Acute insulin deficiency (absolute in DKA; relative in HHNS) precipitates both conditions. Causes include illness, stress, infection and, in patients with DKA, failure to take insulin.

BUILDUP OF GLUCOSE

Inadequate insulin hinders glucose uptake by fat and muscle cells. Because the cells can't take in glucose to convert to energy, glucose accumulates in the blood. At the same time, the liver responds to the demands of the energy-starved cells by converting glycogen to glucose and releasing glucose into the blood, further increasing the blood glucose level. When this level exceeds the renal threshold, excess glucose is excreted in the urine.

Still, the insulin-deprived cells can't utilize glucose. Their response is rapid metabolism of protein, which results in loss of intracellular potassium and phosphorus and excessive liberation of amino acids. The liver converts these amino acids into urea and glucose.

As a result of these processes, blood glucose levels are grossly elevated. The aftermath is increased serum osmolarity and glycosuria (high amounts of glucose in the urine), leading to osmotic diuresis. Glucosuria is higher in HHNS than in DKA because blood glucose levels are higher in HHNS.

A DEADLY CYCLE

The massive fluid loss from osmotic diuresis causes fluid and electrolyte imbalances and dehydration. Water loss exceeds glucose and electrolyte loss, contributing to hyperosmolarity. This, in turn, perpetuates dehydration, decreasing the glomerular filtration rate and reducing the amount of glucose excreted in the urine. This leads to a deadly cycle: Diminished glucose excretion further raises blood glucose levels, producing hyperosmolarity and dehydration and finally causing shock, coma, and death.

DKA complication

All of these steps hold true for DKA and HHNS, but DKA involves an additional, simultaneous process that leads to metabolic acidosis. The absolute insulin deficiency causes cells to convert fats into glycerol and fatty acids for energy. The fatty acids can't be metabolized as quickly as they're released, so they accumulate in the liver, where they're converted into ketones (ketoacids). These ketones accumulate in the blood and urine and cause acidosis. Acidosis leads to more tissue breakdown, more ketosis, more acidosis and, eventually, shock, coma, and death.

- Vascular lesions
- Pregnancy

Pathophysiology

- Decreased ADH reduces the ability of distal and collecting renal tubules to concentrate urine; therefore, filtered water is excreted rather than absorbed
- Copious, dilute urine and intense thirst result

Assessment findings

- Polyuria (greater than 5 L/day)
- Polydipsia (4 to 40 L/day)
- Fatigue
- Hypotension
- Dyspnea
- Dehydration
- Weight loss
- Muscle weakness and pain
- Headache
- Tachycardia
- Almost colorless urine

Diagnostic test findings

- Urine chemistry: specific gravity less than 1.004, osmolality 50 to 200 mOsm/kg
- Blood chemistry: increased sodium and osmolality, BUN, and creatinine; decreased vasopressin
- Water deprivation test: increased urine osmolality after vasopressin administration exceeding 9%

Medical management

- Identification and treatment of underlying cause
- Diet: increased oral fluids
- I.V. therapy: hydration, electrolyte replacement
- Monitoring: vital signs, CVP, I/O, daily weight, and laboratory studies
- Assess fluid balance
- Anticonvulsant: carbamazepine (Tegretol)
- ADH replacements: desmopressin (DDAVP), vasopressin (Pitressin)
- Diuretics: amiloride (Midamor), hydrochlorothiazide (HydroDIURIL)
- Anti-inflammatory: indomethacin (Indocin)
- Antilipemic: clofibrate
- Hypoglycemic: chlorpropamide (Diabinese)

Nursing interventions

- Assess fluid balance
- Encourage fluids
- Administer I.V. fluids
- Monitor and record vital signs, CVP, I/O, daily weight, specific gravity, and laboratory studies
- Administer medications, as prescribed
- Allay the patient's anxiety and provide emotional support
- Individualize home care instructions

Key signs and symptoms of diabetes insipidus

- Polyuria (greater than 5 L/day)
- Polydipsia (4 to 40 L/day)
- Fatigue

Diagnosing diabetes insipidus

- Specific gravity less than 1.004
- Osmolality 50 to 200 mOsm/kg

Treating diabetes insipidus

- Identification and treatment of underlying cause
- I.V. therapy
- ADH replacements
- Diuretics
- Anti-inflammatory

Key nursing interventions for a patient with diabetes insipidus

- Assess fluid balance.
- Administer I.V. fluids.
- Administer medications.

– Know about the disorder and its treatment
– Follow instructions for medication use, and be aware of possible adverse effects
– Recognize the signs and symptoms of dehydration
– Increase fluid intake in hot weather
– Carry medications on person at all times
– Comply with medical follow-up

● **Complications**
  • Dehydration
  • Arrhythmias
  • Hypovolemic shock

● **Surgical intervention**
  • Hypophysectomy, when the etiology is a tumor

HYPERPITUITARISM (ACROMEGALY)

● **Definition**
  • Chronic, progressive disease marked by hormonal dysfunction that results in skeletal overgrowth

● **Causes**
  • Prolactin-secreting hormone adenomas
  • GH-secreting tumors
  • Cushing's syndrome caused by pituitary dysfunction
  • LH-, FSH-, or TSH-secreting adenomas
  • Adrenalectomy
  • Pregnancy

● **Pathophysiology**
  • Excessive secretion of GH occurs after epiphyseal closing
  • Excessive secretion of GH causes overdevelopment of cartilage, bone, and soft tissue; thickens skin; and enlarges sweat glands, sebaceous glands, and gonads
  • GH-induced hypermetabolism causes hormone alterations

● **Assessment findings**
  • Coarse facial features
  • Enlarged tongue
  • Protruding jaw
  • Skeletal abnormalities
  • Cartilaginous and connective tissue overgrowth
  • Spiderlike fingers
  • Wide hands and feet
  • Weakness
  • Impotence
  • Infertility
  • Oily, thick skin and nails
  • Joint deformities

Key complications of diabetes insipidus

● Dehydration
● Arrhythmias

Key facts about hyperpituitarism

● Chronic, progressive disorder marked by hormonal dysfunction
● Results in skeletal overgrowth

Common causes of hyperpituitarism

● Prolactin-secreting hormone adenomas
● GH-secreting tumors

Key signs and symptoms of hyperpituitarism

● Coarse facial features
● Enlarged tongue
● Protruding jaw
● Skeletal abnormalities

- Pain in joints
- Deepening of the voice
- Diaphoresis
- Headache

● **Diagnostic test findings**
  - GH radioimmunoassay: increased plasma GH levels and levels of insulin-like growth factor I
  - Glucose suppression test: failure to suppress the hormone level to below the accepted norm of 2 ng/ml
  - CT scan: pituitary tumor
  - X-ray: thickened long bones and skull

● **Medical management**
  - Radiation therapy via transphenoidal implant
  - Monitoring: vital signs and I/O
  - Laboratory studies: glucose, potassium, and calcium
  - Somatostatin analogue: octreotide (Sandostatin)
  - Dopaminergics: levodopa (Larodopa), bromocriptine (Parlodel)
  - Hormones: somatotropin (Humatrope), ethinyl estradiol, testosterone (AndroGel), levothyroxine (Synthroid), liothyronine (Cytomel), diethylstilbestrol, cortisone (if entire pituitary is removed)
  - Growth hormone antagonist: pegvisomant (Somavert)

● **Nursing interventions**
  - Monitor and record vital signs, I/O, blood glucose levels, and laboratory studies
  - Administer medications, as prescribed
  - Encourage the patient to express his feelings about the illness
  - Maintain activity, as tolerated
  - Provide skin care
  - Position and support painful joints
  - Protect the patient from falls
  - Monitor for infection
  - Provide postradiation nursing care
    - Provide prophylactic skin and mouth care
    - Monitor dietary intake
    - Provide rest periods
  - Provide postoperative care, as appropriate
    - Assess for signs and symptoms of increased ICP
    - Keep the head of the bed elevated 30 degrees
    - Monitor for signs and symptoms of hormone deficiency
    - Monitor I/O
  - Individualize home care instructions
    - Know about the disorder and its treatment
    - Follow instructions for medication use, and be aware of possible adverse effects
    - Observe for signs and symptoms of complications

Diagnosing hyperpituitarism

- GH radioimmunoassay: increased plasma GH and insulin-like growth factor I levels
- Glucose suppression test: failure to suppress the hormone level to below the accepted norm of 2 ng/ml
- CT scan: pituitary tumor

Treating hyperpituitarism

- Radiation therapy
- Dopaminergics
- Hormones
- Somatostatin analogue
- Growth hormone antagonist
- Transphenoidal hypophysectomy

Key nursing interventions for a patient with hyperpituitarism

- Monitor vital signs, I/O, blood glucose levels, and laboratory studies.
- Provide postradiation care.
- Provide postoperative care.
- Administer medications.

– Carry emergency adrenal hormone replacement drugs
– Wear medical identification jewelry
– Comply with medical follow-up

- **Complications**
  - Blindness
  - Vision disturbances
  - Diabetes mellitus
  - Hypertension
  - Heart failure
  - Arteriosclerosis
  - Cardiomyopathy
  - Arthritis
  - Carpal tunnel syndrome
  - Osteoporosis

- **Surgical intervention**
  - Transphenoidal hypophysectomy

HYPOPITUITARISM (SIMMONDS' DISEASE)

- **Definition**
  - Hypofunction of the anterior pituitary gland (adenohypophysis), resulting in insufficient or absent quantities of anterior pituitary gland hormones or target organ hormones
  - Classified as primary or secondary (resulting from dysfunction of the hypothalamus)

- **Causes**
  - Adenomas or carcinomas of the pituitary gland
  - Infection
  - Idiopathic
  - Head trauma
  - Necrosis of the pituitary gland (Sheehan's syndrome)
  - Partial or total hypophysectomy by surgery, radiation, or chemical agent
  - Insufficient hypothalamic-releasing hormones

- **Pathophysiology**
  - Decreased pituitary function results in decreased amounts of GH, TSH, and corticotropin
  - With progressive loss of pituitary function, levels of FSH and LH decrease

- **Assessment findings**
  - GH deficiency
    - Short stature
    - Delayed secondary tooth eruption
    - Delayed puberty
  - Gonadotropin (FSH and LH) deficiency in women
    - Amenorrhea

- Dyspareunia
- Infertility
- Reduced libido
- Breast atrophy
- Sparse or absent axillary and pubic hair
- Gonadotropin (FSH and LH) deficiency in men
  - Impotence
  - Reduced libido
  - Decreased muscle strength
  - Testicular softening and shrinkage
  - Retarded secondary hair growth
- TSH deficiency
  - Cold intolerance
  - Constipation
  - Menstrual irregularity
  - Lethargy
  - Dry, pale, puffy skin
  - Slow thought process
  - Bradycardia
  - Severe growth retardation in children despite treatment
- Corticotropin deficiency
  - Fatigue
  - Nausea, vomiting, anorexia
  - Hypothermia and hypotension during stress
  - Weight loss
  - Depigmentation of the skin and nipples
- Prolactin deficiency
  - Absent postpartum lactation
  - Amenorrhea
  - Sparse axillary and pubic hair

Diagnostic test findings

- Blood chemistry: decreased cortisol, GH, corticotropin, TSH, LH, FSH, glucose, and gonadotropins
- Oral administration of metyrapone: shows the source of low hydroxycorticosteroid levels
- Administration of gonadotropin-releasing hormone: distinguishes between pituitary and hypothalamic causes of gonadotropin deficiency
- Provocative testing: shows persistently low GH and insulin-like growth factor I levels, confirming GH deficiency
- RAIU: decreased
- Fasting serum glucose: decreased glucose
- CT scan: adenohypophyseal tumor
- Visual fields: hemianopsia and loss of color vision
- Angiography: adenohypophyseal tumor
- Urine chemistry: decreased gonadotropins, 17-OHCS, and 17-KS
- Skull X-ray: adenohypophyseal tumor

Treating hypopituitarism

- Radiation therapy
- Hormones
- Monitoring vital signs, I/O, and laboratory studies

Key nursing interventions for a patient with hypopituitarism

- Administer medications.
- Monitor for infection.
- Maintain a warm environment.
- Provide emotional support.

Key complications of hypopituitarism

- Death
- DI
- Hypothyroidism
- Adrenal insufficiency

● **Medical management**
- Diet: high-protein, high-calorie
- Activity: as tolerated
- Monitoring: vital signs, I/O, and laboratory studies
- Radiation therapy
- Dopaminergics: levodopa (Larodopa), bromocriptine (Parlodel)
- Hormones: somatotropin (Humatrope), ethinyl estradiol, testosterone (Androgel), levothyroxine (Synthroid), liothyronine (Cytomel), cortisone

● **Nursing interventions**
- Monitor and record vital signs, I/O, and laboratory studies
- Maintain the patient's diet
- Administer medications, as prescribed
- Encourage the patient to express his feelings about the illness
- Maintain activity, as tolerated
- Prevent falls
- Monitor for infection
- Maintain a warm environment
- Provide skin care
- Allay the patient's anxiety and provide emotional support
- Provide postradiation nursing care
    - Provide prophylactic skin care
    - Monitor dietary intake
    - Provide rest periods
- Individualize home care instructions
    - Know about the disorder and its treatment
    - Follow instructions for medication use, and be aware of possible adverse effects
    - Recognize the signs and symptoms of dehydration
    - Avoid exposure to people with infections
    - Monitor self for infection
    - Comply with medical follow-up

● **Complications**
- Death
- DI
- Hypothyroidism
- Adrenal insufficiency

● **Surgical interventions**
- Hypophysectomy
- Resection of the pituitary gland for tumor removal

NCLEX CHECKS

It's never too soon to begin your NCLEX preparation. Now that you've reviewed this chapter, carefully read each of the following questions and choose the best answer. Then compare your responses to the correct answers.

1. A client is diagnosed with hyperthyroidism. The nurse should expect to see which clinical signs and symptoms? Select all that apply.

☐ **1.** Anxiety
☐ **2.** Dry, flaky skin
☐ **3.** Hypothermia
☐ **4.** Increased blood pressure
☐ **5.** Tachycardia
☐ **6.** Weight gain

2. A client with thyroid cancer undergoes a thyroidectomy. After surgery, the client develops peripheral numbness, tingling, muscle twitching, and spasms. The nurse should administer:

☐ **1.** a thyroid supplement.
☐ **2.** an antispasmodic.
☐ **3.** a barbiturate.
☐ **4.** I.V. calcium gluconate.

3. A client with intractable asthma develops Cushing's syndrome. This development is most likely attributed to long-term or excessive use of:

☐ **1.** prednisone.
☐ **2.** theophylline.
☐ **3.** metaproterenol (Alupent).
☐ **4.** cromolyn (Intal).

4. Which nursing diagnosis is most likely for a client with an acute episode of DI?

☐ **1.** Imbalanced nutrition: More than body requirements
☐ **2.** Deficient fluid volume
☐ **3.** Impaired gas exchange
☐ **4.** Ineffective tissue perfusion: Cardiopulmonary

5. A client with a PTH deficiency would most likely experience abnormal serum levels of:

☐ **1.** sodium and chloride.
☐ **2.** potassium and glucose.
☐ **3.** urea and uric acid.
☐ **4.** calcium and phosphorous.

6. A client with newly diagnosed type 1 diabetes mellitus is learning about diabetic foot care. The nurse should instruct the client to avoid:

☐ **1.** lotions.
☐ **2.** antiperspirants.
☐ **3.** foot soaks.
☐ **4.** nail files.

TOP 10

Items to study for your next test on the endocrine system

1. Functions of the thyroid gland and pancreas
2. Common diagnostic tests used for endocrine disorders
3. Nursing diagnoses appropriate for a patient with an endocrine disorder
4. Nursing interventions for a patient after thyroidectomy
5. Signs and symptoms of hyperthyroidism and hypothyroidism
6. Why thyrotoxic crisis occurs
7. Assessment findings in Cushing's syndrome
8. The difference between type 1 and type 2 diabetes mellitus
9. Signs and symptoms of hypoglycemia and hyperglycemia
10. Complications of diabetes mellitus, including DKA and HHNS

7. Following transsphenoidal hypophysectomy, a nurse notes clear drainage on a client's nasal dressing. Which action should the nurse take next?

☐ **1.** Have the client blow his nose.
☐ **2.** Reinforce the nasal dressing.
☐ **3.** Test the drainage for glucose.
☐ **4.** Send a nasal culture to the laboratory.

8. Which statement by a client following bilateral adrenalectomy indicates to the nurse that the client understands discharge instructions?

☐ **1.** "I'll take steroids for 2 weeks."
☐ **2.** "I'll take steroids for life."
☐ **3.** "I'll take steroids until my symptoms subside."
☐ **4.** "I'll gradually taper the steroids."

9. Which finding would a nurse expect in a client with hypothyroidism?

☐ **1.** Exophthalmos
☐ **2.** Heat intolerance
☐ **3.** Weight loss
☐ **4.** Alopecia

10. A client with diabetes mellitus exhibits tremors, tachycardia, and cold, clammy skin. The nurse should expect to treat the client for which condition?

☐ **1.** Ketoacidosis
☐ **2.** HHNS
☐ **3.** Hypoglycemia
☐ **4.** Somogyi phenomenon

ANSWERS AND RATIONALES

1. CORRECT ANSWER: 1, 4, 5
Hyperthyroidism is a hypermetabolic state with symptoms including anxiety, increased blood pressure, and tachycardia—all seen in sympathetic nervous system stimulation. Symptoms of dry, flaky skin, hypothermia, and weight gain are associated with a hypometabolic state of hypothyroidism.

2. CORRECT ANSWER: 4
Removal of the thyroid gland can cause hyposecretion of PTH, leading to calcium deficiency. Symptoms of calcium deficiency include muscle spasms, numbness, and tingling. Treatment includes immediate I.V. administration of calcium gluconate. Thyroid supplements are necessary following thyroidectomy but don't correct hypocalcemia. An antispasmodic doesn't treat the problem, and a barbiturate isn't indicated.

3. CORRECT ANSWER: 1
Cushing's syndrome results from long-term or excessive use of a glucocorticoid such as prednisone. Theophylline, metaproterenol, and cromolyn don't cause Cushing's syndrome.

4. CORRECT ANSWER: 2

DI causes a pronounced loss of intravascular volume; therefore, the most prominent risk to the client is deficient fluid volume. The client is at risk for imbalanced nutrition, impaired gas exchange, and ineffective tissue perfusion, but these risks stem from the deficient fluid volume.

5. CORRECT ANSWER: 4

Because PTH regulates calcium and phosphorus metabolism, a PTH deficiency would affect calcium and phosphorus levels. PTH doesn't affect sodium, chloride, potassium, glucose, urea, or uric acid.

6. CORRECT ANSWER: 3

Foot soaks macerate the skin and increase the risk of breaks in the skin. To moisturize the feet, the client should use water-soluble lotions. He should also use nail files instead of nail clippers or scissors, and if foot perspiration exists, use antiperspirants.

7. CORRECT ANSWER: 3

The presence of glucose in the nasal drainage indicates leakage of cerebrospinal fluid. Following hypophysectomy, instruct the client to avoid blowing his nose. You may reinforce the dressing, but not until you test the fluid for glucose. Although infection can occur after surgery, clear drainage isn't indicative of infection.

8. CORRECT ANSWER: 2

Following bilateral adrenalectomy, the client requires lifelong glucocorticoid and mineralocorticoid replacement. The client shouldn't stop taking steroids after 2 weeks or until his symptoms subside following removal of the adrenal glands. Because the client requires steroids for life, they can't be tapered.

9. CORRECT ANSWER: 4

The client with hypothyroidism will have coarse hair and alopecia. Exophthalmos, heat intolerance, and weight loss are all associated with hyperthyroidism.

10. CORRECT ANSWER: 3

Tremors, tachycardia, and cold, clammy skin are all signs of hypoglycemia. Ketoacidosis characteristics include abdominal pain, acetone breath, altered consciousness, Kussmaul's respirations, nausea, vomiting, oliguria, tachycardia, and hot, flushed skin. HHNS characteristics include severe dehydration, severe hypotension, fever, stupor, and seizures. Somogyi phenomenon shows rebound hyperglycemia in which the client awakens with symptoms of hyperglycemia.

Renal and urologic system

---

1. Which nursing diagnosis would be a probable nursing diagnosis for a client with a renal disorder?

- ☐ 1. *Imbalanced nutrition: More than body requirements*
- ☐ 2. *Energy field disturbance*
- ☐ 3. *Toileting self-care deficit*
- ☐ 4. *Risk for imbalanced fluid volume*

CORRECT ANSWER: 4

2. A nurse is caring for a client with cystitis. A key nursing intervention would be:

- ☐ 1. enforce fluid restriction of 1 qt (1 L)/day.
- ☐ 2. encourage increased fluid intake (up to 3 qt (3 L)/day).
- ☐ 3. administer analgesics.
- ☐ 4. teach self-catheterization.

CORRECT ANSWER: 2

3. A diagnosis of benign prostatic hyperplasia is supported by findings from which tests?

☐ 1. Digital rectal examination (DRE) and free prostate-specific antigen (PSA)

☐ 2. PSA and biopsy

☐ 3. DRE and carcinoembryonic antigen (CEA)

☐ 4. CEA and magnetic resonance imaging

CORRECT ANSWER: 1

4. A client is admitted to the facility with a tentative diagnosis of acute pyelonephritis. To assess for risk factors for acute glomerulonephritis, the nurse should ask the client which question?

☐ 1. Have you taken any aspirin recently?

☐ 2. Do you drink a lot of milk?

☐ 3. Do you drink a lot of cranberry juice?

☐ 4. Have you had a sore throat lately?

CORRECT ANSWER: 4

5. After a transuretheral prostatic resection, a client returns to the unit with an indwelling urinary catheter attached to a continuous bladder irrigating system. Which nursing intervention may help prevent bladder spasms?

☐ 1. Administering pain medication every 2 hours

☐ 2. Infusing I.V. fluids rapidly over the first 6 hours after surgery

☐ 3. Maintaining the bladder irrigation flow to prevent blood clot formation in the bladder

☐ 4. Clamping the catheter every hour

CORRECT ANSWER: 3

LEARNING OBJECTIVES

After studying this chapter, you should be able to:

● Describe the psychosocial impact of renal and urologic disorders.

● Differentiate between modifiable and nonmodifiable risk factors in the development of a renal or urologic disorder.

● List three probable and three possible nursing diagnoses for any patient with a renal or urologic disorder.

● Identify nursing interventions for a patient with a renal or urologic disorder.

● Identify three teaching topics for a patient with a renal or urologic disorder.

CHAPTER OVERVIEW

Caring for the patient with a renal or urologic disorder requires a sound understanding of renal and urologic anatomy and physiology and fluid balance. A thorough assessment is essential to planning and implementing appropriate patient care. The assessment includes a complete history, a physical examination, diagnostic testing, identification of modifiable and nonmodifiable risk factors, and information related to the psychosocial impact of the disorder on the patient.

Nursing diagnoses focus primarily on impaired urinary elimination, excess or deficient fluid volume, and disturbed body image. Nursing interventions should include assessing patient fluid balance and fluid intake and urine output, and helping the patient adjust to body image changes and possible sexual dysfunction. Patient teaching—a crucial nursing activity—involves providing information about the disorder and its treatment, medication regimens, signs and symptoms of possible complications, reduction of modifiable risk factors through adherence to dietary and fluid recommendations and restrictions, and medical follow-up.

ANATOMY AND PHYSIOLOGY

- **Kidneys** (see *Reviewing renal and urologic anatomy*)
  - Two bean-shaped organs
  - Four components: cortex, medulla, renal pelvis, and nephron
    - Cortex
      - Makes up the outer layer of the kidney
      - Contains the glomeruli, proximal tubules of the nephron, and distal tubules of the nephron
    - Medulla
      - Makes up the inner layer of the kidney
      - Contains the loop of Henle and the collecting tubules
    - Renal pelvis
      - Collects urine from the calyces
    - Nephron
      - Makes up the functional unit of the kidney
      - Contains Bowman's capsule and the glomerulus
      - Contains the renal tubule, which consists of proximal convoluted tubule, loop of Henle, distal convoluted tubule, and collecting segments

- **Ureter**
  - This tubule extends from the renal pelvis to the bladder floor
  - Transports urine from the kidney to the bladder
  - Ureterovesical sphincter prevents reflux of urine from the bladder into the ureter

- **Bladder**
  - Muscular, distensible sac that stores urine
  - Total capacity of approximately 1 L

Key facts about the kidneys

- Two bean-shaped organs
- Four components:
- Cortex: outer layer; contains glomeruli, proximal tubules, and distal tubules
- Medulla: inner layer; contains loop of Henle and collecting tubules
- Renal pelvis: collects urine
- Nephron: functional unit; contains Bowman's capsule, glomerulus, and renal tubule

Key facts about the ureter

- Extends from renal pelvis to bladder floor
- Transports urine from the kidney to the bladder

Key facts about the bladder

- Muscular, distensible sac
- Stores urine

Reviewing renal and urologic anatomy

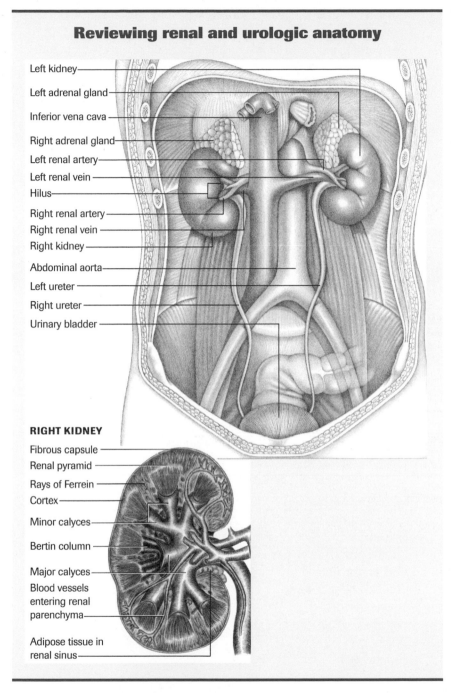

Left kidney
Left adrenal gland
Inferior vena cava
Right adrenal gland
Left renal artery
Left renal vein
Hilus
Right renal artery
Right renal vein
Right kidney
Abdominal aorta
Left ureter
Right ureter
Urinary bladder

RIGHT KIDNEY

Fibrous capsule
Renal pyramid
Rays of Ferrein
Cortex
Minor calyces
Bertin column
Major calyces
Blood vessels entering renal parenchyma
Adipose tissue in renal sinus

Key facts about the urethra

- Extends from the bladder to the urinary meatus
- Transports urine

Key facts about urine formation

- Blood from the renal artery is filtrated.
- Formed filtrate moves through the tubules of the nephron, which reabsorb and secrete electrolytes, water, glucose, amino acids, ammonia, and bicarbonate.
- Antidiuretic hormone and aldosterone control the reabsorption of water and electrolytes.

● **Urethra**
- This tubule extends from the bladder to the urinary meatus
- Urethra transports urine from the bladder to the urinary meatus

● **Urine formation**
- Blood from the renal artery is filtrated across the glomerular capillary membrane in Bowman's capsule

Key facts about blood pressure control

- Blood pressure affects regulation of the kidney's fluid volume
- Decreased blood pressure activates renin-angiotensin system

Key facts about the prostate gland

- Fibrous capsule
- Connected to and surrounds the male urethra
- Contains ducts that secrete seminal fluid

Key assessment findings in a patient with a renal or urologic disorder

- Change in pattern of urination or appearance of urine
- Dysuria
- Pain
- Chills and fever
- Urine output changes

Key physical assessment findings in a patient with a renal or urologic disorder

- Specific gravity abnormalities
- Hematuria

- Filtration requires adequate intravascular volume and adequate cardiac output
- Composition of formed filtrate is similar to blood plasma without proteins
- Formed filtrate moves through the tubules of the nephron, which reabsorb and secrete electrolytes, water, glucose, amino acids, ammonia, and bicarbonate
- Antidiuretic hormone and aldosterone control the reabsorption of water and electrolytes

● **Blood pressure control**
- Blood pressure affects regulation of fluid volume by the kidney
- Decreased blood pressure activates renin-angiotensin system
- Renal disease can alter the renin-angiotensin system

● **Prostate gland**
- This fibrous capsule is connected to and surrounds the male urethra
- Prostate gland contains ducts that secrete the alkaline portion of seminal fluid and that open into the prostatic portion of the urethra

ASSESSMENT FINDINGS

● **History**
- Changes in pattern of urination: frequency, nocturia, hesitancy, urgency, dribbling, incontinence, and retention
- Changes in appearance of urine: dilute, concentrated, hematuria, and pyuria
- Dysuria
- Pain
- Chills and fever
- Urine output changes: polyuria, oliguria, and anuria

● **Physical examination**
- Specific gravity: increased or decreased
- Hematuria
- Periorbital and peripheral edema
- Bladder distention
- Cool skin temperature
- Muscle tremors
- Palpable prostate gland (in men)
- Weight gain
- Hypertension

DIAGNOSTIC TESTS AND PROCEDURES

● **Urinalysis**
- Definition and purpose
  - Laboratory test of urine

– Microscopic examination of urine for color, appearance, pH, specific gravity, protein, glucose, ketones, red blood cells (RBCs), white blood cells (WBCs), and casts
- Nursing interventions
  – Explain the procedure to the patient
  – Instruct the patient to wash the perineal area and obtain first morning urine specimen
  – Use sterile technique to collect from the urinary drainage bag

Urine culture and sensitivity
- Definition and purpose
  – Laboratory test of urine
  – Microscopic examination of urine for bacteria
- Nursing interventions
  – Explain the procedure to the patient
  – Instruct the patient to clean the perineal area and urinary meatus with bacteriostatic solution and collect a midstream specimen in a sterile container
  – Clean the collection port of an indwelling urinary catheter (after clamping the catheter for a short time) and obtain a urine specimen using sterile technique

24-hour urine collection
- Definition and purpose
  – Laboratory test of urine
  – Quantitative analysis of urine collected over 24 hours to determine kidney function (see *Understanding the glomerular filtration rate,* page 342)
- Nursing interventions
  – Explain the procedure to the patient
  – Instruct the patient to void and note time (collection starts with the next voiding)
  – Place urine collection container on ice
  – Measure each voided urine
  – Instruct the patient to void at the end of the 24-hour period

Blood chemistry
- Definition and purpose
  – Laboratory test of blood sample
  – Analysis of blood sample for WBCs, RBCs, erythrocyte sedimentation rate (ESR), platelets, prothrombin time (PT), partial thromboplastin time (PTT), hemoglobin (Hb) and hematocrit (HCT), potassium, sodium, calcium, phosphorus, glucose, bicarbonate, blood urea nitrogen (BUN), creatinine, protein, albumin, and osmolality
- Nursing interventions
  – Explain the procedure to the patient
  – Check the venipuncture site for bleeding after the procedure

Kidneys, ureters, bladder (KUB) X-ray
- Definition and purpose

Key facts about urinalysis

- Laboratory test of urine
- Examines color, appearance, pH, specific gravity, protein, glucose, ketones, RBCs, WBCs, and casts
- Intervention: obtain first morning urine specimen

Key facts about urine culture and sensitivity

- Laboratory test of urine
- Detects bacteria
- Intervention: collect midstream specimen in sterile container

Key facts about 24-hour urine collection

- Laboratory test of urine
- Specimens collected over 24 hours to determine kidney function
- Intervention: instruct the patient to void and note time

Key facts about blood chemistry

- Laboratory test of blood sample
- Analysis for potassium, sodium, calcium, phosphorus, glucose, bicarbonate, BUN, creatinine, protein, albumin, and osmolality
- Intervention: check the site for bleeding after the procedure

Characteristics of the GFR

- The rate at which glomeruli filter blood
- Normal GFR is 120 ml/minute
- Depends on permeability of capillary walls, vascular pressure, and filtration pressure

How GFR affects clearance of substances in the blood

- If tubules neither reabsorb or secrete the substance, clearance equals the GFR.
- If tubules reabsorb the substance, clearance is less than the GFR.
- If tubules secrete the substance, clearance exceeds GFR.
- If tubules reabsorb and secrete the substance, clearance may be less than, equal to, or greater than GFR.

Key facts about KUB X-ray

- Radiographic image of the kidneys, ureters, and bladder
- Intervention: schedule the X-ray before other examinations that require contrast medium

Key facts about CT scan

- Cross-sectional images of various tissue layers
- Intervention: note allergies to iodine, seafood, or radiopaque dyes

Key facts about MRI

- Images of internal organs and tissues
- Intervention: determine if the patient can remain still for 30 to 90 minutes

---

Understanding the glomerular filtration rate

The glomerular filtration rate (GFR) is the rate at which the glomeruli filter blood. The normal GFR is about 120 ml/minute. GFR depends on:
- permeability of capillary walls
- vascular pressure
- filtration pressure.

GFR AND CLEARANCE
Clearance is the complete removal of a substance from the blood. The most accurate measure of glomerular filtration is creatinine clearance. That's because creatinine is filtered by the glomeruli but not reabsorbed by the tubules.

EQUAL TO, GREATER THAN, OR LESS THAN
Here's more about how the GFR affects clearance measurements for a substance in the blood:
- If the tubules neither reabsorb nor secrete the substance—as happens with creatinine—clearance equals the GFR.
- If the tubules reabsorb the substance, clearance is less than the GFR.
- If the tubules secrete the substance, clearance exceeds the GFR.
- If the tubules reabsorb and secrete the substance, clearance may be less than, equal to, or greater than the GFR.

   - Radiographic image of the kidneys, ureters, and bladder
- Nursing interventions
   - Explain the procedure to the patient
   - Schedule the X-ray before other examinations requiring contrast medium
   - Ensure that the patient removes metallic belts

● **Computed tomography (CT) scan of abdomen/pelvis**
- Definition and purpose
   - Cross-sectional radiographic images of various layers of tissue
   - May be done with or without contrast medium
- Nursing interventions
   - Explain the procedure to the patient
   - Note if the patient is allergic to iodine, seafood, or radiopaque dyes
   - Obtain signed informed consent and complete paperwork per facility policy
   - Insert an I.V. catheter if I.V. contrast dye is to be used
   - Tell the patient that he may experience a feeling of warmth or flushing when the contrast dye is administered

● **Magnetic resonance imaging (MRI)**
- Definition and purpose
   - Computerized images of internal organs and tissues through use of magnetic fields and radiofrequency waves
- Nursing interventions
   - Explain the procedure to the patient
   - Obtain a signed informed consent and complete paperwork per facility policy

– Determine if the patient can remain still for 30 to 90 minutes
– Inform the patient that he'll be placed on a narrow, flat table, which is positioned inside a scanner
– Administer a sedative if prescribed

● **Renal ultrasound**
  • Definition and purpose
    – Visualization of the renal system through the use of high-frequency sound waves
  • Nursing interventions
    – Explain the procedure to the patient
    – Tell the patient that he'll need to drink only clear liquids for 2 hours before the procedure and 2 pints of water 1 hour before the procedure

● **Excretory urography**
  • Definition and purpose
    – Fluoroscopic examination of kidneys, ureters, and bladder after injection of a radiopaque dye
  • Nursing interventions before the procedure
    – Explain the procedure to the patient
    – Note the patient's allergies to iodine, seafood, and radiopaque dyes
    – Withhold food and fluids after midnight
    – Administer laxatives as prescribed
    – Insert an I.V. catheter if one isn't already in place
    – Inform the patient about possible throat irritation, flushing of the face, and feelings of warmth when the dye is injected
  • Nursing interventions after the procedure
    – Instruct the patient to drink at least 1 qt (1 L) of fluids
    – Check the venipuncture site for bleeding

● **Cystoscopy**
  • Definition and purpose
    – Direct visualization of the bladder through a cystoscope
  • Nursing interventions before the procedure
    – Explain the procedure to the patient
    – Withhold food and fluids as directed
    – Place obtained written informed consent in the patient's chart
    – Administer enemas and medications, as prescribed
  • Nursing interventions after the procedure
    – Monitor vital signs and intake and output (I/O)
    – Check the patient's urine for blood clots or hematuria
    – Encourage increased oral fluids if not contraindicated

● **Renal angiography**
  • Definition and purpose
    – Radiographic examination of the renal arterial supply after injection of a radiopaque dye through a catheter
  • Nursing interventions before the procedure
    – Explain the procedure to the patient

– Note the patient's allergies to iodine, seafood, and radiopaque dyes
– Inform the patient about a possible warm feeling after dye is injected
– Place obtained written informed consent in the patient's chart
– Withhold food and fluids after midnight
– Instruct the patient to void immediately before the procedure
– Administer enemas as prescribed
• Nursing interventions after the procedure
– Assess vital signs and peripheral pulses
– Inspect the catheter insertion site for bleeding
– Encourage increased oral fluids if not contraindicated

Renal scan
• Definition and purpose
– Visual imaging of blood flow distribution to the kidneys after I.V. injection of a radioisotope
• Nursing interventions before the procedure
– Explain the procedure to the patient
– Insert an I.V. catheter if one isn't already in place
– Assist with administering radioisotope as necessary
– Check the patient's history for allergies
– Obtain a signed consent form before the procedure
• Nursing interventions after the procedure
– Assess the patient for signs of delayed allergic reaction, such as itching and hives
– Wear gloves when caring for incontinent patients, and double-bag linens

Renal biopsy
• Definition and purpose
– Percutaneous procedure to remove a small amount of renal tissue
– Histologic evaluation of specimen
• Nursing interventions before the procedure
– Explain the procedure to the patient
– Obtain baseline clotting studies and vital signs
– Withhold food and fluids after midnight
– Place obtained written informed consent in the patient's chart
• Nursing interventions after the procedure
– Monitor and record vital signs, Hb levels, and HCT
– Check biopsy site for bleeding

Cystourethrography
• Definition and purpose
– Visualization of the bladder and ureters after insertion of a catheter and the introduction of radiopaque dye
• Nursing interventions before the procedure
– Explain the procedure to the patient

Key facts about renal scan
• Procedure using an I.V. injection of a radioisotope
• Visual imaging of blood flow distribution
• Intervention: assess the patient for signs of delayed allergic reaction

Key facts about renal biopsy
• Percutaneous procedure to remove renal tissue
• Histologic evaluation
• Intervention: check biopsy site for bleeding after the procedure

Key facts about cystourethrography
• Procedure in which a catheter and radiopaque dye is inserted
• Visualizes the bladder and ureters
• Intervention: note the patient's allergies before the procedure

– Note the patient's allergies to iodine, seafood, and radiopaque dyes before the procedure
– Obtain a signed consent form per facility policy
– Advise the patient about voiding requirements during the procedure
- Nursing interventions after the procedure
    – Monitor voiding
    – Monitor for urinary tract infection (UTI)

● **Cystometrography**
- Definition and purpose
    – Graphic recording of the pressures exerted at varying phases of filling of the bladder through use of a catheter
    – Evaluation of the bladder's ability to store and release urine
- Nursing interventions before the procedure
    – Explain the procedure to the patient
    – Advise the patient about voiding requirements during the procedure
- Nursing interventions after the procedure
    – Monitor voiding
    – Observe for persistent hematuria
    – Monitor for UTI

PSYCHOSOCIAL IMPACT OF RENAL AND UROLOGIC DISORDERS

● **Developmental impact**
- Negative feelings regarding body image
- Feeling of lack of control over body functions
- Fear of rejection
- Embarrassment from changes in body function and structure
- Decreased self-esteem

● **Economic impact**
- Cost of renal dialysis or organ transplant
- Cost of hospitalizations and follow-up care
- Cost of medications
- Cost of special diet
- Disruption of employment

● **Occupational and recreational impact**
- Restrictions on physical activity
- Changes in leisure activity

● **Social impact**
- Changes in eating patterns
- Social isolation
- Changes in elimination patterns and modes
- Changes in sexual function

Key facts about cystometrography

- Procedure to test urinary bladder
- Records pressures exerted at phases of bladder filling
- Intervention: advise the patient about voiding requirements during the procedure

Key psychosocial impacts of renal and urologic disorders

- Costs associated with hospitalizations, medications, and special diet
- Disruption of employment
- Restrictions on physical activity
- Social isolation
- Changes in activities, eating patterns, elimination patterns, and sexual function

RISK FACTORS

- **Modifiable risk factors**
  - Blood pressure control
  - Diet and fluid intake
  - Exposure to chemical and environmental pollutants
  - Smoking
  - Hygiene
- **Nonmodifiable risk factors**
  - History of renal dysfunction
  - History of diabetes mellitus
  - Aging
  - Family history of renal disease

NURSING DIAGNOSES

- **Probable nursing diagnoses**
  - Risk for imbalanced fluid volume
  - Excess fluid volume
  - Deficient knowledge (disorder and treatment plan)
  - Impaired urinary elimination
  - Acute pain
  - Ineffective sexuality patterns
  - Disturbed body image
  - Situational low self-esteem
  - Anxiety
  - Fear
- **Possible nursing diagnoses**
  - Risk for impaired skin integrity
  - Noncompliance (treatment plan)
  - Risk for activity intolerance
  - Grieving
  - Impaired gas exchange
  - Interrupted family processes
  - Death anxiety
  - Fatigue

KIDNEY TRANSPLANTATION

- **Description**
  - Implantation of a donated kidney in a person with end-stage renal disease
- **Preoperative nursing interventions**
  - Complete patient and family preoperative teaching
    - Explain the procedure to the patient

Key risk factors for renal and urologic disorders
- Diet and fluid intake
- Exposure to pollutants
- Smoking
- History of renal dysfunction

Key probable nursing diagnoses in renal and urologic disorders
- Risk for imbalanced fluid volume
- Excess fluid volume
- Impaired urinary elimination
- Acute pain

Key possible nursing diagnoses in renal and urologic disorders
- Noncompliance (treatment plan)
- Risk for activity intolerance
- Fatigue

Key facts about kidney transplantation
- Implantation of a donated kidney in a person with end-stage renal disease

- Describe the operating room, postanesthesia care unit (PACU), and preoperative and postoperative routines
- Demonstrate postoperative turning, coughing, deep breathing, incentive spirometry, splinting, and range-of-motion (ROM) exercises
- Explain the postoperative need for drainage tubes, surgical dressings, oxygen therapy, I.V. therapy, and pain control
- Complete a preoperative checklist and check that a signed informed consent is in the patient's chart
- Administer preoperative medications as prescribed
- Allay the patient's and his family's anxiety about surgery
- Document the patient's history and physical assessment data
- Verify histocompatibility tests
- Administer immunosuppressive drugs, as prescribed, for 2 days before the transplantation
- Administer transfusion therapy as prescribed
- Administer I.V. therapy as prescribed
- Monitor I/O
- Verify that hemodialysis was completed 24 hours before transplant

- **Postoperative nursing interventions**
  - Assess cardiac and respiratory status and fluid balance
  - Assess pain level, administer postoperative analgesics as prescribed, and evaluate response
  - Assess for return of peristalsis; advance diet as tolerated
  - Administer I.V. fluids and transfusion therapy, as prescribed
  - Allay the patient's anxiety and provide emotional support
  - Provide wound care as directed
  - Encourage turning, coughing, and deep breathing, use of incentive spirometry, and splinting of incision
  - Keep the patient in semi-Fowler's position
  - Encourage activity: as tolerated
  - Monitor and record vital signs, I/O, central venous pressure (CVP), laboratory studies, urine for blood, cardiac rhythm, daily weight, pulse oximetry, and serum creatinine levels
  - Monitor and maintain position and patency of drainage tubes: indwelling urinary catheter, nasogastric (NG), wound drainage
  - Encourage the patient to express his feelings about the illness and surgery
  - Administer antifungals as prescribed
  - Administer immunosuppressive agents with synthetic prostaglandins, as prescribed
  - Administer corticosteroids as prescribed
  - Assess for signs and symptoms of organ rejection
  - Monitor for complications
  - Provide mouth and skin care
  - Administer antibiotics as prescribed
  - Administer antilymphocytic globulin (ALG) and antithymocyte globulin (ATG), as prescribed

---

Key nursing interventions before kidney transplantation

- Verify histocompatibility tests.
- Administer immunosuppressive drugs for 2 days before the transplantation.
- Verify that hemodialysis was completed 24 hours before the transplantation.

Key nursing interventions after kidney transplantation

- Assess cardiac and respiratory status and fluid balance.
- Monitor and record vital signs, I/O, CVP, laboratory studies, urine for blood, cardiac rhythm, daily weight, pulse oximetry, and creatinine levels.
- Monitor and maintain position and patency of drainage tubes.
- Administer immunosuppressive agents with synthetic prostaglandins.
- Administer corticosteroids, as prescribed.
- Monitor for complications.
- Administer ALG and ATG, as prescribed.
- Prepare for hemodialysis.

- Prepare for hemodialysis as directed
- Avoid prolonged periods of sitting
- Assess the allograft site for pain and edema
- Individualize home care instructions
    - Know the facts about your illness and the surgery
    - Follow instructions for medication use and be aware of possible adverse effects
    - Recognize the signs and symptoms of rejection
    - Comply with activity restrictions
    - Perform wound care
    - Adhere to diet and fluid restrictions
    - Monitor stools for occult blood
    - Comply with medical follow-up

● **Surgical complications**
- Renal graft rejection
- Acute renal failure
- Bladder and ureter fistulas
- Candidiasis of mouth
- Hypertension
- Stroke
- Gastric ulcer
- Liver failure
- Depression
- Psychosis
- Heart failure
- Hypovolemia

Key complications of kidney transplantation

- Renal graft rejection
- Acute renal failure
- Gastric ulcer
- Depression
- Heart failure

KIDNEY SURGERY

● **Description**
- Nephrectomy: surgical removal of a kidney
- Lithotomy: surgical removal of renal calculi

Key facts about kidney surgery

- Nephrectomy: surgical removal of the entire kidney
- Lithotomy: surgical removal of renal calculi

● **Preoperative nursing interventions**
- Complete patient and family preoperative teaching
    - Explain the procedure to the patient
    - Describe the operating room, PACU, and preoperative and postoperative routines
    - Demonstrate postoperative turning, coughing, deep breathing, incentive spirometry, splinting, and leg and ROM exercises
    - Explain the postoperative need for drainage tubes, surgical dressings, oxygen therapy, I.V. therapy, and pain control
- Complete a preoperative checklist and make sure a signed informed consent is in the patient's chart
- Administer preoperative medications as prescribed
- Allay the patient's and his family's anxiety about surgery
- Document the patient's history and physical assessment data

Key nursing interventions before kidney surgery

- Complete patient and family preoperative teaching.
- Administer preoperative medications as prescribed.

● Postoperative nursing interventions
- Assess cardiac, respiratory, and neurologic status and fluid balance
- Assess pain level, administer analgesics, as prescribed, and evaluate response
- Assess for return of peristalsis; advance diet, as tolerated, with increased fluids
- Administer I.V. fluids and transfusion therapy, as prescribed
- Allay the patient's anxiety and provide emotional support
- Provide wound care as directed
- Encourage turning, coughing, and deep breathing, use of incentive spirometry, and splinting of incision
- Keep the patient in semi-Fowler's position
- Encourage activity, as tolerated, active and passive ROM exercises, and ambulation
- Monitor and record vital signs, I/O, CVP, laboratory studies, urine for blood, daily weight, and pulse oximetry
- Monitor and maintain position and patency of drainage tubes: NG, indwelling urinary catheter, wound drainage, nephrostomy, suprapubic, ureteral
- Encourage the patient to express his feelings about the illness and surgery
- Administer antibiotics and stool softeners as prescribed
- Don't irrigate or manipulate the nephrostomy tube
- Apply sequential compression stockings while in bed
- Individualize home care instructions
    - Know the facts about your illness and surgery
    - Follow instructions for medication use and be aware of possible adverse effects
    - Recognize the signs and symptoms of complications
    - Perform wound care
    - Avoid using over-the-counter medications unless approved by physician
    - Increase fluid intake as directed
    - Comply with activity restrictions
    - Comply with medical follow-up

● Surgical complications
- Hemorrhage
- Atelectasis
- Pneumothorax
- Pneumonia
- Paralytic ileus
- Infection

PROSTATE SURGERY

● Description
- Transurethral resection of prostate (TURP): insertion of a resectoscope into the urethra to excise prostatic tissue

---

Key nursing interventions after kidney surgery
- Assess cardiac, respiratory, and neurologic status and fluid balance.
- Administer I.V. fluids and transfusion therapy, as prescribed.
- Monitor and record vital signs, I/O, CVP, laboratory studies, urine for blood, daily weight, and pulse oximetry.
- Monitor and maintain position and patency of drainage tubes: NG, indwelling urinary catheter, wound drainage, nephrostomy, suprapubic, ureteral.
- Administer antibiotics as prescribed.
- Individualize home care instructions.

Key complications of kidney surgery
- Atelectasis
- Pneumonia
- Infection

Key facts about prostate surgery

- TURP: insertion of rectoscope into urethra to excise tissue
- Suprapubic prostatectomy: low abdominal incision into bladder to anterior prostate to remove large tumor
- Retropubic prostatectomy: low midline incision below bladder into prostatic capsule to remove mass
- Perineal prostatectomy: incision through perineum to remove prostate and surrounding tissue

Key nursing interventions before prostate surgery

- Complete patient and family preoperative teaching.
- Administer preoperative medications as prescribed.

Key nursing interventions after prostate surgery

- Assess cardiac and respiratory status and fluid balance.
- Monitor and record vital signs, I/O, laboratory studies, stool counts, and pulse oximetry.
- Monitor and maintain position and patency of drainage tubes: NG, indwelling urinary catheter, wound drainage, suprapubic.
- Evaluate appearance of urine and maintain closed continuous bladder irrigation.
- Administer antibiotics as prescribed.
- Monitor urinary patterns after removal of catheter.

- Suprapubic prostatectomy: low abdominal incision into the bladder to the anterior aspect of the prostate to remove large tumors of the prostate
- Retropubic prostatectomy: low midline incision below the bladder into prostatic capsule to remove a mass in the pelvic area
- Perineal prostatectomy: incision through the perineum to remove the prostate and surrounding tissue

● **Preoperative nursing interventions**
- Complete patient and family preoperative teaching
  - Explain the procedure to the patient
  - Describe the operating room, PACU, and preoperative and postoperative routines
  - Demonstrate postoperative turning, coughing, deep breathing, incentive spirometry, splinting, and leg and ROM exercises
  - Explain the postoperative need for drainage tubes, surgical dressings, oxygen therapy, I.V. therapy, and pain control
- Complete a preoperative checklist and make sure a signed informed consent is in the patient's chart
- Administer preoperative medications as prescribed
- Allay the patient's and his family's anxiety about surgery
- Document the patient's history and physical assessment data

● **Postoperative nursing interventions**
- Assess cardiac and respiratory status and fluid balance
- Assess pain level, administer postoperative analgesics, as prescribed, and evaluate response
- Assess for return of peristalsis; advance diet, as tolerated, with increased fluids
- Administer I.V. fluids
- Allay the patient's anxiety and provide emotional support
- Provide wound care as directed
- Encourage turning, coughing, and deep breathing, use of incentive spirometry, and splinting of incision
- Keep the patient in semi-Fowler's position
- Encourage activity, as tolerated, with progressive ambulation
- Monitor and record vital signs, I/O, laboratory studies, stool counts, and pulse oximetry
- Monitor and maintain position and patency of drainage tubes: NG, indwelling urinary catheter, wound drainage, suprapubic
- **Encourage the patient to express his feelings about the surgery and his fear of sexual dysfunction**
- Administer stool softeners as prescribed
- Evaluate appearance of urine and maintain closed continuous bladder irrigation, as directed
- Monitor urinary patterns after removal of catheter
- Administer antibiotics, anticholinergics, antispasmodics, and urinary antiseptics, as prescribed
- **Avoid giving enemas and taking temperature rectally**

- Individualize home care instructions
  - Know about your illness and surgery
  - Follow instructions for medication use and be aware of possible adverse reactions
  - Recognize the signs and symptoms of complications, such as bleeding and urinary tract obstruction
  - Perform wound care
  - Avoid Valsalva's maneuver, lifting, exercising vigorously, or prolonged sitting in the car
  - Increase fluid intake but avoid alcohol and caffeine
  - Comply with medical follow-up

- **Surgical complications**
  - Hemorrhage
  - Shock
  - Infection
  - Epididymitis
  - Impotence
  - Urinary obstruction

URINARY DIVERSION

- **Description**
  - Ureterosigmoidostomy: ureters are excised from the bladder and implanted into the sigmoid colon; urine flows through the colon and is excreted through the rectum
  - Nephrostomy: percutaneous insertion of catheter into kidney
  - Ileal conduit: ureters are implanted into a segment of the ileum that has been resected from the intestinal tract with the formation of an abdominal stoma
  - Cutaneous ureterostomy: ureters are excised from the bladder and brought through the abdominal wall to create a stoma

- **Preoperative nursing interventions**
  - Complete patient and family preoperative teaching
    - Explain the procedure to the patient
    - Describe the operating room, PACU, and preoperative and postoperative routines
    - Demonstrate postoperative turning, coughing, deep breathing, incentive spirometry, splinting, and ROM exercises
    - Explain the postoperative need for drainage tubes, surgical dressings, oxygen therapy, I.V. therapy, and pain control
  - Complete a preoperative checklist and make sure a signed informed consent is in the patient's chart
  - Administer preoperative medications as prescribed
  - Allay the patient's and his family's anxiety about surgery
  - Document the patient's history and physical assessment data
  - Administer bowel preparation as prescribed

Key nursing interventions after urinary diversion

- Assess renal status and fluid balance.
- Encourage the patient to express his feelings about the surgery and his illness.
- Administer antibiotics as prescribed.
- Apply and change ostomy bags.
- Provide skin care, particularly around the stoma.

Key complications of urinary diversion

- Chronic renal failure
- Infection
- Urinary and rectal fistulas
- Hemorrhage

● **Postoperative nursing interventions**
- Assess renal status and fluid balance
- Assess pain level, administer postoperative analgesics, as prescribed, and evaluate response
- Assess for return of peristalsis; advance diet, as tolerated, with increased fluids; avoid giving milk and dairy products
- Administer I.V. fluids
- Allay the patient's anxiety and provide emotional support
- Provide wound care as directed
- Encourage turning, coughing, deep breathing, use of incentive spirometry, and splinting of incision
- Keep the patient in semi-Fowler's position
- Encourage activity, as tolerated, with ambulation
- Monitor and record vital signs, I/O, laboratory studies, daily weight, and pulse oximetry
- Monitor and maintain position and patency of drainage tubes: NG, indwelling urinary catheter, wound drainage
- Encourage the patient to express his feelings about his illness and surgery
- Administer antibiotics and antispasmodics, as prescribed
- Apply and change ostomy bags, as needed
- Assess skin integrity; provide skin care, particularly around the stoma
- Apply sequential compression stockings while in bed
- Individualize home care instructions
  - Know the facts about your illness and surgery
  - Follow instructions for medication use and be aware of possible adverse effects
  - Recognize the signs and symptoms of complications such as stomal stenosis
  - Complete stoma and skin care daily
  - Follow instructions on the use of ostomy bags and leg bags
  - Increase fluid intake
  - Avoid enemas and laxatives
  - Comply with medical follow-up

● **Surgical complications**
- Chronic renal failure
- Infection
- Urinary and rectal fistulas
- Hemorrhage
- Peritonitis
- Ureteral obstruction
- Stomal stenosis
- Bowel obstruction
- Renal calculi

CYSTITIS

- **Definition**
  - Inflammation of the urinary bladder related to a superficial infection that doesn't extend to the bladder mucosa
  - Also known as UTI

- **Causes**
  - Bacteria entering the urethra and then the bladder
  - *Escherichia coli:* most common (70% to 95%)

- **Risk factors**
  - Urinary stasis
  - Renal calculi
  - Sexual intercourse
  - Bladder catheterization
  - Poor perineal hygiene
  - Prostate enlargement
  - Immobility
  - Urinary tract abnormality
  - Diabetes mellitus
  - Pregnancy
  - Menopause

- **Pathophysiology**
  - Bacterial infection from a secondary source spreads to the bladder, causing an inflammatory response
  - Cell destruction from trauma to the bladder wall, particularly the trigone area, initiates an acute inflammatory reaction

- **Assessment findings**
  - Frequency of urination
  - Urgency of urination
  - Burning or pain on urination
  - Lower abdominal discomfort
  - Dark, odoriferous urine
  - Flank tenderness or suprapubic pain
  - Nocturia
  - Low-grade fever
  - Urge to bear down on urination
  - Dribbling

- **Diagnostic test findings**
  - Urine culture and sensitivity: positive identification of organisms (*Escherichia coli, Proteus vulgaris, Streptococcus faecalis*)
  - Urine chemistry: hematuria, pyuria; increased protein, leukocytes, specific gravity
  - Cystoscopy: obstruction or deformity

Key facts about cystitis

- Inflammation of the urinary bladder related to a superficial infection that doesn't extend to the bladder mucosa
- Also known as UTI

Common causes of cystitis

- Poor perineal hygiene
- Urinary stasis
- Bladder catheterization

TOP 3

Signs and symptoms of cystitis

1. Frequency of urination
2. Urgency of urination
3. Burning or pain on urination

Diagnosing cystitis

- Urine culture and sensitivity: positive identification of organisms
- Urine chemistry: hematuria, pyuria, increased protein, leukocytes, specific gravity

Key teaching topics for a patient with a renal or urologic disorder

- Smoking cessation
- Medication therapy
- Infection control measures
- Dietary restrictions
- Fluid intake recommendations and restrictions
- Keeping follow-up appointments

Treating cystitis

- Increased intake of fluids
- Antibiotics

Key nursing interventions for a patient with cystitis

- Encourage fluids to 3 qt/day.
- Encourage voiding every 2 to 3 hours.
- Administer medications.

TIME-OUT FOR TEACHING

Patients with renal or urologic disorders

Be sure to include the following topics in your teaching plan for patients with renal or urologic disorders.

- Medication therapy, including the action, adverse effects, and scheduling of medications
- Infection control measures, including avoiding exposure to people with infections and monitoring self for infection
- Dietary recommendations and restrictions
- Fluid intake recommendations and restrictions
- Signs and symptoms of renal failure
- Rest and activity patterns, including limitations or restrictions
- Signs and symptoms of urinary tract infection
- Community agencies and resources for supportive services
- Smoking cessation
- Optimal body weight maintenance
- Follow-up appointments

● Medical management

- Antibiotics: trimethoprim (Proloprim), co-trimoxazole (Bactrim)
- Antipyretic: acetaminophen (Tylenol)
- Diet: increased intake of fluids
- Activity: as tolerated
- Monitoring: vital signs and I/O
- Laboratory studies: urine culture and sensitivity, WBC count
- Urinary antiseptic: phenazopyridine (Pyridium)

● Nursing interventions

- Encourage fluids to 3 qt (3 L)/day
- Assess renal status
- Monitor and record vital signs, I/O, and laboratory studies
- Administer medications as prescribed
- Allay the patient's anxiety and provide emotional support
- Encourage voiding every 2 to 3 hours
- Individualize home care instructions (for teaching tips, see *Patients with renal or urologic disorders*)
  - Know about the disorder and its treatment
  - Follow instructions for medication use and be aware of possible adverse effects
  - Increase fluid intake to 3 qt (3 L)/day
  - Void every 2 to 3 hours and after intercourse
  - Perform perineal care correctly
  - Avoid bubble baths, vaginal deodorants, and tub baths

● Complications

- Recurrent infection

- Urethritis
- Pyelonephritis
- **Surgical intervention**
  - None

ACUTE GLOMERULONEPHRITIS

- **Definition**
  - Inflammation of the capillary loops in the glomeruli of the kidney
- **Causes**
  - Group A beta-hemolytic streptococcal infection
  - Injected serum proteins
  - Systemic lupus erythematosus (SLE)
- **Pathophysiology**
  - Antigen-antibody complexes are filtered and trapped within the glomeruli, causing inflammation
  - Inflammation occludes the glomeruli, causing decreased glomerular filtration and retention of protein wastes and electrolytes
- **Assessment findings**
  - History of pharyngitis and tonsillitis
  - Peripheral and periorbital edema
  - Hypertension
  - Lethargy and malaise
  - Pallor
  - Anorexia
  - Elevated temperature
  - Tea-colored urine
  - Flank pain
  - Dyspnea
  - Oliguria
- **Diagnostic test findings**
  - Urine chemistry: increased RBCs, WBCs, protein, casts, specific gravity
  - Blood chemistry: increased BUN, creatinine; decreased protein, creatinine clearance, C-reactive protein, albumin
  - Antistreptolysin-O titer: increased titers confirm recent streptococcal infection
  - Hematology: decreased Hb, HCT; increased ESR
  - Renal biopsy: inflammation of the glomerular capillaries
- **Medical management**
  - Antibiotics: penicillin V (Pen-Vee K), ampicillin (Omnipen)
  - Diuretics: chlorthalidone (Hygroton), furosemide (Lasix)
  - Vasodilators: nitroprusside (Nipride)
  - Calcium channel blockers: nifedipine (Procardia), hydralazine (Apresoline)
  - Monitoring: vital signs, I/O, and cardiac rhythm

Treating acute glomerulonephritis

- Antibiotics
- Diuretics

Key nursing interventions for a patient with acute glomerulonephritis

- Assess renal, respiratory, cardiovascular, and neurologic status.
- Monitor and record vital signs, I/O, cardiac rhythm, laboratory studies, and daily weight.
- Enforce dietary and fluid restrictions.
- Administer medications.

Key complications of acute glomerulonephritis

- Metabolic acidosis
- Heart failure
- Hypertension

Key facts about acute pyelonephritis

- Inflammation of renal pelvis
- Occurs when a bacterial infection spreads causing cell destruction from trauma

Common cause of acute pyelonephritis

- Enteric bacteria

Key risk factors for acute pyelonephritis

- Urinary tract obstruction
- Trauma
- UTI

- Diet: restricted intake of sodium, protein, potassium, and fluids until condition resolves
- I.V. therapy: as needed
- Activity: bed rest during acute phase
- Laboratory studies: BUN, creatinine, sodium, potassium, Hb, and HCT

● **Nursing interventions**
- Assess renal, respiratory, cardiovascular, and neurologic status
- Monitor and record vital signs, I/O, cardiac rhythm, laboratory studies, and daily weight
- Administer medications as prescribed
- Enforce dietary and fluid restrictions
- Encourage turning, coughing, and deep breathing
- Encourage the patient to express his feelings about his illness
- Provide skin and mouth care
- Apply sequential compression stocking while in bed
- Individualize home care instructions
  - Know about the disorder and its treatment
  - Follow instructions for medication use and be aware of possible adverse effects
  - Comply with activity restrictions
  - Restrict protein and sodium intake
  - Monitor blood pressure
  - Observe for signs and symptoms of complications
  - Comply with medical follow-up

● **Complications**
- Metabolic acidosis
- Renal failure (rare)
- Hypertensive encephalopathy
- Heart failure
- Hypertension
- Pulmonary edema

● **Surgical interventions**
- None

ACUTE PYELONEPHRITIS

● **Definition**
- Inflammation of renal pelvis

● **Cause**
- Enteric bacteria

● **Risk factors**
- Ureterovesical reflux
- Urinary tract obstruction
- Pregnancy
- Trauma

- UTI
- Urinary catheter
- Diabetes mellitus
- Staphylococcal or streptococcal infections

Pathophysiology
- Bacterial infection from a secondary source spreads to the renal pelvis, causing an inflammatory response
- Cell destruction from trauma to the renal pelvis initiates an inflammatory reaction

Assessment findings
- Burning on urination
- Frequency and urgency of urination
- Elevated temperature
- Chills
- Flank pain
- Dysuria, hematuria, nocturia
- Chronic fatigue
- Anorexia
- Odoriferous, concentrated urine

Diagnostic test findings
- Urine culture and sensitivity: bacteria
- Urine chemistry: pyuria, hematuria; leukocytes, WBCs, and casts; specific gravity greater than 1.025; albuminuria
- Hematology: increased WBCs
- CT scan: calculi, cysts, tumors in kidney or urinary tract
- Excretory urography: atrophy, blockage, or deformity of kidney

Medical management
- Antibiotics: cefazolin (Ancef), cefoxitin (Mefoxin), co-trimoxazole (Bactrim)
- Urinary antiseptic: phenazopyridine (Pyridium)
- Treatment of underlying cause
- Diet: increased fluid intake to 3 qt (3 L)/day
- I.V. therapy: electrolyte and fluid replacement
- Activity: as tolerated
- Monitoring: vital signs and I/O
- Laboratory studies: WBCs, urine protein, and urine culture and sensitivity
- Analgesic: meperidine (Demerol)

Nursing interventions
- Assess renal status and fluid balance
- Encourage fluids to 3 qt (3 L)/day
- Monitor and record vital signs, I/O, laboratory studies, and daily weight
- Administer medications as prescribed
- Allay the patient's anxiety and provide emotional support
- Provide rest periods
- Provide skin, mouth, and perineal care

Key signs and symptoms of acute pyelonephritis
- Burning on urination
- Frequency and urgency of urination
- Flank pain
- Dysuria, hematuria, nocturia

Diagnosing acute pyelonephritis
- Urine culture and sensitivity: bacteria
- Urine chemistry: pyuria, hematuria; leukocytes, WBCs, and casts; specific gravity greater than 1.025; albuminuria

Treating acute pyelonephritis
- Antibiotics
- Increased fluid intake to 3 qt/day
- Treatment of underlying cause

Key nursing interventions for a patient with acute pyelonephritis
- Encourage fluids to 3 qt/day.
- Assess renal status and fluid balance.
- Monitor and record vital signs, I/O, laboratory studies, and daily weight.
- Encourage frequent voiding.

Key facts about chronic pyelonephritis

- Persistent kidney inflammation
- Can lead to chronic renal failure
- Clinical signs: flank pain, anemia, proteinuria, leukocytes in urine, and hypertension
- Treatment: control hypertension, eliminate obstruction, long-term antibiotics

Key complications of acute pyelonephritis

- Recurrent infection
- Chronic renal failure
- Hypertension

Key facts about renal calculi

- Stones in kidneys, ureters, or bladder

Common cause of renal calculi

- Unknown

Chronic pyelonephritis

Chronic pyelonephritis is a persistent kidney inflammation that can scar the kidneys and lead to chronic renal failure. Its etiology may be bacterial, metastatic, or urogenous. This disease most frequently occurs in patients who are predisposed to recurrent acute pyelonephritis, such as those with urinary obstructions or vesicoureteral reflux.

ASSESSMENT AND DIAGNOSIS
Patients with chronic pyelonephritis may have a childhood history of unexplained fevers or enuresis. Clinical signs and symptoms include flank pain, anemia, low urine specific gravity, proteinuria, leukocytes in urine, and hypertension. Uremia seldom develops unless structural abnormalities exist in the excretory system. Intermittent bacteriuria may occur.

When no bacteria are found in the urine, diagnosis depends on excretory urography (the patient's renal pelvis may appear small and flattened) and renal biopsy.

TREATMENT
Effective treatment of chronic pyelonephritis requires control of hypertension, elimination of the obstruction (when possible), and long-term antimicrobial therapy.

- Encourage frequent voiding
- Individualize home care instructions
  - Know about the disorder and its treatment
  - Follow instructions for medication use and be aware of possible adverse effects
  - Void frequently
  - Observe for signs and symptoms of recurrent infection or complications
  - Comply with medical follow-up

● **Complications**
- Recurrent infection
- Chronic renal failure (see *Chronic pyelonephritis*)
- Hypertension
- Septicemia

● **Surgical intervention**
- None

RENAL CALCULI

● **Definition**
- Stones in kidneys, ureters, or bladder

● **Cause**
- Unknown

A close look at renal calculi

Renal calculi vary in size and type. Small calculi may remain in the renal pelvis or pass down the ureter as shown below. A staghorn calculus, shown in the second illustration, is a cast of the innermost part of the kidney — the calyx and renal pelvis. A staghorn calculus may develop from a calculus that stays in the kidney.

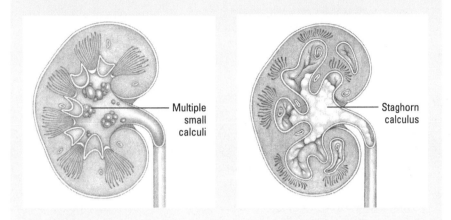

Multiple small calculi

Staghorn calculus

● **Risk factors**
- Metabolic factors
- Infection
- Urinary stasis
- Dehydration
- Immobility
- Family history
- Hypercalcemia
- Urinary tract obstruction

● **Pathophysiology**
- Crystalline substances that normally are dissolved and excreted in the urine form precipitates (see *A close look at renal calculi*)
- Stones are composed of calcium phosphate, oxalate, or uric acid

● **Assessment findings**
- Renal colic
- Costovertebral tenderness
- Flank pain
- Cool, moist skin
- Frequency of urination
- Urgency of urination
- Diaphoresis
- Hypertension
- Tachycardia
- Chills and fever

Key risk factors for renal calculi

- Metabolic factors
- Urinary stasis
- Immobility
- Hypercalcemia

TOP 3

Signs and symptoms of renal calculi

1. Renal colic
2. Costovertebral tenderness
3. Flank pain

Diagnosing renal calculi

- KUB: stones
- Excretory urography: stone size and location

Treating renal calculi

- I.V. therapy: fluid replacement
- Ultrasonic lithotripsy or ESWL
- Analgesics
- Diet restrictions based on stone composition
- Cystoscopy

Key nursing interventions for a patient with renal calculi

- Encourage fluids to 3 qt/day.
- Assess renal status.
- Strain urine.
- Assess pain level, administer analgesics, and evaluate response.

- Pallor
- Nausea and vomiting
- Syncope
- Dysuria, hematuria

● **Diagnostic test findings**
- KUB: stones
- Excretory urography: stone size and location
- Urine chemistry: acidic or alkaline urine, pyuria, proteinuria, hematuria, presence of WBCs, increased specific gravity
- CT scan: stones
- 24-hour urine collection: increased uric acid, oxalate, calcium, phosphorus, creatinine

● **Medical management**
- I.V. therapy: fluid replacement
- Ultrasonic lithotripsy
- Laser impulse
- Extracorporeal shock wave lithotripsy (ESWL)
- Percutaneous nephrostolithotomy
- Encourage fluids to 3 qt (3 L)/day
- Diet: restrictions based on stone composition
    - For calcium stones—acid-ash with limited intake of calcium and milk products
    - For oxalate stones—alkaline-ash with limited intake of foods high in oxalate (cola, tea)
    - For uric acid stones—alkaline-ash with limited intake of foods high in purine
- Activity: as tolerated
- Monitoring: vital signs and I/O
- Laboratory studies: creatinine, BUN, phosphorus, calcium, protein, and urine pH
- Straining of urine
- Antigout agent: sulfinpyrazone (Anturane)
- Analgesic: meperidine (Demerol)
- Antibiotics: cefazolin (Ancef), cefoxitin (Mefoxin)
- Acidifiers: ammonium chloride, methenamine (Mandelamine)
- Alkalinizers: potassium acetate, sodium bicarbonate
- Chemolysis
- Electrohydraulic lithotripsy
- Prevention of cystinuria: tiopronin (Thiola)

● **Nursing interventions**
- Assess renal status
- Encourage fluids to 3 qt/day
- Monitor and record vital signs, I/O, daily weight, and laboratory studies
- Administer medications as prescribed
- Allay the patient's anxiety and provide emotional support
- Strain urine

- Assess pain level, administer analgesics, as prescribed, and evaluate response
- Individualize home care instructions
  - Know about the disorder and its treatment
  - Follow instructions for medication use and be aware of possible adverse effects
  - Increase fluid intake, especially during hot weather, illness, and exercise
  - Void when urge is felt
  - Observe for signs and symptoms of complications
  - Comply with medical follow-up

● **Complications**
- Renal obstruction
- Ureterovesical reflux
- Hydronephrosis
- Pyelonephritis

● **Surgical interventions**
- Ureteral stent
- Cystoscopy
- Percutaneous nephrostomy

ACUTE RENAL FAILURE

● **Definition**
- Sudden inability of the kidneys to regulate fluid and electrolyte balance and remove toxic products from the body
- Classified as prerenal, intrarenal, or postrenal
- Occurs in three phases: oliguric, diuretic, and recovery

● **Causes**
- Various conditions (see *Causes of acute renal failure,* page 362)

● **Pathophysiology**
- Prerenal failure
  - Decreased perfusion of the kidney results in decreased blood flow and glomerular filtrate, ischemia, and oliguria
- Intrarenal failure
  - Damaged nephrons result from ischemia-generated toxic, oxygen-free radicals and anti-inflammatory medications
  - Nephrons are then unable to absorb and secrete water, electrolytes, glucose, amino acids, ammonia, and bicarbonate
- Postrenal failure
  - Usually occurs with urinary obstruction that affects the kidneys bilaterally

● **Assessment findings**
- Urine output less than 400 ml/day for 1 to 2 weeks followed by diuresis (3 to 5 L/day) for 2 to 3 weeks

Causes of acute renal failure

Acute renal failure can be classified as prerenal, intrarenal, or postrenal. All conditions that lead to prerenal failure impair renal perfusion, resulting in decreased glomerular filtration rate and increased proximal tubular reabsorption of sodium and water. Intrarenal failure results from damage to the kidneys themselves; postrenal failure, from obstruction of urine flow.

PRERENAL FAILURE	INTRARENAL FAILURE	POSTRENAL FAILURE
Cardiovascular disorders ● Arrhythmias ● Cardiac tamponade ● Cardiogenic shock ● Heart failure ● Myocardial infarction ● Pulmonary embolism **Hypovolemia** ● Burns ● Dehydration ● Diuretic abuse ● Hemorrhage ● Hypovolemic shock ● Liver failure ● Trauma **Peripheral vasodilation** ● Antihypertensive drugs ● Sepsis **Renovascular obstruction** ● Arterial embolism ● Arterial or venous thrombosis ● Tumor **Severe vasoconstriction** ● Disseminated intravascular coagulation ● Eclampsia ● Malignant hypertension ● Vasculitis	**Acute tubular necrosis** ● Ischemic damage to renal parenchyma from unrecognized or poorly treated prerenal failure ● Nephrotoxins—analgesics (such as phenacetin), anesthetics (such as methoxyflurane), antibiotics (such as gentamicin), heavy metals (such as lead), radiographic contrast media, organic solvents ● Obstetric complications—eclampsia, postpartum renal failure, septic abortion, uterine hemorrhage ● Pigment release—crush injury, myopathy, sepsis, transfusion reaction **Other parenchymal disorders** ● Acute glomerulonephritis ● Acute interstitial nephritis ● Acute pyelonephritis ● Bilateral renal vein thrombosis ● Malignant nephrosclerosis ● Papillary necrosis ● Periarteritis nodosa ● Renal myeloma ● Sickle cell disease ● Systemic lupus erythematosus ● Vasculitis	**Bladder obstruction** ● Anticholinergic drugs ● Autonomic nerve dysfunction ● Infection ● Tumor **Ureteral obstruction** ● Blood clots ● Calculi ● Edema or inflammation ● Necrotic renal papillae ● Retroperitoneal fibrosis or hemorrhage ● Surgery (accidental ligation) ● Tumor ● Uric acid crystals **Urethral obstruction** ● Prostatic hyperplasia or tumor ● Strictures

Key signs and symptoms of acute renal failure

● Urine output less than 400 ml/day for 1 to 2 weeks followed by diuresis (3 to 5 L/day) for 2 to 3 weeks
● Altered LOC
● Uremic breath odor
● Peripheral edema
● Altered mental status (drowsiness, confusion)
● Irritability
● Altered level of consciousness (LOC)
● Bleeding abnormality
● Tachycardia
● Bibasilar crackles
● Dry mucous membranes
● Uremic breath odor
● Peripheral edema

- **Diagnostic test findings**
  - Blood chemistry: increased potassium, phosphorus, magnesium, BUN, creatinine, and uric acid; decreased calcium, carbon dioxide, and sodium
  - Hematology: decreased Hb, HCT, erythrocytes; increased PT and PTT
  - Urine chemistry: albuminuria, proteinuria, increased sodium; casts, RBCs, and WBCs; specific gravity greater than 1.025, then fixed at less than 1.010
  - Arterial blood gas (ABG) analysis: metabolic acidosis
  - CT scan, MRI: may show underlying cause
- **Medical management**
  - I.V. therapy: electrolyte replacement, hypertonic glucose and insulin to treat hyperkalemia
  - Monitoring: vital signs, I/O, cardiac rhythm, and CVP
  - Cation exchange resins: sodium polystyrene sulfonate (Kayexalate) for hyperkalemia
  - Diuretics: furosemide (Lasix), mannitol (Osmitrol)
  - Alkalinizing agent: sodium bicarbonate (with severe metabolic acidosis)
  - Dialysis: hemodialysis or continuous renal replacement therapy (see *Continuous renal replacement therapy*, page 364)
  - Diet: low-protein, increased-carbohydrate, with fluid restrictions and with potassium, sodium, and phosphorus intake regulated according to serum levels
  - Position: semi-Fowler's
  - Activity: bed rest, active and passive ROM and isometric exercises
  - Laboratory studies: BUN, creatinine, phosphorus, calcium, potassium, sodium, Hb, HCT, and specific gravity
  - Treatments: indwelling urinary catheter, incentive spirometry, hypothermia blanket
  - Transfusion therapy: packed RBCs
- **Nursing interventions**
  - Assess fluid balance, respiratory, cardiovascular, and neurologic status
  - Monitor and record vital signs, I/O, CVP, daily weight, cardiac rhythm, and laboratory studies
  - Administer medications as prescribed
  - Restrict fluids
  - Administer I.V. fluids and electrolyte supplements, as indicated
  - Keep the patient in semi-Fowler's position
  - Encourage the patient to express his feelings about his illness
  - Provide rest periods and maintain a quiet environment
  - Monitor the patient for complications
  - Prepare the patient for dialysis if indicated
  - Encourage turning, coughing, and deep breathing
  - Allay the patient's anxiety and provide emotional support
  - Provide skin and mouth care using plain water
  - Individualize home care instruction
    - Know about the disorder and its treatment
      Follow instructions for medication use and be aware of possible adverse effects

Diagnosing acute renal failure

- Blood chemistry: increased potassium, phosphorus, magnesium, BUN, creatinine, and uric acid
- ABG analysis: metabolic acidosis

Treating acute renal failure

- I.V. therapy: electrolyte replacement, hypertonic glucose and insulin
- Diuretics
- Kayexalate
- Dialysis

Key nursing interventions for a patient with acute renal failure

- Restrict fluids.
- Monitor and record vital signs, I/O, CVP, daily weight, laboratory studies, and cardiac rhythm.
- Prepare the patient for dialysis.

Continuous renal replacement therapy

Continuous renal replacement therapy (CRRT) methods vary in complexity. The techniques include the following:

- Slow continuous ultrafiltration (SCUF) uses arteriovenous access and the patient's blood pressure to circulate blood through a hemofilter. Because the goal with this therapy is the removal of fluids, the patient doesn't receive replacement fluids.
- Continuous arteriovenous hemofiltration (CAVH) uses the patient's blood pressure and arteriovenous access to circulate blood through a flow resistance hemofilter. However, to maintain the patency of the filter and the systemic blood pressure, the patient receives replacement fluids.
- Continuous venovenous hemofiltration (CVVH) fuses SCUF and CAVH. A double-lumen catheter is used to provide access to a vein and a pump moves blood through the hemofilter.
- Continuous arteriovenous hemodialysis (CAVH-D) combines hemodialysis with hemofiltration. In this technique, the infusion pump moves dialysate solution concurrent to blood flow, adding the ability to continuously remove solute while removing fluid. Like CAVH, it can also be performed in patients with hypotension and fluid overload.
- Continuous venovenous hemodialysis (CVVH-D) is similar to CAVH-D, except that a vein provides the access while a pump is used to move dialysate solution concurrent with blood flow.

Note: CVVH or CVVH-D is being used instead of CAVH or CAVH-D in many facilities to treat critically ill patients. CVVH has several advantages over CAVH:
- It doesn't require arterial access.
- CVVH can be performed in patients with low mean arterial pressures.
- CVVH has a better solute clearance than CAVH.

NURSING INTERVENTIONS

- Because blood flows through an extracorporeal circuit during CAVH and CVVH, the blood in the hemofilter may need to be anticoagulated. To do this, infuse heparin in low doses as appropriate through the setup.
- To prevent infection, perform skin care at the catheter insertion sites every 48 hours, using sterile technique. Cover the sites with an occlusive dressing.
- Obtain serum electrolyte levels every 4 to 6 hours or as ordered; anticipate adjustments in replacement fluid or dialysate based on the results.

- Observe for signs and symptoms of complications
- Comply with medical follow-up

● **Complications**
- Chronic renal failure
- Electrolyte imbalance
- Hypertensive crisis
- Infection
- Pulmonary edema
- Heart failure
- Metabolic acidosis

● **Surgical interventions**
- Insertion of vascular device for dialysis

CHRONIC RENAL FAILURE

- **Definition**
  - Progressive, irreversible destruction of kidneys, resulting in loss of renal function
- **Causes**
  - Chronic glomerular disease
  - Urinary tract obstructions
  - Diabetes mellitus
  - Vascular diseases
  - Congenital abnormalities such as polycystic kidney disease
  - Collagen diseases
  - Nephrotoxins
- **Pathophysiology**
  - Scarred nephrons can't absorb and secrete water, glucose, amino acids, ammonia, bicarbonate, and electrolytes
  - First stage: renal reserve is diminished, but metabolic wastes don't accumulate although renal damage exists
  - Second stage: renal insufficiency occurs and metabolic wastes begin to accumulate; kidneys are less able to correct metabolic imbalances
  - Third stage (renal failure): uremia occurs with decreased urine output; increased accumulation of metabolic wastes; and disturbed fluid, electrolyte, and acid-base balances
- **Assessment findings**
  - Decreased urine output
  - Hypotension or hypertension
  - Altered LOC
  - Peripheral edema
  - Cardiac arrhythmias
  - Bibasilar crackles
  - Abdominal pain on palpation
  - Poor skin turgor
  - Uremic fetor
- **Diagnostic test findings**
  - Urine chemistry: proteinuria; glycosuria, RBCs and leukocytes, casts and crystals
  - Blood chemistry: increased BUN, creatinine, sodium, and potassium
  - ABG analysis: metabolic acidosis
  - Hematology: decreased Hb, HCT, platelets
  - Renal biopsy: histologic identification of underlying cause
- **Medical management**
  - Monitoring: vital signs and I/O
  - Laboratory studies: BUN, creatinine, potassium, sodium, Hb, HCT, glucose, albumin, and platelets
  - Diuretic: furosemide (Lasix)

Key facts about chronic renal failure

- Progressive, irreversible destruction of kidneys
- Results in loss of renal function
- Occurs in three stages
- First stage: renal reserve is diminished but metabolic wastes don't accumulate
- Second stage: renal insufficiency occurs and metabolic wastes begin to accumulate
- Third stage: uremia occurs with decreased urine output and metabolic waste accumulation increases

Common causes of chronic renal failure

- Chronic glomerular disease
- Urinary tract obstructions
- Diabetes mellitus

Key signs and symptoms of chronic renal failure

- Decreased urine output
- Hypotension or hypertension
- Peripheral edema
- Cardiac arrhythmias

Diagnosing chronic renal failure

- Blood chemistry: increased BUN, creatinine, sodium, and potassium
- ABG analysis: metabolic acidosis

Treating chronic renal failure

- Fluid restrictions
- Diuretics
- Peritoneal dialysis or hemodialysis
- Erythropoietin
- Kidney transplantation

Key nursing interventions for a patient with chronic renal failure

- Restrict fluids.
- Assess renal, respiratory, and cardiovascular status and fluid balance.
- Monitor and record vital signs, I/O, cardiac rhythm, daily weight, and laboratory studies.
- Assist with hemodialysis or peritoneal dialysis.

TOP 5

Complications of chronic renal failure

1. Electrolyte imbalance
2. Arrhythmias
3. Heart failure
4. Pulmonary edema
5. Anemia

- Peritoneal dialysis or hemodialysis
- Diet: low-protein, low-sodium, low-potassium, low-phosphorus, high-calorie, with fluid restrictions
- I.V. therapy: fluids as needed
- Activity: as tolerated
- Transfusion therapy: platelets
- Cation exchange resin: sodium polystyrene sulfonate (Kayexalate)
- Erythropoietin
- Alkalinizing agent: sodium bicarbonate
- Cardiac glycoside: digoxin (Lanoxin)
- Antianemics: ferrous sulfate (Feosol), iron dextran (InFeD), epoetin alfa (recombinant human erythropoietin, Epogen)
- Vitamins: pyridoxine (vitamin B_6), ascorbic acid (vitamin C)
- Calcium supplement: calcium carbonate (Os-Cal)

● **Nursing interventions**
- Assess renal, respiratory, and cardiovascular status and fluid balance
- Monitor and record vital signs, I/O, cardiac rhythm, daily weight, and laboratory studies
- Restrict fluids
- Administer medications as prescribed
- Assist with hemodialysis or peritoneal dialysis
- Encourage the patient to express his feelings about chronicity of illness
- Maintain a cool and quiet environment
- Provide skin and mouth care using plain water
- Monitor for complications
- Individualize home care instructions
    - Know about the disorder and its treatment
    - Follow instructions for medication use and be aware of possible adverse effects
    - Observe for signs and symptoms of complications
    - Maintain dialysis schedule
    - Comply with medical follow-up

● **Complications**
- Electrolyte imbalance
- Arrhythmias
- Heart failure
- Pulmonary edema
- Anemia
- Platelet dysfunction
- Sexual dysfunction

● **Surgical interventions**
- Kidney transplantation
- Insertion of dialysis access device

BLADDER CANCER

● **Definition**
  • Malignant tumor that ulcerates mucosal lining of the bladder

● **Cause**
  • Exact cause unknown

● **Risk factors**
  • Environmental exposure to carcinogens, such as 2-naphthylamine, nitrates
  • Cigarette smoking
  • Chronic bladder irritation or infection
  • Radiation
  • Occupational exposure to carcinogens, especially industrial dyes and solvents
  • Drug induced: cyclophosphamide (Cytoxan)

● **Pathophysiology**
  • Unregulated cell growth and uncontrolled cell division in bladder's transitional epithelium around trigone result in the development of a neoplasm
  • Tumor metastasizes to ureters, prostate gland, vagina, rectum, and periaortic lymph nodes

● **Assessment findings**
  • Painless hematuria
  • Dysuria
  • Frequency and urgency of urination
  • Weight loss
  • Bone pain
  • Urinary incontinence
  • Abdominal pain
  • Fatigue

● **Diagnostic test findings**
  • Cystoscopy: bladder mass
  • Cytologic exam: cytology positive for malignant cells
  • Bladder tumor marker studies: positive
  • CT scan: size, shape, and position of tumor
  • MRI: identifies metastasis
  • Excretory urography: mass or obstruction
  • KUB: mass or obstruction
  • Urine chemistry: hematuria
  • Hematology: decreased RBCs, Hb, HCT

● **Medical management**
  • Radiation therapy
  • Antineoplastics: gemcitabine (Gemzar) and cisplatin (CDDP), paclitaxel (Onxol) and carboplatin (Paraplatin), thiotepa (Thioplex), doxorubicin (Adriamycin)

Key facts about bladder cancer

• Tumor that ulcerates mucosal lining of the bladder
• Tumor metastasizes to ureters, prostate gland, vagina, rectum, and periaortic lymph nodes

Common cause of bladder cancer

• Unknown

Key risk factors for bladder cancer

• Environmental carcinogens
• Cigarette smoking

Key signs and symptoms of bladder cancer

• Painless hematuria
• Frequency and urgency of urination

Diagnosing bladder cancer

• Cystoscopy: bladder mass
• Cytologic exam: positive for malignant cells

Treating bladder cancer

• Radiation therapy
• Antineoplastics
• Analgesics
• Bladder removal
• Ileal conduit

- Analgesic: hydromorphone (Dilaudid)
- Immunotherapy: bacille Calmette-Guérin (BCG)
- I.V. therapy: fluids as needed
- Monitoring: vital signs and I/O
- Laboratory studies: Hb and HCT
- Transfusion therapy: packed RBCs
- Antiemetics: ondansetron (Zofran)

● **Nursing interventions**

- Assess renal status
- Monitor and record vital signs, I/O, and laboratory studies
- Administer medications as prescribed
- Encourage fluids
- Administer I.V. fluids
- Provide emotional support and encourage the patient to express his feelings about his illness
- Provide postchemotherapeutic and postradiation nursing care
    - Provide prophylactic skin, mouth, and perineal care
    - Monitor dietary intake
    - Administer antiemetics and antidiarrheals, as prescribed
    - Monitor the patient for bleeding, infection, and electrolyte imbalance
    - Provide rest periods
- Assess pain level, administer analgesics, as prescribed, and evaluate response
- Provide wound care
- Provide teaching on urinary diversions
- Individualize home care instructions
    - Know about the disorder and its treatment
    - Follow instructions for medication use and be aware of possible adverse effects
    - Observe for signs and symptoms of complications
    - Perform wound care if appropriate
    - Obtain information from the American Cancer Society
    - Seek help from community agencies and resources for supportive services
    - Comply with medical follow-up

● **Complications**

- Ureteral obstruction
- Vesicorectal and vesicovaginal fistulas
- Metastasis

● **Surgical interventions**

- Ileal conduit
- Continent urinary reservoir
- Orthotopic neobladder
- Transurethral resection of bladder
- Bladder removal

BENIGN PROSTATIC HYPERPLASIA

- **Definition**
  - Hyperplasia of the lateral and subcervical lobes of the prostate gland that results in enlargement of the structure
  - Also known as BPH

- **Causes**
  - Unknown
  - Possible link to hormonal activity

- **Risk factors**
  - Age
  - Intact testes

- **Pathophysiology**
  - Enlarged prostate gland compresses urethra, resulting in urinary obstruction and retention
  - Obstruction causes hydroureter and hydronephrosis

- **Assessment findings**
  - Decreased force and amount of urine stream
  - Nocturia, hematuria
  - Urinary hesitancy and urgency
  - Interrupted urine stream
  - Urine retention
  - Dribbling, incontinence
  - Distended bladder
  - International Prostate Symptom Score–evaluates symptoms and response to treatment

- **Diagnostic test findings**
  - Digital rectal examination (DRE): enlarged prostate gland by palpation, distended bladder
  - Urine chemistry: bacteria, hematuria
  - Blood chemistry: increased BUN, creatinine
  - Free PSA: increased
  - International Prostate Symptom Score: determines severity
  - Transrectal ultrasound: enlarged prostate
  - Cystoscopy: enlarged prostate gland, obstructed urine flow, urinary stasis
  - Cystomitrogram: abnormal pressure recordings
  - Urinary flow rate determination: volume small, flow pattern prolonged, peak flow low

- **Medical management**
  - Alpha-adrenergic blocker: phenoxybenzamine (Dibenzyline), prazosin (Minipress), terazosin (Hytrin)
  - 5-alpha-reductase inhibitors: finasteride (Proscar), dutasteride (Avodart)
  - Diet: encourage fluids
  - Monitoring: vital signs and I/O

Key facts about BPH
- Hyperplasia of the lateral and subcervical lobes of the prostate gland
- Results in enlargement of the structure

Common causes of BPH
- Unknown
- Possible link to hormonal activity

TOP 3

Signs and symptoms of BPH
1. Decreased force and amount of urine stream
2. Urinary hesitancy and urgency
3. Interrupted urine stream

Diagnosing BPH
- DRE: enlarged prostate gland by palpation
- Free PSA: increased
- Cystoscopy: enlarged prostate gland, obstructed urine flow, and urinary stasis

Treating BPH
- Alpha-adrenergic blockers
- 5-alpha-reductase inhibitors
- TURP
- Prostatectomy

- Laboratory studies: BUN and creatinine
- Antibiotics: co-trimoxazole (Bactrim), cephalexin (Keflex) (if UTI present)
- Analgesic (after surgery): oxycodone (Tylox)
- Urinary antiseptic (after surgery): phenazopyridine (Pyridium)

● **Nursing interventions**
- Monitor and record: vital signs, I/O, and laboratory studies
- Administer medications as prescribed
- Assess urine output for amount and appearance
- Encourage fluids
- Provide preoperative and postoperative teaching, as appropriate
- Encourage the patient to express his feelings about his illness
- Provide postoperative care if appropriate
    - Maintain position and patency of indwelling urinary catheter and continuous bladder irrigation
    - Assess pain level, administer analgesics, as prescribed, and evaluate response
    - Monitor for bladder spasms
    - Assess urine for color and amount; note presence of blood clots, maintain strict I/O
    - Monitor for signs and symptoms of complications, such as urinary obstruction or UTI
- Individualize home care instructions
    - Know about the disorder and its treatment
    - Follow instructions for medication use and be aware of possible adverse effects
    - Recognize the signs and symptoms of urine retention
    - Comply with medical follow-up
    - Perform intermittent self-catheterization and document time and amount on flow sheet

● **Complications**
- Chronic renal failure
- Renal calculi
- Cystitis

● **Surgical interventions**
- TURP
- Prostatectomy
- Transurethral incision of prostate gland
- Transurethral needle ablation
- Transurethral microwave therapy
- Laser therapy

PROSTATE CANCER

● **Definition**
- Malignant tumor of the prostate gland

Key nursing interventions for a patient with BPH

- Monitor vital signs, I/O, and laboratory studies.
- Administer medications.
- Provide postoperative care.

Key complications of BPH

- Chronic renal failure
- Renal calculi
- Cystitis

Key facts about prostate cancer

- Malignant tumor of the prostate gland
- Metastasis commonly occurs to bone, lymph nodes, brain, and lungs

Cause
- Unknown
- Associated risk factors: family history, age, black race, increased dietary fat, cadmium exposure

Pathophysiology
- Unregulated cell growth and uncontrolled cell division result in the development of a neoplasm
- Obstruction of urine flow occurs when the tumor encroaches on the bladder neck
- Metastasis commonly occurs to bone, lymph nodes, brain, and lungs

Assessment findings
- Urinary hesitancy
- Urine retention
- Decreased size and force of urine stream
- Dribbling
- Dysuria, hematuria
- Weight loss
- Fatigue
- Palpable firm nodule in gland or diffuse induration in posterior lobe (on DRE)

Diagnostic test findings
- PSA: increased
- Prostate cancer markers (investigations): positive for AMACR (x-methyla-cyl-CoA racemase)
- Transrectal ultrasound (TRUS): increased size of prostate or abnormal growth
- CT scan or MRI: defines extent of tumor
- Prostate biopsy: cytology positive for cancer cells

Medical management
- Luteinizing hormone–releasing agonists: leuprolide (Lupron), goserelin (Zoladex)
- Androgen antagonists: bicalutamide (Casodex), flutamide (Eulexin)
- Radiation therapy or implant
- Antineoplastics: paclitaxel (Taxol), estramustine (Emcyt)
- Bisphosphonates: zoledronic acid (Zometa)
- Antifungals: ketoconazole (Nizoral)
- Diet: low-fat
- Activity: as tolerated
- Monitoring: vital signs and I/O
- Laboratory studies: BUN, creatinine, PSA
- I.V. therapy: fluids as needed
- Analgesics: oxycodone (Tylox), meperidine (Demerol)
- Corticosteroid: prednisone (Deltasone)
- Antiemetics: ondansetron (Zofran)

Common cause of prostate cancer
- Unknown

Key risk factors for prostate cancer
- Family history
- Age
- Black race

Key signs and symptoms of prostate cancer
- Urinary hesitancy
- Urine retention
- Decreased size and force of urine stream
- Hematuria
- Palpable firm nodule (on DRE)

Diagnosing prostate cancer
- PSA: increased
- TRUS: increased prostate size or abnormal growth
- Biopsy: positive for cancer cells

Treating prostate cancer
- Luteinizing hormone–releasing agonists
- Androgen antagonists
- Radiation therapy; radiation implant
- Antineoplastics
- Radical prostatectomy
- TURP

Key nursing interventions for a patient with prostate cancer

- Assess renal and fluid status.
- Assess pain level.
- Provide postchemotherapeutic, postradiation, and postoperative care.
- Provide emotional support.

Key complications of prostate cancer

- Metastasis
- Impotence

Key facts about neurogenic bladder

- An interruption of normal bladder innervation
- Three types: flaccid, spastic, and mixed

● **Nursing interventions**
- Assess renal and fluid status
- Monitor and record vital signs, I/O, and laboratory studies
- Administer medications as prescribed
- Maintain the patient's diet
- Monitor fluid intake
- Allay the patient's anxiety and provide emotional support
- Encourage the patient to express his feelings about his illness
- Assess pain level, administer analgesics as prescribed, and evaluate response
- Provide postchemotherapeutic and postradiation nursing care
    - Provide prophylactic skin, mouth, and perineal care
    - Monitor dietary intake
    - Administer antiemetics as prescribed
    - Provide rest periods
- Provide postoperative nursing care
    - Monitor vital signs, I/O, and pain level
    - Provide wound care
    - Monitor urine for blood and clots
- Individualize home care instructions
    - Know about the disorder and its treatment
    - Follow instructions for medication use and be aware of possible adverse effects
    - Observe for signs and symptoms of complications
    - Obtain information from the American Cancer Society
    - Seek help from community agencies and resources for supportive services
    - Comply with follow-up

● **Complications**
- Metastatic cancer (bone, lymph nodes, brain, and lung)
- Impotence
- Urinary incontinence

● **Surgical interventions**
- Radical prostatectomy
- Bilateral orchiectomy
- Cryosurgery
- TURP

NEUROGENIC BLADDER

● **Definition**
- An interruption of normal bladder innervation
- Three types of neurogenic bladder may occur: flaccid, spastic, and mixed

● **Causes**
- Acute infectious diseases such as transverse myelitis

- Cerebral disorders (stroke, brain tumor, Parkinson's disease, multiple sclerosis, dementia)
- Chronic alcoholism
- Collagen diseases such as SLE
- Heavy metal toxicity
- Herpes zoster
- Metabolic disturbances (hypothyroidism, porphyria, or uremia)
- Sacral agenesis
- Spinal cord disease or trauma
- Vascular diseases such as atherosclerosis

● Pathophysiology

- Flaccid neurogenic bladder: caused by a lower motor neuron lesion (below S2 to S4), with decreased intravesical pressure, increased bladder capacity and large residual urine retention, and poor detrusor contraction
- Spastic neurogenic bladder: caused by an upper motor neuron (above S2 to S4), with spontaneous contractions of detrusor muscles, elevated intravesical voiding pressure, bladder wall hypertrophy with trabeculation, and urinary sphincter spasms
- Mixed neurogenic bladder: the result of cortical damage from some disorder or trauma (see *Types of neurogenic bladder,* page 374)

● Assessment findings

- Flaccid neurogenic bladder
  - Overflow incontinence
  - Diminished anal sphincter tone
  - Greatly distended bladder with an accompanying feeling of bladder fullness
- Spastic neurogenic bladder
  - Involuntary or frequent scanty urination without a feeling of bladder fullness
  - Possible spontaneous spasms of the arms and legs
  - Increased anal sphincter tone
- Mixed neurogenic bladder
  - Dulled perception of bladder fullness
  - Diminished ability to empty the bladder
  - Urgency that can't be controlled

● Diagnostic test findings

- Voiding cystourethrography: evaluates bladder neck function, vesicoureteral reflux, and continence
- Urodynamic studies: consist of cystometry, uroflometry, urethral pressure profiles, and sphincter electromyelography; evaluates how well the bladder stores urine, bladder emptying, and the rate of urine movement out of the bladder during voiding
- Retrograde urethrography: reveals presence of strictures and diverticula
- Urine flow studies: diminished or impaired urine flow

Common causes of neurogenic bladder

- Acute infectious diseases
- Cerebral disorders
- Metabolic disturbances
- Spinal cord disease or trauma

Key signs and symptoms of neurogenic bladder

Flaccid
- Overflow incontinence
- Diminished anal sphincter tone

Spastic
- Involuntary or frequent scanty urination
- Increased anal sphincter tone

Mixed
- Dulled perception of bladder fullness
- Diminished ability to empty bladder

Diagnosing neurogenic bladder

- Urodynamic studies: cystometry, uroflometry, urethral pressure profiles, and sphincter electromyelography
- Voiding cystourethrography

Types of neurogenic bladder

NEURAL LESION	TYPE	CAUSE
Upper motor	Uninhibited	• Lack of voluntary control in infancy • Multiple sclerosis
	Reflex or automatic	• Spinal cord transection • Cord tumors • Multiple sclerosis
Lower motor	Autonomous	• Sacral cord trauma • Tumors • Herniated disk • Abdominal surgery with transection of pelvic parasympathetic nerves
	Motor paralysis	• Lesions at levels S2, S3, S4 • Poliomyelitis • Trauma • Tumors
	Sensory paralysis	• Posterior lumbar nerve roots • Diabetes mellitus • Tabes dorsalis

Treating neurogenic bladder

- Valsalva's maneuver, indwelling or intermittent self-catheterization, Credé's maneuver, bladder training
- Antispasmodics
- Alpha-adrenergic blockers
- Anticholinergics

Key nursing interventions for a patient with neurogenic bladder

- Assess renal status.
- Administer medications.
- Assess for signs and symptoms of infection.
- Teach self-catheterization.

● Medical management

- Treatments: Valsalva's maneuver, indwelling or intermittent self-catheterization, Credé's maneuver, incontinence products, ureteral occlusive device, bladder training (to improve bladder function)
- Monitoring: vital signs and I/O
- Antispasmodics: oxybutynin (Ditropan), tolterodine (Detrol)
- Alpha-adrenergic blockers: terazosin (Hytrin), doxazosin (Cardura)
- Anticholinergics: darifenacin (Enablex), hyoscyamine (Levbid)
- Estrogen derivatives: conjugated estrogen (Premarin)
- Tricyclic antidepressants: imipramine (Tofranil), amitriptyline (Elavil)
- Diet: avoidance of stimulants (spicy foods, chocolate, caffeine); controlled fluid intake
- Activity: pelvic muscle exercises

● Nursing interventions

- Assess renal status
- Monitor and record vital signs, I/O, and laboratory studies
- Administer medications as prescribed
- Monitor fluid intake and assist with dietary modifications
- Allay the patient's anxiety and provide emotional support
- Maintain indwelling urinary catheter; teach self-catheterization if appropriate
- Assess for signs and symptoms of infection
- Individualize home care instructions
  - Know about the disorder and its treatment

- Follow instructions for medication use and be aware of possible adverse effects
- Recognize and report signs and symptoms of infection
- Follow bladder training program
- Comply with diet and fluid modifications
- Take measures to prevent UTI
- Perform Credé's maneuver, pelvic exercises, and intermittent self-catheterization
- Comply with medical follow-up

● **Complications**
  - UTI
  - Urolithiasis
  - Renal failure

● **Surgical interventions**
  - Transurethral resection of the bladder neck, urethral dilation, or external sphincterotomy
  - Urinary diversion

NCLEX CHECKS

It's never too soon to begin your NCLEX preparation. Now that you've reviewed this chapter, carefully read each of the following questions and choose the best answer. Then compare your responses to the correct answers.

1. A nurse is caring for a client with acute renal failure. The nurse should expect hypertonic glucose and insulin infusions to be used to treat:
- ☐ **1.** hypernatremia.
- ☐ **2.** hypokalemia.
- ☐ **3.** hyperkalemia.
- ☐ **4.** hypercalcemia.

2. A client with fever and urinary urgency is asked to provide a urine specimen for culture and sensitivity. The nurse should instruct the client to collect the specimen from the:
- ☐ **1.** first stream of urine from the bladder.
- ☐ **2.** middle stream of urine from the bladder.
- ☐ **3.** final stream of urine from the bladder.
- ☐ **4.** full volume of urine from the bladder.

3. A nurse is teaching a client with chronic renal failure about foods to avoid. It would be accurate for her to teach the client to avoid foods high in:
- ☐ **1.** monosaccharides.
- ☐ **2.** disaccharides.
- ☐ **3.** iron.
- ☐ **4.** protein.

Key complications of neurogenic bladder

- UTI
- Urolithiasis

TOP 10

Items to study for your next test on the renal and urologic system

1. Structures of the kidneys and their functions
2. Glomerular filtration rate
3. Nursing interventions for the patient undergoing kidney transplantation
4. Types of urinary diversion surgeries
5. Signs and symptoms of renal calculi
6. How acute renal failure and chronic renal failure happen
7. Nursing interventions for the patient with bladder or prostate cancer
8. Probable nursing diagnoses for the patient with a renal or urologic disorder
9. Treatment of BPH
10. Risk factors for renal calculi

4. A nurse is developing a care plan for a 36-year-old male client hospitalized with renal calculi. Which intervention should she include in his plan?

- ☐ **1.** Maintain bed rest.
- ☐ **2.** Increase dietary purines.
- ☐ **3.** Restrict fluids.
- ☐ **4.** Strain all urine.

5. A client with anemia caused by chronic renal failure is ordered to receive 50 units/kg I.V. of epoetin alfa (Epogen). The client weighs 165 lb. The drug is available with 4,000 units/ml. How many milliliters would the nurse administer? Round your answer to one decimal place.

_____ milliliters

6. Which factor can contribute to renal calculi formation?

- ☐ **1.** Hypocalcemia
- ☐ **2.** Changes in urine pH
- ☐ **3.** Hypothyroidism
- ☐ **4.** Hypertension

7. For a client with renal calcium stones, the nurse should provide instruction on which of the following diets?

- ☐ **1.** Limited intake of calcium and milk products
- ☐ **2.** Limited intake of foods high in oxalate
- ☐ **3.** Limited intake of foods high in purine
- ☐ **4.** Low-cholesterol diet with limited intake of saturated fats

8. Which assessment finding should the nurse expect in a client with flaccid neurogenic bladder?

- ☐ **1.** Greatly distended bladder with a feeling of bladder fullness
- ☐ **2.** Involuntary or frequent scanty urination without a feeling of bladder fullness
- ☐ **3.** Dulled perception of bladder fullness
- ☐ **4.** Spontaneous spasms of the arms and legs

9. A client is scheduled to perform a 24-hour urine test beginning at 8 a.m. on the first day and ending at 8 a.m. on the second day. The nurse should instruct the client to:

- ☐ **1.** discard the second-day 8 a.m. specimen.
- ☐ **2.** discard the first and last specimens.
- ☐ **3.** discard the first-day 8 a.m. specimen.
- ☐ **4.** retain the first-day 8 a.m. specimen.

10. A client is scheduled for an ileal conduit. The nurse knows the client understands the procedure when he states:

- ☐ **1.** "I'll pass urine from my rectum."
- ☐ **2.** "Urine will flow out a catheter."
- ☐ **3.** "Urine will come out an abdominal stoma."
- ☐ **4.** "Urine will flow from my urethra."

ANSWERS AND RATIONALES

1. CORRECT ANSWER: 3

Hyperkalemia is a common complication of acute renal failure. The administration of glucose and regular insulin infusions can temporarily prevent cardiac arrest by moving potassium into the cells and reducing serum potassium levels. Hypernatremia, hypokalemia, and hypercalcemia don't usually occur with acute renal failure and aren't treated with glucose and insulin infusions.

2. CORRECT ANSWER: 2

A midstream specimen is recommended because it's less likely to be contaminated with microorganisms from the external genitalia than other specimens. It isn't necessary to collect a full volume of urine for a urine culture and sensitivity.

3. CORRECT ANSWER: 4

Proteins are typically restricted in clients with chronic renal failure because of their metabolites. Iron and carbohydrates aren't restricted.

4. CORRECT ANSWER: 4

All urine should be strained through gauze or a urine strainer to catch any stones passed. The stone's composition can then be analyzed. Ambulation may aid the movement of the stone down the urinary tract. A client at risk for uric acid stones should follow a low-purine diet to reduce uric acid levels. Encourage fluid intake to help flush the stones out of the urinary tract.

5. CORRECT ANSWER: 0.9

First convert the client's weight to kilograms:

$$165 \text{ lb} \div 2.2 \text{ kg/lb} = 75 \text{ kg}$$

Then determine the dose:

$$50 \text{ units} \times 75 = 3{,}750 \text{ units}$$

$$\frac{4{,}000 \text{ units}}{1 \text{ ml}} = \frac{3{,}750 \text{ units}}{X}$$

$$4{,}000X = 3{,}750 \text{ ml}$$

$$X = \frac{3{,}750 \text{ ml}}{4{,}000}$$

$$X = 0.93 \text{ or } 0.9 \text{ ml}$$

6. CORRECT ANSWER: 2

Urine that's consistently acidic or alkaline provides a favorable medium for stone formation.

7. CORRECT ANSWER: 1

A client with calcium stones should follow a diet with limited intake of calcium and milk products. A limited intake of foods high in oxalate is appropriate for a client with oxalate stones. A client with uric acid stones should limit intake of foods high in purine. A client with coronary artery disease should follow a low-cholesterol diet with limited intake of saturated fats.

8. CORRECT ANSWER: 1

A client with flaccid neurogenic bladder will have a greatly distended bladder with an accompanying feeling of bladder fullness, overflow incontinence, and diminished anal sphincter tone. With spastic neurogenic bladder, the client will experience involuntary or frequent scanty urination without a feeling of bladder fullness, possible spontaneous spasms of the arms and legs, and increased anal sphincter tone. With mixed neurogenic bladder, the client has a dulled perception of bladder fullness, a diminished ability to empty the bladder, and urgency that can't be controlled.

9. CORRECT ANSWER: 3

With a 24-hour urine test, discard the first specimen and retain the last specimen. Therefore, the nurse should instruct the client to discard the first-day 8 a.m. urine specimen and retain the second-day 8 a.m. specimen.

10. CORRECT ANSWER: 3

With an ileal conduit, the ureters are implanted into a segment of the ileum that has been resected from the intestinal tract with the formation of an abdominal stoma. With a ureterosigmoidostomy, the ureters are excised from the bladder and implanted into the sigmoid colon. Urine then flows through the colon and is excreted through the rectum. With a nephrostomy, a catheter is inserted percutaneously into the kidney. Normal urine flow occurs through the urethra.

8

Musculoskeletal system

PRETEST

1. A possible complication of osteogenic sarcoma and osteoporosis is:

- ☐ 1. kyphosis.
- ☐ 2. metastasis.
- ☒ 3. pathologic fracture.
- ☐ 4. carpal tunnel syndrome.

CORRECT ANSWER: 3

2. Which assessment findings are indicative of a herniated lumbosacral disk?

- ☐ 1. Tinel sign and Phalen's sign
- ☒ 2. Straight-leg-raising test and Lasègue sign
- ☐ 3. Flick sign and Phalen's sign
- ☐ 4. Homans' sign and Lasèque sign

CORRECT ANSWER: 2

3. A client who was hospitalized for osteomyelitis is being prepared for discharge. Which statement by the client indicates an understanding of the nurse's instructions?

- ☒ 1. "I should try to avoid anyone with an infection."
- ☐ 2. "I should only take my antibiotics when I get a fever."
- ☐ 3. "I no longer have to worry about infection because I was already treated with antibiotics."
- ☐ 4. "I can resume all former activities immediately."

CORRECT ANSWER: 1

4. A female client, age 36, complains of fatigue, weight loss, and a low-grade fever. She also complains of pain in her fingers, elbows, wrists, ankles, and knees. Which of the following conditions should the nurse suspect?

- ☐ 1. Gout
- ☐ 2. Osteomyelitis
- ☐ 3. Systemic lupus erythematosus
- ☒ 4. Rheumatoid arthritis

CORRECT ANSWER: 4

5. A client is complaining of chest pain and shortness of breath, with decreased pulse oximetry readings after surgery for a fractured hip. The nurse suspects that the client is experiencing:

- ☐ 1. a panic attack.
- ☒ 2. fat embolism.
- ☐ 3. incisional pain.
- ☐ 4. an asthma attack.

CORRECT ANSWER: 2

LEARNING OBJECTIVES

After studying this chapter, you should be able to:

- Describe the psychosocial impact of musculoskeletal disorders.
- Differentiate between modifiable and nonmodifiable risk factors in the development of a musculoskeletal disorder.
- List three probable and three possible nursing diagnoses for a patient with a musculoskeletal disorder.
- Identify nursing interventions for a patient with a musculoskeletal disorder.
- Identify three teaching topics for a patient with a musculoskeletal disorder.

CHAPTER OVERVIEW

Caring for the patient with a musculoskeletal disorder requires a sound understanding of musculoskeletal anatomy and physiology as well as body mechanics. A thorough assessment is essential to planning and implementing appropriate patient care. The assessment includes a complete history, physical examination, diagnostic testing, identification of modifiable and nonmodifiable risk factors, and information related to the psychosocial impact of the disorder on the patient and his family.

Nursing diagnoses focus primarily on impaired physical mobility and altered peripheral tissue perfusion. Nursing interventions are designed to maintain or improve the patient's ability to carry out the activities of daily living (ADLs) and prevent further injury. Patient teaching—a crucial nursing activity—involves providing information about the disorder and its treatment, medication regimens, signs and symptoms of possible complications, reduction of modifiable risk factors (such as using proper body mechanics, preventing falls, participating in body flexibility and strength regimens), and medical follow-up.

ANATOMY AND PHYSIOLOGY REVIEW

- **Skeleton**
  - Consists of 206 bones (long, short, flat, or irregular)
  - Stores calcium, magnesium, phosphorus, and carbonate; marrow produces red blood cells (RBCs)
  - Works with muscles to provide support, locomotion, and protection of internal organs (see *Anatomy of a bone,* page 382)

- **Skeletal muscles**
  - Provide body movement and posture by tightening and shortening
  - Attach to bones by tendons
  - Begin contracting with the stimulus of a muscle fiber by a motor neuron
  - Derive energy for muscle contraction from hydrolysis of adenosine triphosphate to adenosine diphosphate and phosphate
  - Retain some contraction to maintain muscle tone
  - Relax with the breakdown of acetylcholine by cholinesterase (see *Anatomy of a muscle,* page 383)

- **Ligaments**
  - Tough bands of collagen fibers that connect bones
  - Encircle a joint to add strength and stability

- **Tendons**
  - Nonelastic collagen cords
  - Connect muscles to bones

- **Joints**
  - Articulation of two bone surfaces
  - Provide stabilization and permit locomotion; degree of joint movement is called *range of motion* (ROM) (see *Basic joint movements,* page 384)

Key facts about the skeleton

- 206 bones
- Stores calcium, magnesium, phosphorus, and carbonate
- Marrow produces RBCs
- Functions include support, locomotion, and protection of internal organs

Key facts about skeletal muscles

- Provide body movement and posture
- Attach to bones by tendons
- Retain some contraction for muscle tone

Key facts about joints

- Articulation of two bone surfaces
- Provide stabilization
- Permit locomotion
- ROM is degree of joint movement

Anatomy of a bone

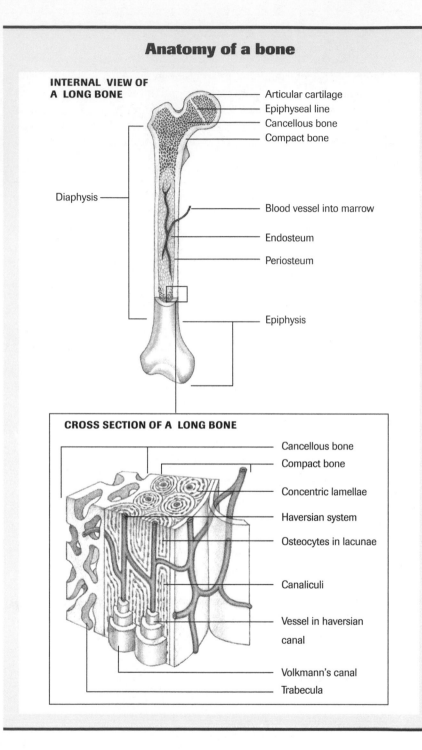

INTERNAL VIEW OF A LONG BONE

- Articular cartilage
- Epiphyseal line
- Cancellous bone
- Compact bone
- Diaphysis
- Blood vessel into marrow
- Endosteum
- Periosteum
- Epiphysis

CROSS SECTION OF A LONG BONE

- Cancellous bone
- Compact bone
- Concentric lamellae
- Haversian system
- Osteocytes in lacunae
- Canaliculi
- Vessel in haversian canal
- Volkmann's canal
- Trabecula

Key facts about synovium

- Lines a joint's inner surfaces
- Secretes synovial fluid
- Reduces friction

● Synovium

- Membrane that lines a joint's inner surfaces
- Secretes synovial fluid and antibodies
- Reduces friction in joints (in conjunction with cartilage)

Anatomy of a muscle

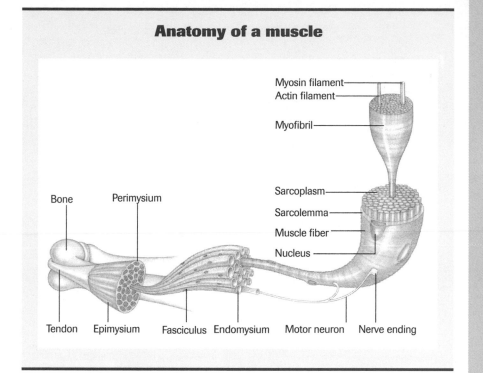

Myosin filament
Actin filament
Myofibril
Sarcoplasm
Sarcolemma
Muscle fiber
Nucleus
Bone
Perimysium
Tendon
Epimysium
Fasciculus
Endomysium
Motor neuron
Nerve ending

Key facts about cartilage
- Composed of fibers embedded in firm gel
- Smooth surface for articulating bones
- Absorbs shocks to joints

● **Cartilage**
- Composed of fibers embedded in firm gel
- Serves as a smooth surface for articulating bones
- Absorbs shock to joints
- Atrophies with limited ROM or in the absence of weight bearing

Key facts about the bursa
- Fluid-filled sac
- Serves as padding
- Facilitates motion of body structures

● **Bursa**
- Fluid-filled sac
- Serves as padding to reduce friction
- Facilitates the motion of body structures that rub against each other

ASSESSMENT FINDINGS

● **History**
- Pain
- Numbness, tingling
- Joint stiffness
- Swelling
- Fatigue
- Fever
- Difficulty with movement

Key assessment findings in disorders of the musculoskeletal system
- Pain
- Numbness, tingling
- Joint stiffness
- Difficulty with movement

● **Physical examination**
- Abnormal vital signs
- Inflammation

Types of joint movements

- Circumduction
- Flexion and extension
- Adduction and abduction
- Retraction and protraction
- Pronation and supination
- Internal and external rotation
- Eversion and inversion

Basic joint movements

Diarthrodial joints permit 13 angular and circular motions. (All are evaluated in a musculoskeletal assessment.) The shoulder demonstrates circumduction; the elbow, flexion and extension; the arm, abduction and adduction; the jaw, retraction and protraction; the hand, pronation and supination; the hip, internal and external rotation; and the foot, eversion and inversion.

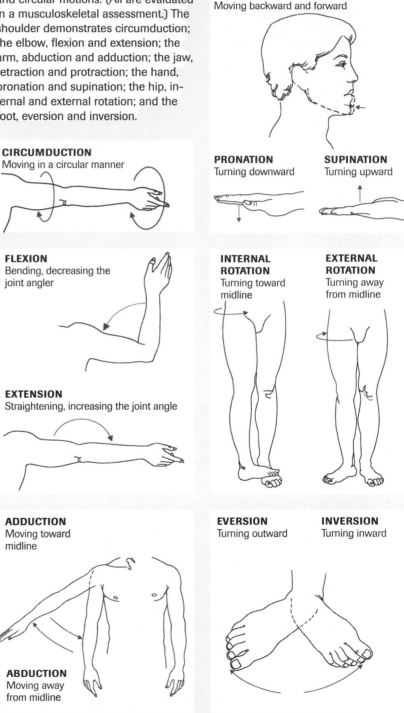

CIRCUMDUCTION
Moving in a circular manner

RETRACTION AND PROTRACTION
Moving backward and forward

PRONATION
Turning downward

SUPINATION
Turning upward

FLEXION
Bending, decreasing the joint angler

EXTENSION
Straightening, increasing the joint angle

INTERNAL ROTATION
Turning toward midline

EXTERNAL ROTATION
Turning away from midline

ADDUCTION
Moving toward midline

ABDUCTION
Moving away from midline

EVERSION
Turning outward

INVERSION
Turning inward

- Edema
- Skin breakdown
- Skeletal deformity
- Limited ROM
- Poor posture
- Muscle weakness
- Muscle stiffness and rigidity
- Abnormal skin color and temperature
- Paresthesia
- Nodules
- Erythema
- Tophi
- Abnormal peripheral pulses
- Muscle spasms or tremors
- Gait abnormalities

DIAGNOSTIC TESTS AND PROCEDURES

- ● **Electromyography (EMG)**
  - Definition and purpose
    - Test of muscle activity
    - Graphical recording of the muscle at rest and during contraction
  - Nursing interventions
    - Explain that the patient will be asked to flex and relax muscles during the procedure
    - Explain that the procedure may cause some minor discomfort but isn't painful
    - Administer analgesics as prescribed, after the procedure

- ● **Arthroscopy**
  - Definition and purpose
    - Direct visualization of a joint through use of a fiber-optic telescope (arthroscope) after injection of local anesthesia
  - Nursing interventions before the procedure
    - Explain the procedure, skin preparation, and use of local anesthetics
    - Administer prophylactic antibiotics as prescribed
  - Nursing interventions after the procedure
    - Apply a pressure dressing to the injection site
    - Monitor neurovascular status (see *Neurovascular checks,* page 386)
    - Apply ice to the affected joint
    - Limit weight bearing or joint use until allowed by the physician
    - Administer analgesics as prescribed

- ● **Arthrocentesis**
  - Definition and purpose
    - Needle aspiration of synovial fluid from a joint under local anesthesia to examine a specimen or remove the fluid

5 Ps of assessing a neurovascular injury

- Pain
- Pallor
- Paralysis
- Paresthesia
- Pulselessness

Key facts about arthrocentesis

- Needle aspiration of synovial fluid from a joint
- Used to examine a specimen or remove fluid
- Intervention: maintain a pressure dressing on the aspiration site after the procedure

Key facts about a bone scan

- Procedure using an I.V. injection of an isotope
- Provides visual imaging of bone metabolism
- Intervention: explain that the patient will be required to drink several glasses of fluid to enhance excretion of isotope not absorbed by bone tissue

Neurovascular checks

Injury may cause nerve or arterial damage, producing any or all of the five Ps: pain, pallor, paralysis, paresthesia, and pulselessness. When performing a neurovascular check, compare findings bilaterally and above and below the injury.

PAIN

Ask the patient if he's having pain. Assess the location, severity, and quality of the pain as well as anything that seems to relieve or worsen it. Pain that's unrelieved by an opioid or that worsens when the limb is elevated (elevation reduces circulation and worsens ischemia) may indicate compartment syndrome.

PALLOR

Paleness, discoloration, and coolness of the injured site may indicate neurovascular compromise from decreased blood supply to the area. Check capillary refill time. Tissues should return to normal color within 3 seconds. Palpate skin temperature with the back of your hand.

PARALYSIS

Note deficits in movement or strength. If the patient can't move the affected area or if movement causes severe pain and muscle spasms, he might have nerve or tendon damage. For a femoral fracture, assess peroneal nerve injury by checking for sensation over the top of the foot between the first and second toes.

PARESTHESIA

Ask the patient about changes in sensation, such as numbness or tingling. Check for loss of sensation by touching the injured area with the tip of an open safety pin or the point of a paper clip. Abnormal sensation or loss of sensation indicates neurovascular involvement.

PULSELESSNESS

Palpate peripheral pulses distal to the injury, noting rate and quality. If a pulse is decreased or absent, blood supply to the area is reduced.

- Nursing interventions before the procedure
  - Explain the procedure to the patient
  - Administer prophylactic antibiotics as prescribed
- Nursing interventions after the procedure
  - Maintain a pressure dressing on the aspiration site
  - Monitor neurovascular status
  - Apply ice to the affected area
  - Limit weight bearing or joint use until allowed by the physician
  - Administer analgesics as prescribed

● **Bone scan**
- Definition and purpose
  - Visual imaging of bone metabolism after I.V. injection of a radioisotope
- Nursing interventions before the procedure
  - Explain the procedure to the patient
  - Determine the patient's ability to lie still during the scan
  - Advise the patient that radioisotope will be injected I.V.

– Explain that the patient will be required to drink several glasses of fluid during the waiting period to enhance excretion of isotope not absorbed by bone tissue

● **Myelogram**
  • Definition and purpose
    – Fluoroscopic visualization of the subarachnoid space, spinal cord, and vertebral bodies after injection of radiopaque dye by lumbar puncture
  • Nursing interventions before the procedure
    – Explain the procedure to the patient
    – Note the patient's allergies to iodine, seafood, and radiopaque dyes
    – Inform the patient about possible throat irritation and flushing of the face from the injection
    – Obtain a signed informed consent
  • Nursing interventions after the procedure
    – Maintain bed rest, with the head of the bed between 15 and 30 degrees
    – Inspect the insertion site for bleeding
    – Monitor neurovital signs
    – Encourage oral fluids

● **X-ray examination**
  • Definition and purpose
    – Noninvasive radiographic examination of bones and joints
  • Nursing interventions
    – Explain the procedure to the patient
    – Use caution when moving a patient with a suspected fracture
    – Make sure the patient isn't pregnant to prevent possible fetal damage from radiation exposure

● **Blood chemistry**
  • Definition and purpose
    – Laboratory test of a blood sample
    – Analysis for potassium, sodium, calcium, phosphorus, glucose, bicarbonate, blood urea nitrogen (BUN), creatinine, protein, albumin, osmolality, creatine kinase, serum aspartate aminotransferase, aldolase, rheumatoid factor, complement fixation, lupus erythematosus (LE) cell preparation test, antinuclear antibody (ANA), anti-deoxyribonucleic acid (DNA), and C-reactive protein
  • Nursing interventions
    – Explain the procedure to the patient
    – Monitor the venipuncture site for bleeding after the procedure

● **Hematologic studies**
  • Definition and purpose
    – Laboratory test of a blood sample
    – Analysis for white blood cells (WBCs), RBCs, platelets, prothrombin time, partial thromboplastin time, erythrocyte sedimentation rate (ESR), hemoglobin (Hb), and hematocrit (HCT)

Key facts about a myelogram

● Fluoroscopic procedure using an injection of radiopaque dye
● Allows visualization of the subarachnoid space, spinal cord, and vertebral bodies
● Intervention: before the procedure, note the patient's allergies

Key facts about X-ray examination

● Noninvasive examination of bones and joints
● Intervention: before the procedure, make sure the patient isn't pregnant to prevent possible fetal damage from radiation exposure

Key facts about blood chemistry

● Blood test
● Analyzes levels of potassium, calcium, BUN, protein, LE, anti-DNA, and other factors
● Intervention: monitor the venipuncture site for bleeding after the procedure

Key facts about hematologic studies

● Blood test
● Analyzes for substances, such as WBCs, RBCs, Hb, and HCT
● Intervention: note current drug therapy to anticipate possible interference with test results

Key psychosocial impacts of musculoskeletal disorders

- Decreased self-esteem
- Dependence
- Economic impact: disruption or loss of employment, cost of hospitalizations, home health care, special equipment
- Restrictions on physical activity

Key modifiable risk factors in musculoskeletal disorders

- Occupations that require heavy lifting, use of machinery, or repetitive motion
- Vegetarian diet
- Contact sports
- Obesity

Key nonmodifiable risk factors in musculoskeletal disorders

- Aging
- Menopause
- Family history

- Nursing interventions
- Explain the procedure to the patient
- Note current drug therapy to anticipate possible effect on test results
- Assess the venipuncture site for bleeding after the procedure

PSYCHOSOCIAL IMPACT OF MUSCULOSKELETAL DISORDERS

- **Developmental impact**
  - Decreased self-esteem
  - Fear of rejection
  - Changes in body image
  - Embarrassment from changes in body structure and function
  - Dependence on others

- **Economic impact**
  - Disruption or loss of employment
  - Cost of vocational retraining
  - Cost of hospitalizations
  - Cost of home health care
  - Cost of special equipment

- **Occupational and recreational impact**
  - Restrictions on work activity
  - Changes in leisure activity
  - Restrictions on physical activity

- **Social impact**
  - Social isolation
  - Changes in role performance

RISK FACTORS

- **Modifiable risk factors**
  - Occupations that require heavy lifting or use of machinery
  - Occupational or recreational activities that include repetitive motion of joints
  - Vegetarian diet
  - Medication history
  - Stress
  - Contact sports
  - Obesity

- **Nonmodifiable risk factors**
  - Aging
  - Menopause
  - Family history of musculoskeletal illness
  - History of musculoskeletal injury
  - History of immune disorders
  - History of osteoporosis

NURSING DIAGNOSES

● **Probable nursing diagnoses**
- Anxiety
- Fear
- Impaired physical mobility
- Ineffective tissue perfusion: Peripheral
- Impaired skin integrity
- Acute pain
- Toileting self-care deficit
- Feeding self-care deficit
- Bathing or hygiene self-care deficit

● **Possible nursing diagnoses**
- Sexual dysfunction
- Powerlessness
- Constipation
- Disturbed body image
- Social isolation
- Risk for disuse syndrome
- Chronic pain
- Interrupted family processes

JOINT SURGERY

● **Description**
- Arthrodesis — surgical removal of cartilage from joint surfaces to fuse a joint into a functional position
- Synovectomy — removal of the synovial membrane from a joint, using an arthroscope, to reduce pain
- Arthroplasty (total joint replacement) — surgical replacement of a joint with a metal, plastic, or porous prosthesis

● **Preoperative nursing interventions**
- Complete patient and family preoperative teaching
  - Explain the procedure to the patient
  - Describe the operating room, postanesthesia care unit (PACU), and preoperative and postoperative routines
  - Demonstrate postoperative turning, coughing, deep breathing, incentive spirometry, splinting, and ROM exercises
  - Explain the postoperative need for drainage tubes, surgical dressings, oxygen therapy, I.V. therapy, pain control, and physical therapy
- Complete a preoperative checklist and make sure a signed informed consent is in the patient's chart
- Administer medications as prescribed
- Provide emotional support to allay the patient's and family's anxiety about surgery
- Document the patient's history and physical assessment data

---

Key probable nursing diagnoses in patients with musculoskeletal disorders

- Impaired physical mobility
- Ineffective tissue perfusion: Peripheral
- Impaired skin integrity

Key facts about joint surgery

- Arthrodesis — surgical removal of cartilage from joint surfaces to fuse a joint into a functional position
- Synovectomy — removal of the synovial membrane from a joint, using an arthroscope, to reduce pain
- Arthroplasty (total joint replacement) — surgical replacement of a joint with a metal, plastic, or porous prosthesis

Key nursing interventions before joint surgery

- Complete preoperative teaching.
- Complete preoperative checklist.
- Administer preoperative medications.
- Document assessment data.

Key nursing interventions after joint surgery

- Assess pain level, administer analgesics, and evaluate response.
- Encourage turning, coughing, deep breathing, and use of incentive spirometer.
- Maintain active and passive ROM for unaffected limbs and isometric exercises.
- Elevate affected extremity.
- Provide specific care for joint involved.

Key complications of joint surgery

- Infection
- Hemorrhage
- Embolus

● **Postoperative nursing interventions**
- Assess cardiac and respiratory status
- Assess pain level, administer analgesics as prescribed, and evaluate response
- Administer I.V. fluids and transfusion therapy as prescribed
- Allay the patient's anxiety and provide emotional support
- Provide wound care as directed
- Encourage turning, coughing, deep breathing, and use of incentive spirometry
- Maintain activity: active and passive ROM for unaffected limbs and isometric exercises as tolerated
- Monitor vital signs, intake and output (I/O), laboratory studies, neurovascular checks, and pulse oximetry
- Monitor and maintain the position and patency of wound drainage tubes
- Encourage the patient to express his feelings about limited mobility
- Assess movement limitations
- Elevate the affected extremity
- Administer medications as prescribed
- Assess for return of peristalsis; advance diet as tolerated
- Provide routine cast care (arthrodesis)
- Provide specific care for total knee replacement
    – Maintain continuous passive motion device
    – Apply a knee immobilizer before getting the patient out of bed
    – Administer anticoagulants as prescribed
- Provide specific care for total hip replacement
    – Maintain hips in abduction
    – Limit hip flexion to 90 degrees when sitting
    – Turn to the affected or unaffected side as ordered
    – Avoid sitting in low or soft chairs
    – Don't allow the patient to cross his legs; possible dislodgment of the prosthesis or dislocation may occur
    – Have the patient use an elevated toilet seat
    – Administer anticoagulants, as prescribed
- Individualize home care instructions
    – Know about your surgery and recovery time
    – Comply with activity restrictions
    – Perform wound care
    – Observe for signs and symptoms of complications
    – Continue cast care as directed
    – Comply with medical follow-up

● **Surgical complications**
- Infection
- Hemorrhage
- Joint injury
- Embolus

EXTERNAL FIXATION

● **Description**
  • Fracture immobilization in which transfixing pins are inserted through the bone above and below the fracture and then attached to a rigid external metal frame

● **Preoperative nursing interventions**
  • Complete patient and family preoperative teaching
    – Explain the procedure to the patient
    – Describe the operating room, PACU, and preoperative and postoperative routines
    – Demonstrate postoperative turning, coughing, deep breathing, incentive spirometry, splinting, and ROM exercises
    – Explain the postoperative need for drainage tubes, surgical dressings, oxygen therapy, I.V. therapy, pain control, and physical therapy
  • Complete a preoperative checklist and make sure that a signed informed consent is in the patient's chart
  • Administer medications as prescribed
  • Provide emotional support to allay the patient's and family's anxiety about surgery
  • Document the patient's history and physical assessment data
  • Monitor for fracture complications
  • Maintain the position of the affected extremity with sandbags and pillows, traction, or a splint

● **Postoperative nursing interventions**
  • Monitor vital signs, I/O, laboratory studies, and neurovascular checks
  • Assess pain level, administer analgesics as prescribed, and evaluate response
  • Assess for return of peristalsis; advance diet as tolerated
  • Administer I.V. fluids
  • Allay the patient's anxiety and provide emotional support
  • Encourage turning, coughing, deep breathing, and use of incentive spirometry
  • Keep the patient in semi-Fowler's position
  • Maintain activity: active and passive ROM for unaffected limbs, isometric exercises (strengthening and increasing muscle tone by contracting muscles against resistance either from other muscles or a stationary object), and quadriceps setting as tolerated
  • Encourage the patient to express his feelings about limited mobility
  • Provide wound care as directed
  • Maintain balanced suspension traction
  • Individualize home care instructions
    – Know about your surgery and recovery time
    – Follow instructions for medication use and be aware of possible adverse effects

Key complications of external fixation

- Infection
- Hemorrhage
- Chronic pain

Key facts about amputation

- Surgical removal of all or part of a limb
- Two types: closed and open

Key nursing interventions before amputation

- Complete patient and family preoperative teaching.
- Prepare the patient for the possibility of phantom limb sensation or phantom pain.
- Provide emotional support to allay the patient's and family's anxiety about surgery.

– Attend physical therapy sessions
– Maintain fixator as set
– Complete pin care daily as directed
– Comply with activity restrictions
– Comply with medical follow-up

● **Surgical complications**
- Infection of wound and pin sites
- Osteomyelitis
- Hemorrhage
- Chronic pain

AMPUTATION

● **Description**
- Surgical removal of all or part of a limb
- Two types of amputation
  – Closed (flap)
  – Open (guillotine)

● **Preoperative nursing interventions**
- Complete patient and family preoperative teaching
  – Explain the procedure to the patient
  – Describe the operating room, PACU, and preoperative and postoperative routines
  – Demonstrate postoperative turning, coughing, deep breathing, incentive spirometry, splinting, and ROM exercises
  – Explain the postoperative need for drainage tubes, surgical dressings, oxygen therapy, I.V. therapy, pain control, and physical therapy
- Complete a preoperative checklist and make sure that a signed informed consent is in the patient's chart
- Administer medications as prescribed
- Provide emotional support to allay the patient's and family's anxiety about surgery
- Document the patient's history and physical assessment data
- Prepare the patient for the possibility of phantom limb sensation or phantom pain

● **Postoperative nursing interventions**
- Assess cardiac and respiratory status
- Assess pain level, administer analgesics as prescribed, and evaluate response
- Administer I.V. fluids and transfusion therapy as prescribed
- Provide emotional support to allay the patient's and family's anxiety
- Provide wound care as directed
- Encourage turning, coughing, deep breathing, and use of incentive spirometry
- Assess for return of peristalsis; advance diet as tolerated

- Maintain activity: active and passive ROM for unaffected limbs and isometric exercises as tolerated
- Monitor vital signs, I/O, laboratory studies, neurovascular checks, and pulse oximetry
- Monitor and maintain the position and patency of wound drainage tubes
- **Encourage the patient to express his feelings about changes in his body image and phantom limb sensation and pain**
- Administer medications as prescribed
- Elevate the affected extremity as directed
- Inspect the stump for bleeding, infection, and edema
- Maintain a rigid dressing for the stump prosthesis
- Reinforce physical therapy participation
- Provide trapeze as appropriate
- Encourage participation in ADLs
- Individualize home care instructions
    - Know the facts about your surgery and recovery time
    - Follow instructions for medication use and be aware of possible adverse effects
    - Recognize the signs and symptoms of complications
    - Complete stump care daily
    - Follow instructions for use of a prosthesis
    - Maintain a physical therapy regimen
    - Make use of contact information for local support groups and services
    - Comply with medical follow-up
- **Surgical complications**
    - Hemorrhage
    - Infection
    - Contractures
    - Skin breakdown
    - Depression

CARPAL TUNNEL RELEASE

- **Description**
    - Surgical ligation of the transverse carpal ligament to relieve compression of the median nerve in the carpal canal of the wrist
    - May be performed endoscopically or open
- **Preoperative nursing interventions**
    - Complete patient and family preoperative teaching
        - Explain the procedure to the patient
        - Describe the operating room, PACU, and preoperative and postoperative routines
        - Demonstrate postoperative turning, coughing, deep breathing, incentive spirometry, splinting, and ROM exercises
        - Explain the postoperative need for drainage tubes, surgical dressings, oxygen therapy, I.V. therapy, and pain control

Key nursing interventions after amputation

- Assess cardiac and respiratory status.
- Assess pain level and administer postoperative analgesics as prescribed.
- Provide wound care as directed.
- Monitor vital signs, I/O, laboratory studies, neurovascular checks, and pulse oximetry.
- Elevate the affected extremity as directed.
- Inspect the stump for bleeding, infection, and edema.
- Maintain a rigid dressing for the stump prosthesis.
- Provide trapeze.
- Encourage the patient to express his feelings about changes in his body image and phantom limb sensation and pain.

Key complications of amputation

- Infection
- Skin breakdown
- Depression

Key facts about carpal tunnel release

- Surgical ligation of the transverse carpal ligament
- Performed to relieve compression of the median nerve in the carpal canal of the wrist

Key nursing interventions before carpal tunnel release

- Demonstrate postoperative turning, coughing, deep breathing, incentive spirometry, splinting, and ROM exercises.
- Administer preoperative medications as prescribed.

Key nursing interventions after carpal tunnel release

- Assess pain level and administer postoperative analgesics as prescribed.
- Provide wound care as directed.
- Elevate the hand and apply ice.

Key complications of carpal tunnel release

- Infection
- Paralysis

Key facts about ORIF of the hip

- Surgical reduction and stabilization of a fracture using orthopedic devices or hardware
- Types of orthopedic devices and hardware include Austin Moore prosthesis, Smith-Petersen nail, Jewett nail, intramedullary nails, and compression screws

- Complete a preoperative checklist and make sure a signed informed consent is in the patient's chart
- Administer medications as prescribed
- Provide emotional support to allay the patient's and family's anxiety about surgery
- Document the patient's history and physical assessment data

● **Postoperative nursing interventions**
- Assess pain level, administer analgesics as prescribed, and evaluate response
- Assess for return of peristalsis; advance diet as tolerated
- Administer I.V. fluids
- Provide emotional support to allay the patient's anxiety
- Provide wound care as directed
- Maintain activity; encourage ambulation and activity to affected extremity per neurosurgeon's orders
- Monitor vital signs and neurovascular checks
- Elevate the affected hand and apply ice
- Administer medications, as prescribed
- Assist with ADLs as needed
- Apply splint as directed
- Encourage movement of the fingers to decrease swelling
- Individualize home care instructions
    - Know about your surgery and recovery plan
    - Follow instructions for medication use and be aware of possible adverse effects
    - Continue active ROM exercises of the affected hand and follow activity restrictions
    - Use a splint as directed
    - Monitor the affected hand for return of sensation and motor function
    - Perform wound care as directed
    - Comply with medical follow-up

● **Surgical complications**
- Infection
- Paralysis

OPEN REDUCTION INTERNAL FIXATION (ORIF) OF THE HIP

● **Description**
- Surgical reduction and stabilization of a fracture, using orthopedic devices or hardware, such as Austin Moore prosthesis, Smith-Petersen nail, Jewett nail, intramedullary nails, and compression screws

● **Preoperative nursing interventions**
- Complete patient and family preoperative teaching
    - Explain the procedure to the patient

– Describe the operating room, PACU, and preoperative and postoperative routines

– Demonstrate postoperative turning, coughing, deep breathing, incentive spirometry, splinting, and ROM exercises

– Explain the postoperative need for drainage tubes, surgical dressings, oxygen therapy, I.V. therapy, and pain control

- Complete a preoperative checklist and make sure a signed informed consent is in the patient's chart
- Administer medications as prescribed
- Provide emotional support to allay the patient's and family's anxiety about surgery
- Document the patient's history and physical assessment data
- Monitor the patient for fracture complications
- Keep the affected extremity in position with sandbags and pillows or traction

● Postoperative nursing interventions

- Assess cardiac and respiratory status
- Assess pain level, administer analgesics as prescribed, and evaluate response
- Assess for return of peristalsis; advance diet as tolerated
- Administer I.V. fluids and transfusion therapy as prescribed
- Provide emotional support to allay the patient's and family's anxiety
- Provide wound care as directed
- Encourage turning, coughing, deep breathing, and use of incentive spirometry
- Keep the patient in semi-Fowler's position: no higher than 30 degrees
- Maintain activity: active and passive ROM for unaffected limbs, isometric exercises, and progressive ambulation per physical therapist's directions
- Monitor vital signs, laboratory studies, neurovascular checks, and pulse oximetry
- Monitor and maintain the position and patency of drainage tubes
- Use abductor pillow and trochanter rolls
- Apply sequential compression or pneumatic stockings
- Administer anticoagulants as prescribed
- Administer antibiotics as prescribed
- Administer stool softeners as prescribed
- Individualize home care instructions

– Know about your surgery and recovery plan

– Follow instructions for medication use and be aware of possible adverse effects

– Comply with activity restrictions and follow physical therapy plan

– Perform wound care

– Observe for signs and symptoms of complications

– Apply sequential compression stockings

– Use an elevated toilet seat

– Comply with medical follow-up

Key nursing interventions before ORIF of the hip

- Monitor the patient for fracture complications.
- Keep the affected extremity in position with sandbags and pillows.

Key nursing interventions after ORIF of the hip

- Assess cardiac and respiratory status.
- Assess pain level and administer analgesics as prescribed.
- Provide wound care as directed.
- Keep the patient in semi-Fowler's position: no higher than 30 degrees.
- Monitor vital signs, laboratory studies, neurovascular checks, and pulse oximetry.
- Use abductor pillow and trochanter rolls.
- Apply sequential compression or pneumatic stockings.
- Administer anticoagulants as prescribed.
- Administer stool softeners as prescribed.

Key complications of ORIF of the hip

- Hemorrhage
- Thrombophlebitis
- Pulmonary embolism

Key facts about laminectomy

- Surgical excision of vertebral posterior arch

Key nursing interventions before laminectomy

- Complete patient and family preoperative teaching.
- Administer medications as ordered
- Teach the patient the logrolling technique.

Key nursing interventions after laminectomy

- Assess neurologic and neurovascular status.
- Inspect surgical dressings for drainage of CSF and blood.
- Keep the patient in a flat position.
- Turn the patient by logrolling.
- Prevent flexion of the neck after cervical laminectomy.
- Administer muscle relaxants, corticosteroids, and stool softeners, as prescribed.

● **Surgical complications**
- Osteomyelitis
- Hemorrhage
- Thrombophlebitis
- Pneumonia
- Avascular necrosis
- Pulmonary embolism

LAMINECTOMY

● **Description**
- Surgical excision of vertebral posterior arch

● **Preoperative nursing interventions**
- Complete patient and family preoperative teaching
  - Explain the procedure to the patient
  - Describe the operating room, PACU, and preoperative and postoperative routines
  - Demonstrate postoperative turning, coughing, deep breathing, incentive spirometry, splinting, and ROM exercises
  - Explain the postoperative need for drainage tubes, surgical dressings, oxygen therapy, I.V. therapy, and pain control
- Complete a preoperative checklist and make sure a signed informed consent is in the patient's chart
- Administer medications as ordered
- Provide emotional support to allay the patient's and family's anxiety about surgery
- Document the patient's history and physical assessment data
- Teach the patient the logrolling technique

● **Postoperative nursing interventions**
- Assess neurologic and neurovascular status
- Assess pain level, administer analgesics as prescribed, and evaluate response
- Assess for return of peristalsis; give solid foods and liquids as tolerated
- Administer I.V. fluids
- Provide emotional support to allay the patient's and family's anxiety
- Inspect surgical dressings for drainage of cerebrospinal fluid (CSF) and blood; provide wound care as directed
- Encourage turning, coughing, deep breathing, and use of incentive spirometry
- Keep the patient in a flat position as directed and turn the patient by logrolling
- Maintain activity: active and passive ROM and isometric exercises
- Monitor vital signs, I/O, laboratory studies, and neurovascular checks
- Prevent flexion of the neck after cervical laminectomy
- Administer muscle relaxants as prescribed
- Administer corticosteroids as prescribed

- Administer stool softeners as prescribed
- Individualize home care instructions
  - Know about your surgery and recovery plan
  - Follow instructions for medication use and be aware of possible adverse effects
  - Comply with activity restrictions and maintain physical therapy plan
  - Use a supportive brace
  - Sleep on a firm mattress
  - Monitor lower extremities for numbness and decreased circulation
  - Monitor ability to void
  - Perform wound care as directed
  - Comply with medical follow-up
- **Surgical complications**
  - Urine retention
  - Motor and sensory deficits
  - Infection
  - Muscle spasms
  - Paralytic ileus

SPINAL FUSION

- **Description**
  - Stabilization of spinous processes with bone chips from iliac crest or Harrington rod metallic implant
- **Preoperative nursing interventions**
  - Complete patient and family preoperative teaching
    - Explain the procedure to the patient
    - Describe the operating room, PACU, and preoperative and postoperative routines
    - Demonstrate postoperative turning, coughing, deep breathing, incentive spirometry, splinting, and ROM exercises
    - Explain the postoperative need for drainage tubes, surgical dressings, oxygen therapy, I.V. therapy, and pain control
  - Complete a preoperative checklist and make sure a signed informed consent is in the patient's chart
  - Administer medications as prescribed
  - Provide emotional support to allay the patient's and family's anxiety about surgery
  - Document the patient's history and physical assessment data
  - Teach the patient the logrolling technique
- **Postoperative nursing interventions**
  - Assess cardiac, respiratory, and neurologic status
  - Check neurovascular status: color, temperature, pulses, movement, and sensation in extremities
  - Assess pain level, administer analgesics as prescribed, and evaluate response

Key nursing interventions after spinal fusion

- Assess cardiac, respiratory, and neurologic status.
- Provide wound care as directed.
- Check neurovascular status: color, temperature, pulses, movement, and sensation in extremities.
- Administer antibiotics, corticosteroids, and stool softeners, as prescribed.
- Reposition the patient every 2 hours using the logrolling technique.

Key complications of spinal fusion

- Infection
- Muscle spasms
- Motor and sensory deficits

Key facts about RA

- Systemic inflammatory disease that affects the synovial lining of the joints
- Inflammation is followed by formation of pannus and destruction of cartilage, bone, and ligaments
- Pannus is replaced by fibrotic tissue and calcification

Common causes of RA

- Unknown
- Autoimmune disease

- Assess for return of peristalsis; advance diet as tolerated
- Administer I.V. fluids
- Provide emotional support to allay the patient's and family's anxiety
- Provide wound care as directed
- Encourage turning, coughing, deep breathing, and use of incentive spirometry
- Maintain the patient in the supine position
- Maintain activity: active and passive ROM and isometric exercises
- Monitor vital signs, I/O, and laboratory studies
- Administer antibiotics as prescribed
- Administer corticosteroids as prescribed
- **Reposition the patient every 2 hours using the logrolling technique**
- Administer muscle relaxants as prescribed
- Administer stool softeners as prescribed
- Individualize home care instructions
    - Know about your surgery and recovery plan
    - Follow instructions for medication use and be aware of possible adverse effects
    - Comply with activity restrictions and follow physical therapy plan
    - Note spinal flexion limitations
    - Complete exercises for the lower back daily
    - Sleep on a firm mattress
    - Monitor lower extremities for numbness and decreased circulation
    - Monitor ability to void
    - Perform wound care as directed
    - Comply with medical follow-up

● Surgical complications

- Urine retention
- Infection
- Muscle spasms
- Motor and sensory deficits
- Paralytic ileus

RHEUMATOID ARTHRITIS (RA)

● Definition

- Systemic inflammatory disease that affects the synovial lining of the joints

● Causes

- Unknown
- Autoimmune disease
- Genetic transmission (increases susceptibility to the disease)

● Pathophysiology

- Inflammation of the synovial membranes is followed by formation of pannus, an inflammatory exudate, and destruction of cartilage, bone, and ligaments

- Pannus is replaced by fibrotic tissue and calcification, which causes subluxation of the joint

Assessment findings

- Fatigue
- Anorexia
- Malaise
- Elevated body temperature
- Painful, swollen joints
- Limited ROM due to deformity
- Subcutaneous nodules
- Symmetrical joint swelling (mirror image of affected joints)
- Morning stiffness
- Paresthesia of the hands and the feet
- Crepitus
- Pericarditis
- Splenomegaly
- Leukopenia
- Enlarged lymph nodes

Diagnostic test findings

- X-rays: joint space narrowing, bone erosions
- Rheumatoid factor: positive
- Hematology: increased ESR, WBCs, platelets
- Gamma globulin: increased immunoglobulin (Ig) M, IgG
- Synovial fluid analysis: increased WBCs, decreased viscosity, opaque
- Latex fixation test: positive rheumatoid factor
- Tumor necrosis factor: elevated
- ANA test: positive

Medical management

- Activity: as tolerated; physical therapy, occupational therapy
- Monitoring: vital signs and I/O
- Disease-modifying antirheumatic drugs: leflunomide (Arava), methotrexate (Rheumatrex), infliximab (Remicade), etanercept (Enbrel), hydroxychloroquine (Plaquenil)
- Gold therapy: gold sodium thiomalate (Aurolate)
- Analgesic: acetaminophen (Tylenol)
- Nonsteroidal anti-inflammatory drugs (NSAIDs): indomethacin (Indocin), ibuprofen (Motrin), sulindac (Clinoril), piroxicam (Feldene), flurbiprofen (Ansaid), diclofenac (Voltaren), naproxen (Naprosyn), diflunisal (Dolobid)
- Glucocorticoids: prednisone (Deltasone), hydrocortisone (Cortef)
- Immunomodulators: anakinra (Kineret), abatacept (Orencia)
- Heat therapy, cold therapy
- Plasmapheresis
- Antimetabolite: methotrexate (Rheumatrex)

TOP 4

Signs and symptoms of RA

1. Painful, swollen joints
2. Symmetrical joint swelling
3. Morning stiffness
4. Crepitus

Diagnosing RA

- Rheumatoid factor: positive
- Latex fixation test: positive rheumatoid factor
- ANA test: positive

Treating RA

- Disease-modifying antirheumatic drugs
- NSAIDs
- Glucocorticoids
- Heat therapy, cold therapy
- Joint replacement

Key teaching topics for a patient with a musculoskeletal disorder

- Disorder and its implications
- Medication therapy
- Rest and activity patterns
- Proper body mechanics
- Exercises for extremities

Key nursing interventions for a patient with RA

- Assess neuromuscular status.
- Administer medications as prescribed.
- Check joints for swelling, pain, and redness.
- Keep joints extended and provide passive ROM to affected joints

Key complications of RA

- Depression
- Peripheral neuropathy
- Keratoconjunctivitis

TIME-OUT FOR TEACHING
Patients with musculoskeletal disorders

Be sure to include the following topics in your teaching plan when caring for patients with musculoskeletal disorders.

- Disorder and its implications
- Medication therapy, including the action, adverse effects, and scheduling
- Use of assistive and adaptive devices, such as crutches, a walker, or a cane
- Signs and symptoms of soft tissue and bone infection
- Rest and activity patterns, including activity limitations or restrictions
- Signs and symptoms of motor, sensory, and circulatory deficits
- Safe environment

- Optimal body weight maintenance
- Change in activities of daily living to compensate for limited range-of-motion
- Proper body mechanics and correct posture
- Exercises for extremities
- Dietary recommendations and restrictions
- Community agencies and resources for supportive services
- Signs and symptoms of skin breakdown and contractures
- Follow-up appointments

● Nursing interventions

- Assess neuromuscular status
- Assess pain level, administer analgesics as prescribed, and evaluate response
- Keep joints extended; provide passive ROM exercises to affected joints
- Administer medications as prescribed
- Encourage the patient to express his feelings about changes in mobility and function
- Assist with ADLs
- Check joints for swelling, pain, and redness; provide heat therapy or cold therapy, as ordered
- Individualize home care instructions (for teaching tips, see *Patients with musculoskeletal disorders*)
  - Know about the disorder and its treatment
  - Follow instructions for medication use and be aware of possible adverse effects
  - Follow physical therapy recommendations
  - Avoid cold, stress, and infection
  - Complete skin and foot care daily
  - Contact the Arthritis Foundation and community services, as appropriate
  - Comply with medical follow-up

● Complications

- Depression
- Peripheral neuropathy
- Osteoporosis
- Keratoconjunctivitis

● **Surgical interventions**
  - Joint replacement
  - Synovectomy

OSTEOARTHRITIS (DEGENERATIVE JOINT DISEASE)

● **Definition**
  - Degeneration of articular cartilage, usually affecting the weight-bearing joints (spine, knees, hips)

● **Causes**
  - Aging
  - Obesity
  - Joint trauma
  - Congenital abnormalities

● **Pathophysiology**
  - Cartilage softens with age, narrowing the joint space
  - Normal use thins and erodes cartilage
  - Cartilage flakes enter the synovial lining, which fibroses, thus limiting joint movement (see *Understanding osteoarthritis*, page 402)

● **Assessment findings**
  - Pain relieved by resting joints
  - Joint stiffness
  - Heberden's nodes and Bouchard's nodes (see *Digital joint deformities*, page 403)
  - Limited ROM
  - Crepitation (a grating sensation associated with degenerative joint disease that can be heard or felt; it's best detected by palpation of the affected joint)
  - Increased pain in damp, cold weather
  - Enlarged, edematous joints
  - Smooth, taut, shiny skin

● **Diagnostic test findings**
  - X-rays: joint deformity, narrowing of joint space, bone spurs
  - Arthroscopy: bone spurs, narrowing of joint space
  - Hematology: increased ESR

● **Medical management**
  - Heat therapy
  - Cold therapy
  - Analgesic: aspirin
  - NSAIDs: indomethacin (Indocin), ibuprofen (Motrin), sulindac (Clinoril), piroxicam (Feldene), flurbiprofen (Ansaid), diclofenac (Voltaren), naproxen (Naprosyn), diflunisal (Dolobid)
  - Activity: as tolerated, based on joints affected
  - Isometric exercises, strengthening exercises, aerobic exercises

Key facts about osteoarthritis
- Degeneration of articular cartilage
- Cartilage flakes enter the synovial lining, which fibroses and limits joint movement
- Usually affects the weight-bearing joints (spine, knees, hips)

Common causes of osteoarthritis
- Aging
- Obesity
- Joint trauma

TOP 3

Signs and symptoms of osteoarthritis
1. Enlarged, edematous joints
2. Joint stiffness
3. Heberden's nodes and Bouchard's nodes

Diagnosing osteoarthritis
- X-rays: joint deformities or bone spurs
- Hematology: increased ESR

Treating osteoarthritis
- Heat therapy
- Cold therapy
- NSAIDs
- Exercises

Characteristics of osteoarthritis

- Cartilage may break down before symptoms surface
- Early symptoms: mild, dull ache or stiffness in affected joint
- Later symptoms: pain that worsens throughout day with limited movement, and persistent stiffness

Understanding osteoarthritis

The characteristic breakdown of articular cartilage is a gradual response to aging or predisposing factors, such as joint abnormalities or traumatic injury. The illustrations below will help you understand how osteoarthritis progresses.

NORMAL ANATOMY

Normally, bones fit together. Cartilage—a smooth, fibrous tissue—cushions the end of each bone, and synovial fluid fills the joint space. This fluid lubricates the joint and eases movement, much like brake fluid functions in a car.

EARLY STAGE

Cartilage may begin to break down long before symptoms surface. In early osteoarthritis, the patient typically has no symptoms or has a mild, dull ache when he uses the joint. Rest relieves the discomfort. Or he may feel stiffness in the affected joint, especially in the morning. The stiffness usually lasts 15 minutes or less.

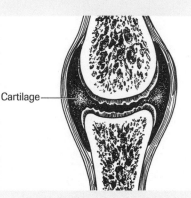

Cartilage

LATER STAGE

As the disease progresses, whole sections of cartilage may disintegrate, osteophytes (bony spurs) form, and fragments of cartilage and bone float freely in the joint. More common now, pain may be present even during rest. It typically worsens throughout the day. Movement becomes increasingly limited, and stiffness may persist even after limbering exercises.

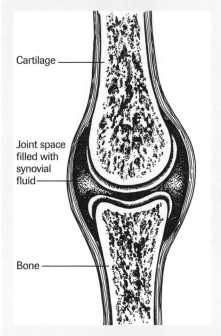

Cartilage

Joint space filled with synovial fluid

Bone

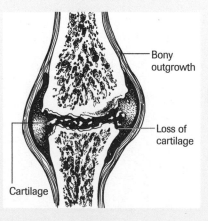

Bony outgrowth

Loss of cartilage

Cartilage

Digital joint deformities

Osteoarthritis of the interphalangeal joints produces irreversible changes in the distal joints (Heberden's nodes) and proximal joints (Bouchard's nodes). Initially painless, these nodes gradually progress to or suddenly flare up as redness, swelling, tenderness, and impaired sensation and dexterity.

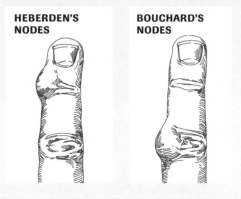

HEBERDEN'S NODES

BOUCHARD'S NODES

- Weight reduction
- Canes, walkers, as appropriate

● **Nursing interventions**
- Assess musculoskeletal status; determine degree of joint mobility
- Assess pain level, administer analgesics as prescribed, and evaluate response
- Administer medications as prescribed
- Urge the patient to express his feelings about changes in his mobility
- Provide rest periods as needed
- Maintain calorie count
- Provide moist compresses and paraffin baths (heat therapy) as prescribed
- Teach proper body mechanics
- Provide passive ROM exercises
- Individualize home care instructions
  - Know about the disorder and its treatment
  - Follow instructions for medication use and be aware of possible adverse effects
  - Contact the Arthritis Foundation and community resources, as appropriate
  - Comply with activity restrictions; follow exercise recommendations
  - Observe dietary recommendations if weight loss is indicated
  - Comply with medical follow-up

● **Complications**
- Contractures
- GI bleeding
- Injury

● **Surgical interventions**
- Synovectomy
- Arthrodesis
- Joint replacement

Key facts about gout

- Inflammatory joint disease
- Caused by the deposit of uric acid crystals

Common causes of gout

- Genetics
- Decreased uric acid excretion
- Chronic renal failure

Key signs and symptoms of gout

- Joint pain
- Redness and swelling in joints
- Tophi in great toe, ankle, and outer ear

Diagnosing gout

- Hematology: increased ESR
- Blood chemistry: increased uric acid
- Synovial fluid analysis: sodium urate crystals

Treating gout

- Low-purine, alkaline-ash diet
- Uricosuric agents
- Antigout agents
- Xanthine-oxidase inhibitor

GOUT

- **Definition**
  - Inflammatory joint disease caused by the deposit of uric acid crystals
- **Causes**
  - Genetics
  - Decreased uric acid excretion
  - Chronic renal failure
  - Myxedema
  - Polycythemia vera
  - Hyperparathyroidism
- **Pathophysiology**
  - End product of purine metabolism is uric acid
  - Abnormal purine metabolism results in decreased secretion of urates and increased blood levels of uric acid
  - Uric acid forms a precipitate in areas where blood flow is slowest
  - Genetic defect in purine metabolism can cause overproduction of uric acid
- **Assessment findings**
  - Joint pain
  - Redness and swelling in joints
  - Tophi in great toe, ankle, and outer ear (see *Gouty deposits*)
  - Malaise
  - Tachycardia
  - Elevated skin temperature
- **Diagnostic test findings**
  - Hematology: increased ESR
  - Blood chemistry: increased uric acid
  - Synovial fluid analysis: sodium urate crystals
- **Medical management**
  - Uricosuric agents: probenecid (Benemid), sulfinpyrazone (Anturane)
  - Xanthine-oxidase inhibitor: allopurinol (Zyloprim)
  - Antigout: colchicine
  - Analgesic: aspirin
  - NSAIDs: indomethacin (Indocin), ibuprofen (Motrin), sulindac (Clinoril), piroxicam (Feldene), flurbiprofen (Ansaid), diclofenac (Voltaren), naproxen (Naprosyn), diflunisal (Dolobid)
  - Diet: low-purine, alkaline-ash; increase fluid intake to 3 qt (3 L)/day; limit alcohol consumption
  - Activity: as tolerated
  - Exercise program, including passive and active ROM exercises and ambulation as tolerated
  - Laboratory studies: uric acid, ESR

Gouty deposits

The final stage of gout is marked by painful polyarthritis, with large, subcutaneous, tophaceous deposits in cartilage, synovial membranes, tendons, and soft tissue. The skin over the tophus is shiny, thin, and taut.

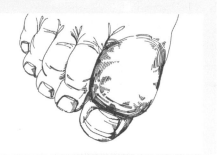

● **Nursing interventions**
- Assess pain level, administer analgesics as prescribed, and evaluate response
- Encourage fluids to 3 qt (3 L)/day
- Assess integumentary status
- Administer medications as prescribed
- Demonstrate proper joint exercises
- Provide a bed cradle
- Allay the patient's anxiety and provide emotional support
- Individualize home care instructions
  - Know about the disorder and its treatment
  - Follow instructions for medication use and be aware of possible adverse effects
  - Contact the Arthritis Foundation and community resources, as appropriate
  - Recognize signs and symptoms of gout flare-up
  - Limit alcohol intake
  - Avoid fasting
  - Identify ways to reduce stress
  - Comply with medical follow-up

● **Complications**
- Renal calculi
- Cartilage damage
- GI bleeding

● **Surgical interventions**
- None

OSTEOMYELITIS

● **Definition**
- Bacterial infection of bone and soft tissue

Common causes of osteomyelitis

- *S. aureus*
- Hemolytic streptococcus

Key signs and symptoms of osteomyelitis

- Bone pain
- Localized edema, redness, and warmth
- Increased pain with movement

Diagnosing osteomyelitis

- Blood cultures: positive identification of organism
- Hematology: increased WBCs, ESR
- Wound culture: positive identification of organism
- C-reactive protein: elevated

Treating osteomyelitis

- Antibiotics
- Cast or splint for the affected body part
- Wound care

● **Causes**
- *Staphylococcus aureus*
- Hemolytic streptococcus

● **Risk factors**
- Open wound
- Infection

● **Pathophysiology**
- Organism reaches bone through an open wound or via the bloodstream
- Infection causes bone destruction
- Bone fragments necrose (sequestra)
- New bone cells form over the sequestrum during healing, resulting in nonunion

● **Assessment findings**
- Malaise
- Elevated body temperature
- Bone pain
- Tachycardia
- Localized edema, redness, and warmth
- Muscle spasms
- Increased pain with movement
- Nausea

● **Diagnostic test findings**
- Ultrasound: soft-tissue abscess or fluid collection
- Blood cultures: positive identification of organism
- C-reactive protein: elevated (first 7 days)
- Hematology: increased WBCs, ESR
- Wound culture: positive identification of organism
- Bone biopsy: positive
- Bone scan: positive

● **Medical management**
- Antibiotic: specific for bacteria causing infection; nafcillin (Unipen), cefazolin (Ancef), clindamycin (Cleocin)
- Analgesic: oxycodone (Tylox)
- Monitoring: vital signs, I/O, and neurovascular checks
- Diet: high-calorie, high-vitamin C and D, high-protein, and high-calcium
- I.V. therapy: fluids as needed
- Activity: bed rest
- Laboratory studies: WBCs, ESR
- Wound care
- Heat therapy
- Cast or splint for the affected body part
- Antipyretic: aspirin, acetaminophen (Tylenol)

● **Nursing interventions**
- Assess integumentary status and neurovascular status of affected extremity

- Monitor and record vital signs, I/O, and laboratory studies
- Assess pain level, administer analgesics as prescribed, and evaluate response
- Administer medications as prescribed
- Encourage fluids to 3 qt (3 L)/day
- Administer I.V. fluids as ordered
- Provide wound care as directed
- Encourage the patient to express his feelings about his illness
- Reposition the patient every 2 hours; immobilize the affected body part
- Individualize home care instructions
    - Know about the disorder and its treatment
    - Follow instructions for medication use and be aware of possible adverse effects
    - Perform wound care
    - Observe for signs and symptoms of complications
    - Adhere to activity restrictions
    - Avoid exposure to people with infections
    - Comply with medical follow-up

● **Complications**
- Bone necrosis
- Amputation
- Chronic osteomyelitis
- Pathologic fractures
- Sepsis

● **Surgical interventions**
- Incision and drainage of bone abscess
- Sequestrectomy
- Bone graft
- Bone segment transfer

OSTEOPOROSIS

● **Definition**
- A metabolic bone dysfunction that results in reduced bone mass and increased porosity
- Metabolic illnesses or medications that cause osteoporosis increase the risk of skeletal fracture

● **Causes**
- Liver disease
- Calcium deficiency
- Vitamin D deficiency
- Protein deficiency
- Bone marrow disorders
- Cushing's syndrome
- Hyperthyroidism

Key nursing interventions for a patient with osteomyelitis

- Monitor and record vital signs, I/O, and laboratory studies.
- Provide wound care.
- Assess pain level, administer analgesics, and evaluate response.

Key complications of osteomyelitis

- Bone necrosis
- Amputation
- Sepsis

Key facts about osteoporosis

- A metabolic bone dysfunction that results in reduced bone mass and increased porosity
- Illnesses or medications that cause osteoporosis increase the risk of skeletal fracture

Common causes of osteoporosis

- Calcium deficiency
- Bone marrow disorders

Key risk factors for osteoporosis

- Age
- Postmenopause
- Immobility
- Corticosteroid use

Key signs and symptoms of osteoporosis

- Dowager's hump (kyphosis)
- Back pain: thoracic and lumbar
- Loss of height
- Joint pain
- Pathologic fracture

Diagnosing osteoporosis

- X-ray: thin, porous bone
- DEXA scan: decreased bone mineral density

Treating osteoporosis

- Calcium supplement
- Exercise program with weight bearing
- Bisphosphonates

Key nursing interventions for a patient with osteoporosis

- Assess musculoskeletal status.
- Assist with planning an exercise program with weight bearing.
- Prevent falls.

● **Risk factors**
- Family history
- Age
- Female gender
- Postmenopause
- Smoking
- Immobility
- Corticosteroid use

● **Pathophysiology**
- Rate of bone resorption exceeds the rate of bone formation
- Increased phosphate stimulates parathyroid activity, which increases bone resorption
- Estrogens decrease bone resorption

● **Assessment findings**
- Dowager's hump (kyphosis)
- Back pain: thoracic and lumbar
- Loss of height
- Unsteady gait
- Joint pain
- Weakness
- Pathologic fracture

● **Diagnostic test findings**
- X-ray: thin, porous bone; increased vertebral curvature; possible fracture
- Dual energy X-ray absorptiometry (DEXA) scan: decreased bone mineral density

● **Medical management**
- Diet: high in calcium, protein, vitamins, minerals, and boron
- Dietary restrictions: limit caffeine and alcohol
- Activity: exercise program with weight bearing
- Laboratory studies: calcium, phosphorus
- Hormone replacement: estradiol (Estrace), conjugated estrogen (Premarin)
- Bisphosphonates: alendronate sodium (Fosamax), ibandronate (Boniva)
- Calcium supplement: calcium carbonate (Os-Cal)
- Calcitonin (Miacalcin)
- Parathyroid hormone: teriparatide (Forteo)
- Analgesic: acetaminophen (Tylenol)

● **Nursing interventions**
- Assess musculoskeletal status
- Administer medications as prescribed
- Encourage the patient to express feelings about diagnosis
- Prevent falls
- Assist the patient in planning an exercise program with weight bearing
- Individualize home care instructions
  - Know about the disorder and its treatment
  - Follow instructions for medication use and be aware of possible adverse effects

– Follow an exercise program with weight bearing
– Follow safety measures to prevent fractures
– Contact the Osteoporosis Foundation

● **Complication**
  • Pathologic fractures

● **Surgical intervention**
  • Fracture repair

OSTEOGENIC SARCOMA (OSTEOSARCOMA)

● **Definition**
  • Malignant bone tumor that invades the ends of long bones

● **Causes**
  • Osteoblastic activity
  • Osteolytic activity

● **Pathophysiology**
  • Unregulated cell growth and uncontrolled cell division result in the development of a neoplasm
  • Tumor arises from osteoblasts and dissolves the bone and soft tissue
  • Tumor may spread to the lung

● **Assessment findings**
  • Pain
  • Limited movement
  • Pathologic fractures
  • Soft tissue mass over the tumor site
  • Warm tissue over the tumor site
  • Elevated body temperature

● **Diagnostic test findings**
  • Bone scan: mass
  • Biopsy: cytology positive for cancer cells
  • Computed tomography (CT) scan: mass
  • Blood chemistry: increased alkaline phosphatase
  • Bone marrow aspiration: cancer cells

● **Medical management**
  • Radiation therapy
  • Analgesics: oxycodone (Tylox), meperidine (Demerol)
  • Antineoplastics: cyclophosphamide (Cytoxan), vincristine (Oncovin)
  • Diet: high-protein
  • I.V. therapy: fluids as needed
  • Activity: as tolerated
  • Monitoring: vital signs and I/O
  • Laboratory studies: calcium, phosphorus
  • Antiemetics: ondansetron (Zofran)
  • Antidiarrheals: attapulgite (Kaopectate), loperamide (Imodium)

Key nursing interventions for a patient with osteogenic sarcoma

- Assess integumentary and musculoskeletal status.
- Assess pain level, administer analgesics, and evaluate response.
- Provide postchemotherapeutic nursing care.

Key complications of osteogenic sarcoma

- Metastasis
- Pathologic fractures

Key facts about carpal tunnel syndrome

- Chronic compression neuropathy of the median nerve at the wrist
- Median nerve supplies motor innervation to the wrist and fingers

Key causes of carpal tunnel syndrome

- Strenuous and repetitive use of the hands
- Fractures or dislocations of the wrist
- Tenosynovitis

● **Nursing interventions**
- Assess integumentary and musculoskeletal status
- Assess pain level, administer analgesics as prescribed, and evaluate response
- Monitor and record vital signs, I/O, and laboratory studies
- Administer medications as prescribed
- Maintain the patient's diet
- Encourage the patient to express his feelings about his diagnosis
- Provide postchemotherapeutic nursing care
    - Provide prophylactic skin, mouth, and perineal care
    - Monitor dietary intake
    - Administer antiemetics and antidiarrheals as prescribed
    - Monitor for bleeding, infection, and electrolyte imbalance
    - Provide rest periods as needed
- Individualize home care instructions
    - Know about the disorder and its treatment
    - Follow instructions for medication use and be aware of possible adverse effects
    - Observe for signs and symptoms of complications
    - Avoid exposure to people with infections
    - Monitor pain control interventions
    - Complete skin care daily
    - Contact the American Cancer Society and community resources, as appropriate
    - Comply with medical follow-up

● **Complications**
- Metastasis
- Pathologic fractures
- Depression

● **Surgical intervention**
- Amputation

CARPAL TUNNEL SYNDROME

● **Definition**
- Chronic compression neuropathy of the median nerve at the wrist

● **Causes**
- Strenuous and repetitive use of the hands
- Fractures or dislocations of the wrist
- Bruising of the wrist
- Menopause
- Genetics
- Pregnancy
- Tenosynovitis
- RA
- Acromegaly

- Hyperparathyroidism
- Obesity
- Gout
- Amyloidosis

● **Pathophysiology**
- Median nerve supplies sensory innervation to the palmar surface of the thumb and the first three fingers (see *The carpal tunnel*, page 412)
- Median nerve also supplies motor innervation to the wrist and finger flexion
- Compression of the median nerve in the space between the inelastic transverse carpal ligament and the bones of the wrist (carpal tunnel) leads to pain and numbness in the thumb, index, middle, and one-half of the ring finger

● **Assessment findings**
- Nocturnal pain and paresthesia in the thumb and first three fingers, relieved by shaking the hand (flick sign)
- Burning and tingling of the hand
- Impaired sensation in the hand
- Pain radiating to forearm, shoulder, neck, and chest
- Thenar atrophy (mound on palm of hand at the base of the thumb)
- Loss of fine motor movement of the hand
- Weakness
- Positive Tinel's sign; positive Phalen's test (see *Eliciting signs of carpal tunnel syndrome*, page 413)

● **Diagnostic test findings**
- Motor nerve velocity studies: segmental, distal, median, and motor conduction delay, and conduction block at wrist

● **Medical management**
- Position: avoid flexion of the wrist; use a splint for immobilization; elevate the hand
- Monitoring: neurovascular checks
- Analgesic: acetaminophen (Tylenol)
- Glucocorticoid: cortisone (Cortone)
- NSAIDs: indomethacin (Indocin), ibuprofen (Motrin), sulindac (Clinoril), piroxicam (Feldene), flurbiprofen (Ansaid), diclofenac (Voltaren), naproxen (Naprosyn), diflunisal (Dolobid)
- Vitamin: pyridoxine (Vitamin B_6)

● **Nursing interventions**
- Assess neurovascular status
- Elevate the patient's hand
- Administer medications as prescribed
- Encourage the patient to express his feelings about his diagnosis and its effect on his activities or job
- Provide ROM exercises to the splinted hand and wrist

Key signs and symptoms of carpal tunnel syndrome

- Nocturnal pain and paresthesia in the thumb and first three fingers
- Burning and tingling of the hand
- Weakness
- Tinel's sign: positive
- Phalen's test: positive

Diagnosing carpal tunnel syndrome

- Motor nerve velocity studies: conduction delay and block at wrist

Treating carpal tunnel syndrome

- Avoid flexion of the wrist
- Carpal tunnel release
- Hand splint
- Glucocorticoids
- NSAIDs

Parts of the hand and wrist involved in carpal tunnel syndrome

- Carpal tunnel
- Radial nerve
- Median nerve
- Ulnar nerve
- Flexor tendons of fingers
- Transverse carpal ligament

Key nursing interventions for a patient with carpal tunnel syndrome

- Assess neurovascular status.
- Instruct the patient to:
- provide ROM to the splinted hand and wrist
- avoid manual activity that includes dorsiflexion and volar flexion of the wrist.

The carpal tunnel

The carpal tunnel is clearly visible in this palmar view and cross section of a right hand. Note the median nerve flexor tendons of fingers, and blood vessels passing through the tunnel on their way from the forearm to the hand.

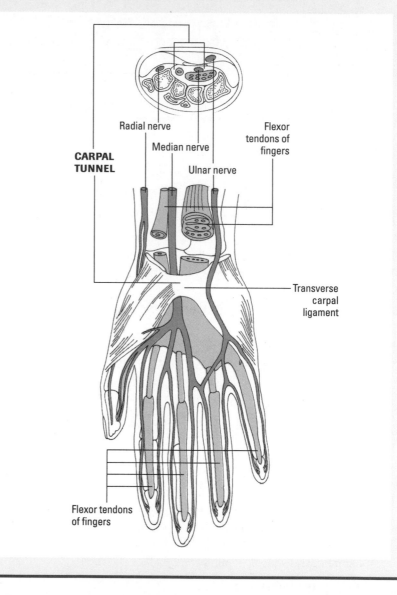

- Protect the hand from cold, burns, abrasions, local trauma, and chemical irritations
- Instruct the patient to avoid manual activity that includes dorsiflexion and volar flexion of the wrist
- Individualize home care instructions
  - Know about the disorder and its treatment

Eliciting signs of carpal tunnel syndrome

Two simple tests—for Tinel's sign and Phalen's sign—may confirm the diagnosis of carpal tunnel syndrome. The tests prove that certain wrist movements compress the median nerve, causing pain, burning, numbness, or tingling in the hand and fingers.

TINEL'S SIGN
Lightly percuss the transverse carpal ligament over the median nerve where the patient's palm and wrist meet. If this action produces discomfort, such as numbness or tingling shooting into the palm and fingers, the patient has Tinel's sign.

PHALEN'S SIGN
If flexing the patient's wrist for about 30 seconds causes the patient to feel subsequent pain or numbness in her hand or fingers, she has Phalen's sign. The more severe the carpal tunnel syndrome, the more rapidly the symptoms develop.

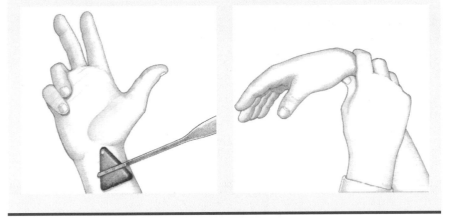

– Follow instructions for medication use and be aware of possible adverse effects
– Comply with activity restrictions
– Maintain ROM exercises for the hand
– Protect the hand from trauma
– Splint the hand as directed
– Consider vocational retraining if appropriate
– Comply with medical follow-up

● **Complications**
  • Contracture
  • Chronic hand pain
  • Loss of thumb abduction and opposition (ape hand)
  • Trophic changes of tips of thumbs and index and middle fingers

● **Surgical intervention**
  • Carpal tunnel release

Key complications of carpal tunnel syndrome
● Contracture
● Loss of thumb abduction and opposition

Key facts about herniated intervertebral disk

- Rupture of intervertebral disk
- Two types: lumbosacral and cervical

Key signs and symptoms of herniated intervertebral disk

Lumbosacral
- Pain in the lower back radiating across the buttock and down the leg
- Weakness, numbness, and tingling of the foot and leg

Cervical
- Neck pain that radiates down the arm to the hand

Diagnosing herniated intervertebral disk

- CT scan: disk displacement
- MRI: disk bulges or protrusions
- X-ray: narrowing of disk space

HERNIATED INTERVERTEBRAL DISK

● **Definition**
- Rupture of intervertebral disk
- Two types of ruptured disk
  - Lumbosacral (L4, L5)
  - Cervical (C5, C6, C7)

● **Causes**
- Back or neck strain
- Congenital bone deformity
- Degeneration of disk
- Weakness of ligaments
- Heavy lifting
- Trauma

● **Pathophysiology**
- Protrusion of the nucleus pulposus into the spinal canal compresses the spinal cord or nerve roots
- Compression of the spinal cord or nerve roots causes pain, numbness, and loss of motor function (see *How a herniated disk develops*)

● **Assessment findings**
- Lumbosacral
  - Pain in the lower back radiating across the buttock and down the leg; may be sudden or gradual
  - Limited ability to bend forward (see *Two tests for a herniated disk*, page 416)
  - Weakness, numbness, and tingling of the foot and leg
  - Pain on ambulation
  - Gait abnormalities
  - Depressed or absent deep tendon upper extremity reflexes or Achilles reflex
- Cervical
  - Neck stiffness
  - Weakness, numbness, and tingling of the hand
  - Neck pain that radiates down the arm to the hand
  - Weakness of affected upper extremity
  - Atrophy of biceps and triceps
  - Straightening of normal lumbar curve with scoliosis away from the affected side

● **Diagnostic test findings**
- X-ray: narrowing of disk space
- CT scan: disk displacement
- Magnetic resonance imaging (MRI): disk bulges or protrusions
- Myelogram: compression of spinal cord
- EMG: spinal nerve involvement

How a herniated disk develops

A spinal disk has two parts: the soft center called the *nucleus pulposus* and the tough, fibrous, surrounding ring called the *anulus fibrosus.* The nucleus pulposus acts as a shock absorber, distributing the mechanical stress applied to the spine when the body moves.

NORMAL VERTEBRA AND INTERVERTEBRAL DISK

Physical stress—usually a twisting motion—can cause the anulus fibrosus to tear or rupture, allowing the nucleus pulposus to push through (herniate) into the spinal canal. This process allows the vertebrae to move closer together as the disk compresses. This, in turn, causes pressure on the nerve roots as they exit between the vertebrae. Pain and, possibly, sensory and motor loss follow.

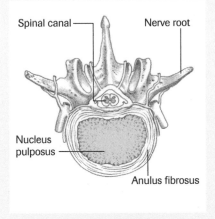

A herniated disk can also occur with intervertebral joint degeneration.

If the disk has begun to degenerate, minor trauma may cause herniation.

Herniation occurs in three stages: protrusion, extrusion, and sequestration.

PROTRUSION

The nucleus pulposus presses against the anulus fibrosus.

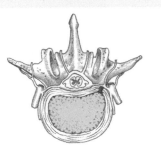

EXTRUSION AND SEQUESTRATION

The nucleus pulposus bulges forcefully through the anulus fibrosus, pushing against the nerve root. Then, the anulus fibrosus gives way as the core of the disk bursts through to press against the nerve root.

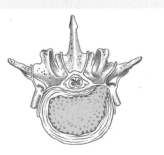

Characteristics of a herniated disk

- Physical stress, which causes the anulus fibrosus to tear or rupture
- Herniation of the nucleus pulposus into the spinal canal
- Pressure on nerve roots, which causes pain
- Three stages of herniation: protrusion, extrusion, and sequestration

Treating herniated intervertebral disk

- Neurovascular checks
- Heating pad; moist, hot compresses
- NSAIDs
- Corticosteroids
- Laminectomy
- Microdiskectomy

● **Medical management**
- Activity: bed rest (initially, if acute); active and passive ROM and isometric exercises
- Monitoring: vital signs, neurovascular checks, and laboratory studies
- Heating pad; moist, hot compresses
- Orthopedic devices: back brace, cervical collar
- Analgesic: oxycodone (Tylox)

Two tests for a herniated disk

The straight-leg-raising test and its variant, Lasègue sign, are perhaps the best tests to perform when a herniated disk is suspected.

STRAIGHT-LEG-RAISING TEST

Have the patient lie in the supine position. Place one hand on the patient's ilium to stabilize the pelvis and the other hand under the patient's ankle. Slowly raise the patient's leg. If the patient complains of posterior leg (sciatic) pain—*not back pain*—suspect a herniated disk.

LASÈGUE SIGN

To do this test, have the patient lie supine with his thigh and knee flexed (to a 90-degree angle). Resistance and pain as well as loss of ankle or knee-jerk reflex indicate spinal root compression.

- Pelvic traction
- Cervical traction
- Muscle relaxants: diazepam (Valium), cyclobenzaprine (Flexeril)
- Chemonucleolysis using chymopapain (Chymodiactin)
- NSAIDs: indomethacin (Indocin), ibuprofen (Motrin), sulindac (Clinoril), piroxicam (Feldene), flurbiprofen (Ansaid), diclofenac (Voltaren), naproxen (Naprosyn), diflunisal (Dolobid)
- Corticosteroid: cortisone (Cortone)
- Transcutaneous electrical nerve stimulation
- Physical therapy
- Deep vein thrombosis (DVT) prophylaxis

● Nursing interventions

- Assess neurovascular status
- Keep the patient in a position of comfort
- Maintain traction, braces, and cervical collar, as appropriate
- Monitor and record vital signs and laboratory studies
- Assess pain level, administer analgesics as prescribed, and evaluate response
- Administer medications as prescribed
- Encourage the patient to express his feelings about his diagnosis
- Provide skin and back care
- Reposition the patient every 2 hours using the logrolling technique (after surgery)
- Individualize home care instructions
  - Know about the disorder and its treatment
  - Follow instructions for medication use and be aware of possible adverse effects
  - Comply with activity restrictions
  - Maintain an exercise program as directed
  - Use a back brace or cervical collar, as appropriate
  - Comply with medical follow-up

Key nursing interventions for a patient with herniated intervertebral disk

- Assess neurovascular status.
- Maintain traction, braces, and cervical collar.
- Assess pain level, administer analgesics, and evaluate response.
- Reposition every 2 hours using the logrolling technique.

● **Complications**
  - Thrombophlebitis
  - Chronic pain
  - Muscle atrophy
  - Progressive paralysis

● **Surgical interventions**
  - Laminectomy
  - Spinal fusion
  - Microdiskectomy
  - Percutaneous lateral diskectomy

FRACTURES

● **Definition**
  - Break in the continuity of bone
  - Types of fractures (see *Classifying fractures,* page 418)
    – Burst
    – Linear
    – Impacted (overriding)
    – Angulated
    – Displaced
    – Segmental
    – Longitudinal
    – Complete
      Incomplete
    – Comminuted
    – Greenstick
    – Simple (closed)
    – Compound (open)
    – Transverse
    – Spiral
    – Oblique
    – Depressed
    – Compression
    – Avulsion
    – Pathologic
    – Stress
  - Types of hip fractures
    – Intracapsular
    – Extracapsular
    – Intertrochanteric

● **Causes**
  - Trauma
  - Force on a bone

Key complications of herniated intervertebral disk

- Thrombophlebitis
- Chronic pain

Key facts about fractures

- Break in the continuity of bone
- Occurs when stress placed on the bone is more than the bone can withstand
- Results in muscle spasm, edema, hemorrhage, compressed nerves, and ecchymosis

Key types of fractures

- Complete
- Incomplete
- Simple
- Compound
- Transverse
- Spiral

Common causes of fractures

- Trauma
- Force on a bone

Key classifications for fractures

- Comminuted
- Impacted
- Nondisplaced
- Overriding
- Angulated
- Displaced
- Segmental
- Avulsed
- Linear
- Spiral
- Longitudinal
- Transverse
- Oblique

Classifying fractures

One of the best-known systems for classifying fractures uses a combination of general terms to describe the fracture (for example, a simple, nondisplaced, oblique fracture).

Here are definitions of the classifications and terms used to describe fractures along with illustrations of fragment positions and fracture lines.

GENERAL CLASSIFICATION OF FRACTURES

Simple (closed): Bone fragments don't penetrate the skin.
Compound (open): Bone fragments penetrate the skin.
Incomplete (partial): Bone continuity isn't completely interrupted.
Complete: Bone continuity is completely interrupted.

CLASSIFICATION OF FRAGMENT POSITION

Comminuted: Bone breaks into separate small pieces.

Impacted: One bone fragment is forced into another.

Nondisplaced: The two sections of bone maintain essentially normal alignment.

Overriding: Fragments overlap, shortening the total bone length.

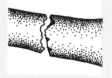

Angulated: Fragments lie at an angle to each other.

Displaced: Fracture fragments separate and are deformed.

Segmental: Fractures occur in two adjacent areas with an isolated central segment.

Avulsed: Fragments are pulled from normal position by muscle contractions or ligament resistance.

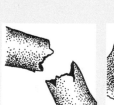

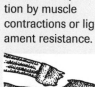

Key risk factors for fractures

- Aging
- Osteoporosis
- Contact sports

● **Risk factors**
- Aging
- Immobility
- Malnutrition
- Osteoporosis
- Contact sports
- Bone tumors
- Previous fracture

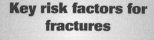

Classifying fractures *(continued)*

CLASSIFICATION OF FRAGMENT POSITION

Linear: The fracture line runs parallel to the bone's axis.

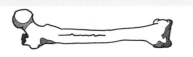

Spiral: The fracture line crosses the bone at an olique angle, creating a spiral pattern.

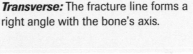

Longitudinal: The fracture line extends in a longitudinal (but not parallel) direction along the bone's axis.

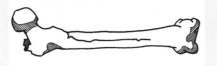

Transverse: The fracture line forms a right angle with the bone's axis.

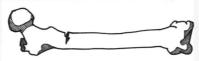

Oblique: The fracture line crosses the bone at roughly a 45-degree angle to the bone's axis.

- **Pathophysiology**
  - Fracture occurs when stress placed on the bone is more than the bone can withstand
  - Localized tissue injury results in muscle spasm, edema, hemorrhage, compressed nerves, and ecchymosis

- **Assessment findings**
  - Pain aggravated by motion
  - Tenderness over the fracture site
  - Loss of function or motion
  - Edema
  - Crepitus
  - Ecchymosis
  - Deformity
  - False motion
  - Paresthesia
  - Affected leg that appears shorter (fractured hip)

Key signs and symptoms of fractures

- Pain aggravated by motion
- Loss of function or motion
- Deformity
- Edema
- Ecchymosis

Diagnosing fractures

- X-ray: break in continuity of bone
- Hematology: decreased Hb and HCT

Treating fractures

- Abductor pillow (fractured hip)
- Analgesics
- Skin traction: Buck's, Bryant's, or Russell
- Skeletal traction
- Cast or closed reduction (fracture)
- ORIF
- External fixation

Key nursing interventions for a patient with a fracture

- Assess neurovascular status.
- Keep the legs abducted (fractured hip).
- Monitor and record vital signs, I/O, and laboratory studies.
- Provide skin, pin, and cast care.
- Keep the hip extended (fractured hip).
- Provide a trapeze.
- Encourage turning, coughing, deep breathing, and incentive spirometry.
- Manage pain.

● Diagnostic test findings
- X-ray: break in continuity of bone
- Hematology: decreased Hb and HCT

● Medical management
- Position: elevate the fractured extremity; keep the patient flat with the leg abducted for a fractured hip
- Activity: as tolerated for extremity fractures; active and passive ROM exercises for unaffected limbs for fractured hip; isometric exercises
- Monitoring: vital signs, I/O, and neurovascular checks
- Laboratory studies: Hb, HCT, phosphorus, and calcium
- Ice packs, abductor pillow (fractured hip)
- Analgesic: oxycodone (Tylox) and acetaminophen (Tylenol)
- Skin traction: Buck's, Bryant's, or Russell
- Skeletal traction: Thomas splint with Pearson attachment, Steinmann pin, Kirschner wire, or Crutchfield tongs (fractured neck)
- Cast or closed reduction (fracture)
- Cast or pin care

● Nursing interventions
- Assess neurovascular status
- Keep the patient in a flat position with legs abducted and the foot of the bed elevated 25 degrees (fractured hip)
- Elevate a fractured extremity and apply ice
- Monitor and record vital signs, I/O, and laboratory studies
- Assess pain level, administer analgesics as prescribed, and evaluate response
- Administer medications as prescribed
- Allay the patient's anxiety and provide emotional support
- Provide skin, pin, and cast care
- Turn the patient to the affected or unaffected side every 2 hours as ordered; keep the hip extended (fractured hip)
- Maintain activity as tolerated (fractures); teach crutch walking when appropriate
- Promote independence in ADLs
- Provide active and passive ROM and isometric exercises for unaffected limbs
- Provide a trapeze if appropriate
- **Maintain traction to ensure proper body alignment and promote healing** (see *Nursing considerations for a patient in skeletal or skin traction*)
- Encourage turning, coughing, and deep breathing, and use of incentive spirometry
- Apply sequential compression stockings while in bed
- Individualize home care instructions
  - Know about the disorder and its treatment
  - Follow instructions for medication use and be aware of possible adverse effects

Nursing considerations for a patient in skeletal or skin traction

NURSING ACTION	RATIONALE
Check ropes, knots, pulleys, freedom of movement, and intactness.	These checks help ensure that the traction is functioning properly.
Check the entire traction setup, pin site, and all suspension apparatus for tightness or signs of loosening.	These actions help ensure that the traction is functioning properly.
Check weights to ensure that they're hanging freely.	These checks help ensure that there's a proper amount of traction.
Make sure the weights aren't "lifted" during care.	This action helps to avoid pain caused by sudden muscle contraction and disrupted fragments of the injured or fractured bone. (Move patients in skeletal traction for position changes without lifting or releasing the weights.)
Take care not to bump the weights or weight holders.	This action helps to avoid pain caused by rope movements, which affect the traction bow and pin.
Check all skin surfaces for signs of tolerance or pressure areas (especially on the occipital area of the head, shoulder blades, elbows, coccyx, and heels).	These checks may uncover signs of pressure that include redness, tenderness or pain, soreness caused by excoriation, and numbness.
Provide physical and psychological comfort. Answer questions honestly, answer the call light promptly, provide prompt and thorough care, encourage patient participation in care, provide diversionary activities, and prepare the patient and family for discharge.	These actions help ensure that the patient participates in and is prepared for self-care.

    – Complete cast or pin care (fracture)
    – Attend physical therapy sessions if prescribed
    – Comply with activity restrictions
    – Observe for signs and symptoms of complications
    – Comply with medical follow-up

● **Complications**
- DVT
- Fat embolism
- Pulmonary embolism
- Pneumonia
- Urinary tract infections
- Compartment syndrome
- Hypovolemic shock
- Osteomyelitis
- Pressure ulcer

- **Surgical interventions**
  - ORIF of the bone
  - External fixation for fractures

SYSTEMIC LUPUS ERYTHEMATOSUS (SLE)

- **Definition**
  - Chronic inflammatory autoimmune disorder that affects connective tissue
- **Cause**
  - Unknown
- **Risk factors**
  - Stress or emotional upset
  - Streptococcal or viral infection
  - Exposure to sunlight or ultraviolet light
  - Injury
  - Surgery
  - Exhaustion
  - Immunization
  - Abnormal estrogen metabolism
- **Pathophysiology**
  - Defect in the body's immunologic mechanism produces serum autoantibodies directed against components of the patient's cell nuclei
  - Deposits of antigen or antibody complexes affect connective cells throughout the body, including blood vessels, mucous membranes, joints, skin, kidneys, muscles, brain, and heart
- **Assessment findings**
  - Painful or swollen joints
  - Muscle pain
  - Oral and nasopharyngeal ulcerations
  - Alopecia
  - Photosensitivity
  - Low-grade fever
  - Butterfly erythema on face
  - Raynaud's phenomenon
  - Abdominal pain
  - Malaise and weakness
  - Weight loss
  - Lymphadenopathy
  - Anorexia
- **Diagnostic test findings**
  - LE cell preparation test: positive
  - ANA test: positive
  - Rheumatoid factor: positive
  - Hematology: decreased Hb, HCT, WBCs, platelets; increased ESR

- Urine chemistry: proteinuria, hematuria
- Blood chemistry: decreased complement fixation

Medical management

- Analgesics, NSAIDs: indomethacin (Indocin), ibuprofen (Motrin), sulindac (Clinoril), piroxicam (Feldene), diclofenac (Voltaren), naproxen (Naprosyn), diflunisal (Dolobid)
- Corticosteroid: prednisone (Deltasone)
- Antimalarial: hydroxychloroquine (Plaquenil)
- Immunosuppressants: azathioprine (Imuran), cyclophosphamide (Cytoxan), mycophenolate mofetil (CellCept), methotrexate (Rheumatrex)
- I.V. therapy: fluids as needed
- Activity: regular exercise program
- Monitoring: vital signs and I/O
- Laboratory studies: Hb, HCT, WBCs, platelets, ESR, BUN, and creatinine
- Plasmapheresis
- Antipyretic: aspirin, acetaminophen (Tylenol)
- Antianemics: ferrous sulfate (Feosol), ferrous gluconate (Fergon)
- Vitamins and minerals

Nursing interventions

- Assess musculoskeletal and renal status
- Monitor and record vital signs, I/O, laboratory studies, and daily weight
- Administer medications as prescribed
- Encourage the patient to express his feelings about his illness and the chronicity of the disease
- Avoid exposing the patient to sunlight
- Minimize environmental stress
- Provide rest periods as needed
- Prevent infection
- Individualize home care instructions
  - Know about the disorder and its treatment
  - Follow instructions for medication use and be aware of possible adverse effects
  - Identify ways to reduce stress
  - Observe for signs and symptoms of complications
  - Avoid exposure to people with infections
  - Avoid over-the-counter medications unless approved by physician
  - Avoid exposure to sunlight
  - Contact local support services as appropriate
  - Comply with medical follow-up

Complications

- Pleurisy
- Pleural effusions
- Pericarditis, myocarditis, endocarditis
- Coronary atherosclerosis
- Renal failure

- Seizures
- Depression
- Infection
- **Surgical intervention**
  - None

NCLEX CHECKS

It's never too soon to begin your NCLEX preparation. Now that you've reviewed this chapter, carefully read each of the following questions and choose the best answer. Then compare your responses to the correct answers.

1. A probable nursing diagnosis for the patient recovering from an amputation is:

☒ **1.** *Disturbed body image*
☐ **2.** *Delayed surgical recovery*
☐ **3.** *Deficient diversional activity*
☐ **4.** *Risk for disuse syndrome*

2. The nurse notes a positive Tinel's sign in a client. Presence of this sign might indicate:

☐ **1.** thrombophlebitis.
☐ **2.** osteoporosis.
☐ **3.** RA.
☒ **4.** carpal tunnel syndrome.

3. A client received a hip prosthesis for a right hip fracture sustained after a fall. In the immediate postoperative period, the nurse should maintain the leg:

☒ **1.** in an abducted position.
☐ **2.** in an adducted position.
☐ **3.** in a neutral position.
☐ **4.** with the hip flexed more than 90 degrees.

4. A 78-year-old client has a history of osteoarthritis. Which signs and symptoms would the nurse expect to find on physical assessment?

☒ **1.** Joint pain, crepitus, Heberden's nodes
☐ **2.** Hot, inflamed joints; crepitus; joint pain
☐ **3.** Tophi, enlarged joints, Bouchard's nodes
☐ **4.** Swelling, joint pain, tenderness on palpation

5. When teaching an elderly female client who has osteoporosis, the nurse should include information about which major complication?

☐ **1.** Loss of estrogen
☒ **2.** Bone fracture
☐ **3.** Negative calcium balance
☐ **4.** Dowager's hump

6. A client with a sports injury undergoes a diagnostic arthroscopy of his left knee. After the procedure, the nurse assesses the client's leg. What are the priority nursing assessment factors?

- ☐ **1.** Wound and skin
- ☐ **2.** Mobility and sensation
- ☐ **3.** Vascular and integumentary
- ☒ **4.** Circulatory and neurologic

7. A client develops L5-S1 herniated nucleus pulposus, which impinges on the left nerve root. Most likely, the client would experience pain that radiates:

- ☐ **1.** up the spinal column.
- ☐ **2.** to the lower abdomen.
- ☒ **3.** down the left leg.
- ☐ **4.** across to the right pelvis.

8. A client is undergoing rehabilitation following a fracture. As part of his regimen, the client performs isometric exercises. Which of the following provides the best evidence that the client understands the proper technique?

- ☐ **1.** Exercising bilateral extremities simultaneously
- ☐ **2.** Periodic monitoring of his heart rate
- ☒ **3.** Forced resistance against stable objects
- ☐ **4.** Swinging of limbs through full ROM

9. A client in balanced suspension traction for a fractured femur needs to be repositioned toward the head of the bed. During repositioning, the nurse should:

- ☐ **1.** place slight additional tension on the traction cords.
- ☐ **2.** release the weights and replace immediately after positioning.
- ☐ **3.** lift the traction and the client during repositioning.
- ☒ **4.** maintain the same degree of traction tension.

10. While assessing a client with osteoarthritis, the nurse palpates a grating sensation as the client bends her fingers. The nurse documents this assessment finding as:

- ☐ **1.** fremitus.
- ☒ **2.** crepitation.
- ☐ **3.** a thrill.
- ☐ **4.** a click.

ANSWERS AND RATIONALES

1. Correct answer: 1
Disturbed body image is a probable nursing diagnosis for the client recovering from an amputation due to the loss of a limb, which changes his appearance, and the change in body function.

2. Correct answer: 4
You may observe a positive Tinel's sign — tingling over the median nerve on light percussion — in a client with carpal tunnel syndrome. A positive Tinel's sign isn't associated with thrombophlebitis, osteoporosis, or RA.

3. CORRECT ANSWER: 1

After receiving a hip prosthesis, the client should keep the affected leg abducted. Adduction may dislocate the hip. Keep the hip in a neutral position if an internal fixation device was used. The hip must not be flexed more than 90 degrees for the first 2 months and even less than that for the first 10 days.

4. CORRECT ANSWER: 1

Signs and symptoms of osteoarthritis include joint pain, crepitus, Heberden's nodes, Bouchard's nodes, and enlarged joints. Hot, inflamed joints rarely occur with osteoarthritis. Tophi are deposits of sodium urate crystals that occur with chronic gout, not osteoarthritis. Swelling, joint pain, and tenderness on palpation occur with a sprain injury.

5. CORRECT ANSWER: 2

Bone fracture is a major complication of osteoporosis that results when loss of calcium and phosphate increases the fragility of bones. Estrogen deficiencies result from menopause, not osteoporosis. Calcium and vitamin D supplements may be used to support bone metabolism, but a negative calcium balance isn't a complication of osteoporosis. Dowager's hump results from bone fractures; it develops when repeated vertebral fractures increase spinal curvature.

6. CORRECT ANSWER: 4

Following a procedure on an extremity, focus assessments on neurovascular status of the extremity. Swelling of the extremity can impair both neurologic and circulatory function of the leg. After establishing the neurovascular stability of the extremity, the nurse can address the other concerns of skin, mobility, and pain.

7. CORRECT ANSWER: 3

The pain associated with herniated nucleus pulposus of L5-S1 primarily affects the lower back with radiation down the leg. Pain that radiates up the spinal column, to the lower abdomen, or across to the right pelvis isn't associated with a lumbar herniation.

8. CORRECT ANSWER: 3

Isometric exercises involve applying pressure against a stable object, such as pressing the hands together or pushing an arm against a wall. Exercising extremities simultaneously isn't characteristic of isometrics. Heart rate monitoring is associated with aerobic exercising. Limb swinging isn't isometric.

9. CORRECT ANSWER: 4

Traction is used to reduce the fracture and must be maintained at all times, including during repositioning. It isn't appropriate to increase traction tension or release or lift the traction during repositioning.

10. CORRECT ANSWER: 2

Crepitation is the grating sensation that can be felt or heard that's associated with degenerative joint diseases such as osteoarthritis.

9

Integumentary system

PRETEST

1. A client received a skin graft on his left hand and wrist following a severe burn. What instructions should the nurse give the client regarding activity?

☐ 1. Keep the extremity dependent to increase blood flow to the area.

☐ 2. Perform range-of-motion exercises every 2 hours while awake.

☐ 3. Keep the extremity elevated and avoid movement of the extremity until the graft site is secure.

☐ 4. Keep the extremity in a sling at all times.

CORRECT ANSWER: 3

2. Which nursing intervention is appropriate to avoid development of a pressure ulcer?

☐ 1. Keep the client flat in bed.

☐ 2. Keep the client in semi-Fowler's position.

☐ 3. Reposition the client every 4 hours.

☐ 4. Reposition the client every 2 hours.

CORRECT ANSWER: 4

3. A probable nursing diagnosis for the client with psoriasis is:

- [ ] 1. *Situational low self-esteem*
- [ ] 2. *Disturbed sensory perception (auditory)*
- [ ] 3. *Disturbed personal identity*
- [ ] 4. *Risk for activity intolerance*

CORRECT ANSWER: 1

4. A 40-year-old golfer presents with a waxy, crusted lesion on his posterior neck. Which of the following conditions is suspected?

- [ ] 1. Herpes zoster
- [ ] 2. Psoriasis
- [ ] 3. Basal cell carcinoma
- [ ] 4. Malignant melanoma

CORRECT ANSWER: 3

5. Which assessment finding is indicative of herpes zoster?

- [ ] 1. Skin vesicles clustered along peripheral sensory nerves
- [ ] 2. Irregular, circular, bordered lesions with hues of tan, black, or blue
- [ ] 3. Erythematous, well-demarcated papules and plaques with silver scales
- [ ] 4. Waxy nodules with telangiectasis on the surface of the face or ears

CORRECT ANSWER: 1

LEARNING OBJECTIVES

After studying this chapter, you should be able to:

- Describe the psychosocial impact of integumentary disorders.
- Differentiate between modifiable and nonmodifiable risk factors in the development of an integumentary disorder.
- List three probable and three possible nursing diagnoses for a patient with an integumentary disorder.
- Identify nursing interventions for a patient with an integumentary disorder.
- Identify three teaching topics for a patient with an integumentary disorder.

CHAPTER OVERVIEW

Caring for the patient with an integumentary disorder requires a sound understanding of integumentary anatomy and physiology as well as the management of modifiable risk factors. A thorough assessment is essential to planning and implementing appropriate patient care. The assessment includes a complete history, physical examination, diagnostic testing, identification of modifiable and nonmodifiable risk factors, and information related to the psychosocial impact of the disorder on the patient.

Nursing diagnoses focus primarily on impaired skin integrity, ineffective tissue perfusion, and body image disturbance. Nursing interventions are designed to support healing of the skin, prevent further injury to the affected area, and help the patient adjust to the change in his body image. Patient teaching—a crucial nursing activity—involves providing information about the disorder and its treatment, medication regimens, signs and symptoms of possible complications, reducing modifiable risk factors to prevent skin damage and infection, and medical follow-up.

What's in your skin

This cross section of the skin illustrates major skin structures.

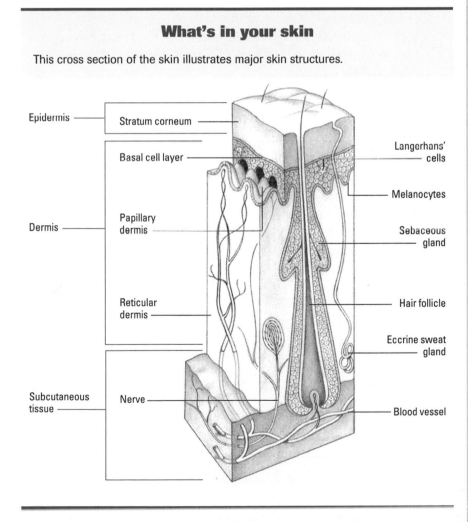

Epidermis — Stratum corneum

Basal cell layer

Papillary dermis

Dermis

Reticular dermis

Subcutaneous tissue — Nerve

Langerhans' cells

Melanocytes

Sebaceous gland

Hair follicle

Eccrine sweat gland

Blood vessel

Parts of the skin

- Stratum corneum
- Basal cell layer
- Langerhans' cells
- Melanocytes
- Papillary dermis
- Sebaceous glands
- Hair follicles
- Reticular dermis
- Eccrine sweat glands
- Nerves
- Blood vessels

3 layers of skin

- Epidermis: outer layer; composed of dense squamous cells
- Dermis: origin of hair, nails, sebaceous glands, eccrine sweat glands, and apocrine sweat glands
- Subcutaneous tissue: third layer of skin; provides heat, insulation, shock absorption, and a reserve of calories

Key functions of the glandular appendages

- Sebaceous glands lubricate hair and epidermis
- Eccrine sweat glands regulate body temperature
- Apocrine sweat glands secrete odorless fluid

Key functions of the hair and nails

- Hair: protects and covers the body
- Nails: protect the tips of the fingers and toes

ANATOMY AND PHYSIOLOGY REVIEW

● **Skin**
  - First line of defense against trauma and microorganisms
  - Prevents loss of water and electrolytes
  - Regulates body temperature through sweat production and evaporation
  - Composed of three layers: epidermis, dermis, and subcutaneous tissue or hypodermis (see *What's in your skin,* page 429)
    - Epidermis
      · Outer avascular layer composed of dense squamous cells that shed constantly
      · Keratinocytes and melanocytes are found in this layer
    - Dermis
      · Origin of hair, nails, sebaceous glands, eccrine sweat glands, and apocrine sweat glands
      · Collagen layer that supports the epidermis and contains nerves and blood vessels
    - Subcutaneous tissue (hypodermis)
      · Composed of loose connective tissue filled with fatty cells
      · Provides heat, insulation, shock absorption, and a reserve of calories

● **Glandular appendages**
  - Three types: sebaceous, eccrine, and apocrine
  - Sebaceous glands (oil)
    - Found primarily in the skin of the scalp, face, upper body, and genital region
    - Lubricate hair and epidermis; stimulated by sex hormones
  - Eccrine sweat glands
    - Located over most of the body
    - Regulate body temperature through water secretion
  - Apocrine sweat glands
    - Located in the axilla and genital areas
    - Secrete odorless fluid; decomposition of this fluid by bacteria causes odor

● **Hair**
  - Formed from keratin and produced by matrix cells in the dermal layer
  - Protects and covers the body, except for the palms, lips, soles of the feet, nipples, and external genitalia
  - Hormones stimulate differential growth

● **Nails**
  - Formed when epidermal cells are converted into hard plates of keratin
  - Protect the tips of the fingers and toes

ASSESSMENT FINDINGS

● **History**
  - Change in skin color, texture, and temperature

Evaluating skin turgor

To assess skin turgor in an adult, gently squeeze the skin on the forearm or sternal area between your thumb and forefinger, as shown. In an infant, roll a fold of loosely adherent abdominal skin between your thumb and forefinger, then release the skin.

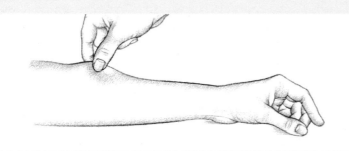

If the skin quickly returns to its original shape, the patient has normal turgor. If the skin doesn't return to its original shape within 30 seconds or if it maintains a tented position as shown, it has poor turgor.

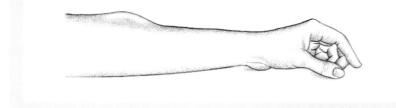

- Perspiration or dryness
- Itching
- Brittle, thick, or soft nails
- Hair loss or gain
- Rash

● Physical examination

- Abnormal pattern of pigmentation and hair distribution
- Altered skin texture, turgor, color, and temperature (see *Evaluating skin turgor*)
- Peripheral edema
- Trophic changes: skin, hair, and nails
- Skin lesions: type, shape, and character
- Nevi and scars
- Erythema
- Petechiae or ecchymosis
- Pressure ulcers

Assessing skin turgor

- Squeeze the skin on the forearm or sternal area.
- If the skin returns to normal shape, the skin has normal turgor.
- If the skin doesn't return to original shape in 30 seconds or if it maintains a tented position, it has poor turgor.

Key signs and symptoms of a disorder of the integumentary system

- Change in skin color, texture, and temperature
- Perspiration or dryness
- Itching
- Skin lesions
- Erythema
- Peripheral edema
- Trophic changes in skin, hair, and nails

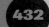

Key facts about blood chemistry

- Blood test
- Analysis for potassium, sodium, calcium, phosphorus and other factors
- Intervention: check the site for bleeding after the procedure

Key facts about hematologic studies

- Blood test
- Analysis for RBCs, WBCs, platelets, Hb, and other factors
- Intervention: check the site for bleeding after the procedure

Key facts about skin biopsy

- Procedure to remove a small amount of skin
- Histologic evaluation
- Intervention: check the site for bleeding and infection after the procedure

Key facts about skin testing

- Procedure using a patch, scratch, or intradermal technique
- Administers allergens to the skin
- Intervention: record date and time for follow-up reading

Key facts about skin scraping

- Procedure in which cells are scraped and covered with potassium hydroxide
- Examines scales, nails, and hair
- Intervention: check the site for bleeding and infection

DIAGNOSTIC TESTS AND PROCEDURES

- ● **Blood chemistry**
  - Definition and purpose
    - Laboratory test of a blood sample
    - Analysis for potassium, sodium, calcium, phosphorus, ketones, glucose, osmolality, chloride, blood urea nitrogen (BUN), and creatinine
  - Nursing interventions
    - Explain the procedure to the patient
    - Check the site for bleeding after the procedure

- ● **Hematologic studies**
  - Definition and purpose
    - Laboratory test of a blood sample
    - Analysis for red blood cell (RBC) count, white blood cell (WBC) count, erythrocyte sedimentation rate, platelets, prothrombin time, partial thromboplastin time, hemoglobin (Hb), and hematocrit (HCT)
  - Nursing interventions
    - Explain the procedure to the patient
    - Check the site for bleeding after the procedure

- ● **Skin biopsy (punch biopsy)**
  - Definition and purpose
    - Procedure using a circular punch instrument to remove a small amount of skin tissue
    - Histologic evaluation
  - Nursing interventions
    - Explain the procedure to the patient
    - Check the site for bleeding and infection after the procedure

- ● **Skin testing**
  - Definition and purpose
    - Procedure using a patch, scratch, or intradermal technique
    - Administration of an allergen to the skin's surface or into the dermis
  - Nursing interventions
    - Explain the procedure to the patient
    - Keep the area dry
    - Record the site, date, and time of test
    - Inspect the site for erythema, papules, vesicles, edema, and induration
    - Record the date and time for follow-up site reading

- ● **Skin scrapings**
  - Definition and purpose
    - Procedure calling for cells scraped by a scalpel and covered with potassium hydroxide
    - Microscopic examination of scales, nails, and hair
  - Nursing interventions
    - Explain the procedure to the patient
    - Check the scraping site for bleeding and infection

- **Wound culture**
  - Definition and purpose
    - Laboratory test
    - Microscopic examination of cells, including Gram stain, culture and sensitivity, cytology, and immunofluorescence
  - Nursing interventions
    - Explain the procedure to the patient
    - Follow laboratory procedure guidelines
    - Note current antibiotic therapy

- **Wood's light examination**
  - Definition and purpose
    - Procedure using ultraviolet (UV) light
    - Direct examination of skin
  - Nursing intervention: Explain the procedure to the patient

PSYCHOSOCIAL IMPACT OF INTEGUMENTARY DISORDERS

- **Developmental impact**
  - Changes in body image
  - Fear of rejection
  - Changes in role performance
  - Decreased self-esteem

- **Economic impact**
  - Cost of medications and treatment
  - Disruption or loss of employment
  - Cost of hospitalizations and follow-up care

- **Occupational and recreational impact**
  - Restrictions in physical activity
  - Changes in leisure activity

- **Social impact**
  - Social isolation
  - Sexual dysfunction

RISK FACTORS

- **Modifiable risk factors**
  - Infection
  - Occupation
  - Exposure to chemical and environmental pollutants
  - Exposure to radiation
  - Exposure to the sun
  - Personal hygiene habits
  - Environment
  - Use of skin products, detergents, and softeners

Key nonmodifiable risk factors for integumentary disorders

- Aging
- History of endocrine, vascular, or immune disorders
- Family history of skin disease or allergies

- Stress
- Diet
- Medications

● **Nonmodifiable risk factors**
  - Aging
  - History of endocrine, vascular, or immune disorders
  - Family history of skin disease or allergies
  - History of allergies
  - Exposure to communicable disease
  - Pregnancy
  - Menopause
  - Skin moles

NURSING DIAGNOSES

Probable nursing diagnoses for a patient with an integumentary disorder

- Impaired skin integrity
- Disturbed body image
- Anxiety

● **Probable nursing diagnoses**
  - Impaired skin integrity
  - Disturbed body image
  - Situational low self-esteem
  - Acute pain
  - Disturbed sensory perception (tactile)
  - Anxiety
  - Ineffective tissue perfusion (peripheral)

Possible nursing diagnoses for a patient with an integumentary disorder

- Ineffective coping
- Risk for infection
- Social isolation

● **Possible nursing diagnoses**
  - Ineffective breathing pattern
  - Ineffective coping
  - Risk for deficient fluid volume
  - Risk for infection
  - Fear
  - Social isolation

SKIN GRAFT

Key facts about a skin graft

- Replacement of damaged skin with healthy skin
- Three types: split-thickness graft, full-thickness graft, and pinch graft

● **Description**
  - Replacement of damaged skin with healthy skin to protect underlying structures or to reconstruct areas for cosmetic or functional purposes
  - Split-thickness graft: graft of one-half of the epidermis, which is removed by a dermatome
  - Full-thickness graft: graft of the entire epidermis
  - Pinch graft: graft of a small piece of skin, obtained by elevating the skin with a needle and removing it with scissors

● **Preoperative nursing interventions**
  - Complete patient and family preoperative teaching
    - Explain the procedure to the patient

– Describe the operating room, postanesthesia care unit, and preoperative and postoperative routines
– Demonstrate postoperative turning, coughing, deep breathing, splinting, and range-of-motion (ROM) exercises
– Explain the postoperative need for drainage tubes, surgical dressings, oxygen therapy, I.V. therapy, and pain control
• Complete a preoperative checklist and make sure a signed informed consent is in the patient's chart
• Administer preoperative medications as prescribed
• Provide emotional support to allay the patient's and family's anxiety about surgery
• Document the patient's history and physical assessment data
• Prepare the donor and graft sites as directed

● **Postoperative nursing interventions**
• Assess pain level, administer analgesics as prescribed, and evaluate response
• Administer I.V. fluids
• Allay the patient's anxiety and provide emotional support
• Provide graft care as directed
• Encourage turning, coughing, deep breathing, and use of incentive spirometry
• Maintain activity as directed; enforce activity restrictions based on location of graft
• Monitor and record vital signs, intake and output (I/O), and neurovascular checks distal to the recipient site
• Elevate and immobilize the graft site, as directed
• Encourage the patient to express his feelings about his surgery
• Administer medications as prescribed
• **Assess the graft site for infection, hematoma, and fluid accumulation under the graft; keep the graft and donor sites free from pressure**
• Maintain room temperature as ordered
• Individualize home care instructions
– Know about the surgery and recovery
– Follow instructions for medication use and be aware of possible adverse effects
– Continue physical therapy
– Perform wound care
– **Protect the graft site from direct sunlight**
– Observe for signs and symptoms of complications
– Comply with medical follow-up

● **Possible surgical complications**
• Infection of the graft or donor sites
• Graft rejection or failure
• Hematoma under the graft
• Fluid accumulation under the graft

Key nursing interventions before a skin graft
● Demonstrate postoperative turning, coughing, deep breathing, splinting, and ROM exercises.
● Complete a preoperative checklist.
● Prepare the donor and graft sites.

Key nursing interventions after a skin graft
● Elevate and immobilize the graft site.
● Administer medications as prescribed.
● Assess the graft site for infection, hematoma, and fluid accumulation under the graft.

Key complications of a skin graft
● Infection of the graft or donor sites
● Graft rejection or failure

Key facts about psoriasis

- Chronic, noninfectious skin inflammation that occurs in patches
- Papules coalesce to form plaques

Common causes of psoriasis

- Epidermal trauma
- Streptococcal infection

Key signs and symptoms of psoriasis

- Pruritus
- Papules and plaques
- Erythema

Diagnosing psoriasis

- Skin biopsy: positive
- Serum uric acid level: increased

Treating psoriasis

- Corticosteroids
- Antipsoriatics
- Antimetabolite
- Photochemotherapy
- Keratolytics
- Antimicrobial

PSORIASIS

● **Definition**
- Chronic, noninfectious skin inflammation that occurs in patches
- Characterized by recurring remissions and exacerbations

● **Causes**
- Epidermal trauma
- Streptococcal infection
- Genetics

● **Risk factors**
- Stress
- Climate changes
- Hormones

● **Pathophysiology**
- Loss of normal regulatory mechanisms of cell division leads to rapid multiplication of epidermal cells that interferes with formation of normal protective layer of skin
- Papules coalesce to form plaques

● **Assessment findings**
- Erythematous, well-demarcated papules and plaques covered with silver scales, typically appearing on the scalp, chest, elbows, knees, back, and buttocks
- Pruritus
- Yellow discoloration and thickening of nails
- Erythema

● **Diagnostic test finding**
- Skin biopsy: positive
- Serum uric acid level: increased

● **Medical management**
- Treatments: bed cradle, daily soaks, and tepid, wet compresses
- Corticosteroids (topical): triamcinolone (Kenalog) covered with occlusive dressing, betamethasone (Valisone)
- UVB light or natural sunlight
- Antipsoriatics: anthralin (Anthra-Derm), coal tar (Estar), followed by exposure to UV light, etretinate (Tegison)
- Antimetabolite (for severe, unresponsive psoriasis): methotrexate (Amethopterin)
- Photochemotherapy (PUVA therapy): methoxsalen (Oxsoralen) followed by exposure to black light
- Keratolytics: benzoyl peroxide (Benzagel), salicylic acid (Keratex gel)
- Antimicrobial: sulfasalazine (Azulfidine)
- Diet: no alcohol

● **Nursing interventions**
- Assess skin integrity
- Administer medications as prescribed

TIME-OUT FOR TEACHING

Patients with integumentary disorders

Be sure to include the following topic areas in your teaching plan when caring for patients with integumentary disorders.

- Medication therapy, including the action, adverse effects, and scheduling
- Prevention of skin damage and irritation, including:
  - avoiding extreme temperatures
  - maintaining comfortable room temperature
  - avoiding known irritants
  - avoiding scratching and rubbing
  - using sunblock
  - maintaining hydration
  - maintaining skin integrity

- Wound care as directed
- Infection control measures
- Cautious use of skin care products
- Daily skin care
- Signs and symptoms of skin infection
- Smoking cessation
- Optimal body weight maintenance
- Community agencies and resources for supportive services
- Fluid intake
- Follow-up appointments

- Provide emotional support; encourage the patient to express his feelings
- Administer UV light and PUVA therapy, as ordered
- Apply occlusive dressings
- Prevent scratching
- Help the patient to remove scales during soaks
- Individualize home care instructions (for teaching tips, see *Patients with integumentary disorders*)
  - Know about the disorder and its treatment
  - Follow instructions for medication use and be aware of possible adverse effects
  - Identify ways to reduce stress
  - Wear light cotton clothing over affected areas
  - Contact the National Psoriasis Foundation
  - Comply with medical follow-up

● **Complications**
  - Depression
  - Infection

● **Surgical interventions**
  - None

HERPES ZOSTER (SHINGLES)

● **Definition**
  - Acute viral infection of nerve structure caused by varicella zoster

● **Causes**
  - Cytotoxic drug–induced immunosuppression
  - Hodgkin's lymphoma

Key teaching topics for a patient with an integumentary disorder

- Medication therapy
- Prevention of skin damage and irritation
- Wound care
- Infection control measures

Key nursing interventions for a patient with psoriasis

- Assess skin integrity.
- Encourage the patient to express his feelings about the disorder.
- Administer UV light and PUVA therapy.
- Prevent scratching.

Key complications of psoriasis

- Depression
- Infection

Key facts about herpes zoster

- Acute viral infection of nerve structure
- Caused by varicella zoster
- Affects spinal and cranial sensory ganglia and posterior gray matter of the spinal cord

Common causes of herpes zoster

- Cytotoxic drug–induced immunosuppression
- Exposure to varicella zoster
- Debilitating disease

Key signs and symptoms of herpes zoster

- Neuralgia
- Unilaterally clustered skin vesicles along peripheral sensory nerves on trunk, thorax, or face

Diagnosing herpes zoster

- Antinuclear antibody: positive
- Skin culture: positive

Treating herpes zoster

- Analgesics
- Antianxiety agents
- Antipruritic
- Corticosteroids
- Antiviral agents

Key nursing interventions for a patient with herpes zoster

- Assess pain level, administer analgesics as prescribed, and evaluate response.
- Encourage the patient to express his feelings about his illness.
- Provide cool compresses, tepid baths, and a bed cradle.
- Prevent scratching and rubbing of affected areas.

- Exposure to varicella zoster
- Debilitating disease

● **Pathophysiology**
- Activation of dormant varicella zoster virus causes an inflammatory reaction
- Affected areas include spinal and cranial sensory ganglia and posterior gray matter of the spinal cord

● **Assessment findings**
- Neuralgia
- Malaise
- Pruritus
- Burning
- Unilaterally clustered skin vesicles along peripheral sensory nerves on trunk, thorax, or face
- Erythema
- Fever
- Anorexia
- Headache
- Paresthesia
- Edematous skin

● **Diagnostic test findings**
- Antinuclear antibody: positive
- Skin cultures and stains: identification of organism

● **Medical management**
- Monitoring: vital signs, seventh cranial nerve function, and neurovascular checks
- Activity: as tolerated
- Treatments: cool compresses, tepid baths, and bed cradle
- Transcutaneous peripheral nerve stimulation (for postherpetic neuralgia)
- Analgesics: acetaminophen (Tylenol), oxycodone (Tylox)
- Antianxiety agents: diazepam (Valium), hydroxyzine (Vistaril)
- Antipruritic: diphenhydramine (Benadryl)
- Corticosteroids: hydrocortisone (Cortef), triamcinolone (Kenalog)
- Antiviral agents: acyclovir (Zovirax), vidarabine (Vira-A), interferon (Roferon-A)
- Laboratory studies: culture and sensitivity
- Demulcent and skin protectant

● **Nursing interventions**
- Assess pain level, administer analgesics as prescribed, and evaluate response
- Monitor and record vital signs, laboratory results, and neurovascular and neurologic status
- Administer medications as directed
- Maintain meticulous hygiene to prevent spread of infection
- Encourage the patient to express his feelings about his illness

- Provide cool compresses, tepid baths, and bed cradle
- Prevent scratching and rubbing of affected areas
- Allay the patient's anxiety and provide emotional support
- Individualize home care instructions
  - Know about the disorder and its treatment
  - Follow instructions for medication use and be aware of possible adverse effects
  - Observe for signs and symptoms of complications
  - Wear lightweight, loose cotton clothing
  - Comply with medical follow-up

● **Complications**
- Infection
- Chronic pain
- Posttherapeutic neuralgia
- Ophthalmic herpes zoster
- Facial paralysis
- Vertigo
- Tinnitus
- Hearing loss
- Visceral dissemination

● **Surgical intervention**
- None

BURNS

● **Definition**
- Heat or chemical injury to tissue
- Described as first-, second-, or third-degree

● **Causes**
- Radiation: X-ray, sun, nuclear reactors
- Mechanical: friction
- Chemical: acids, alkalies, vesicants
- Electrical: lightning, electrical wires
- Thermal: flame, frostbite, scald

● **Pathophysiology**
- Cell destruction causes loss of intracellular fluid and electrolytes
- Amount of cell destruction is directly related to the extent (area) and degree (depth) of burn
- First-degree (superficial partial-thickness) involves epidermal layer (see *Burn classification,* page 440)
- Second-degree (dermal partial-thickness) involves epidermal and dermal layers
- Third-degree (full-thickness) involves epidermal, dermal, subcutaneous layers, and nerve endings

Depth and burn classification

- First-degree: epidermis only
- Second-degree: epidermis, dermis, and possibly some subcutaneous tissue
- Third-degree: subcutaneous tissue and possibly fascia, muscle, and bone

Key signs and symptoms of burns

- First-degree
- Erythema
- Edema
- Pain
- Blanching
- Second-degree
- Pain
- Oozing, fluid-filled vesicles
- Erythema
- Shiny, wet subcutaneous layer after vesicles rupture
- Third-degree
- Eschar
- Edema
- Little or no pain

Burn classification

CHARACTERISTIC	FIRST-DEGREE BURN	SECOND-DEGREE BURN	THIRD-DEGREE BURN
Thickness	Superficial, partial-thickness	Deep, partial-thickness	Full-thickness
Appearance	Dry with no blisters	Weeping, edematous blisters	Dry, leathery, and possibly edematous
Color	Pink	White to pink or red	White to charred
Comfort	Painful	Very painful	Little or no pain
Depth	Epidermis only	Epidermis, dermis, and possibly some subcutaneous tissue	Subcutaneous tissue and possibly fascia, muscle, and bone

● **Assessment findings**
- Visual examination: severity and extent of burn determined by Rule of Nines, Lund and Browder chart
- First-degree
  - Erythema
  - Edema
  - Pain
  - Blanching
- Second-degree
  - Pain
  - Oozing, fluid-filled vesicles
  - Erythema
  - Shiny, wet subcutaneous layer after vesicles rupture
- Third-degree
  - Eschar
  - Edema
  - Little or no pain

● **Diagnostic test findings**
- Blood chemistry: increased potassium; decreased sodium, albumin, complement fixation, immunoglobulins
- Arterial blood gas (ABG) analysis: metabolic acidosis
- 24-hour urine collection: decreased creatinine clearance, negative nitrogen balance
- Hematology: increased Hb, HCT; decreased fibrinogen, platelets, WBCs
- Urine chemistry: hematuria, myoglobinuria

● **Medical management**
- Treatment: based on severity and extent of burn
- Secure airway and provide oxygen therapy

- I.V. therapy: hydration and electrolyte replacement using Evan, Brooke, Parkland, or Massachusetts General Hospital protocols; saline lock
- Withhold oral food and fluids until the patient is stable
- Diet: high-protein, high-calorie, with increased fluids (high-calorie, high-protein drinks)
- Intubation and mechanical ventilation if patient is in respiratory distress
- Activity: bed rest if burn is severe
- Monitoring: vital signs, cardiac rhythm, hemodynamic variables, I/O, and neurovascular checks
- Laboratory studies: potassium, sodium, glucose, osmolality, creatinine, BUN, Hb, HCT, platelets, WBCs, ABG levels, culture and sensitivity
- Nutritional support: total parental nutrition (TPN), nasogastric tube feedings if patient can't take food by mouth
- Treatments: indwelling urinary catheter, postural drainage, chest physiotherapy, incentive spirometry, and bed cradle
- Transfusion therapy: fresh frozen plasma, platelets, packed RBCs, plasma
- Antibiotic: gentamicin sulfate (Garamycin)
- Anti-infectives (topical): mafenide (Sulfamylon), silver sulfadiazine (Silvadene), silver nitrate
- Antianxiety: diazepam (Valium), lorazepam (Ativan)
- Antitetanus: tetanus toxoid
- Analgesic: morphine (Roxanol)
- Colloid: 5% albumin (Albuminar-5)
- Diuretic: mannitol (Osmitrol)
- Wound care
- Pulse oximetry

● **Nursing interventions**
- Administer oxygen and maintain patent airway
- Administer I.V. fluids as directed; assess for signs of hypovolemia
- Assess respiratory status and fluid balance
- Assess pain level, administer analgesics as prescribed, and evaluate response
- Monitor and record vital signs, I/O, laboratory studies, hemodynamic variables, signs and symptoms of infection, daily weight, neurovascular checks, and pulse oximetry
- Maintain the patient's diet; withhold food and fluids, as ordered
- Provide suction; turning, coughing, and deep breathing; chest physiotherapy; and postural drainage
- Provide tracheostomy care or endotracheal care as indicated
- Administer TPN
- Administer medications as prescribed
- **Encourage the patient to express his feelings about his injury**
- Allay the patient's anxiety and provide emotional support
- Elevate affected extremities and provide ROM exercises
- Maintain a warm environment during acute period
- Provide skin and mouth care

- Individualize home care instructions
  - Know about the disorder and its treatment
  - Follow instructions for medication use and be aware of possible adverse effects
  - Perform wound and skin care
  - Observe for signs and symptoms of complications
  - Follow dietary recommendations
  - Avoid wearing restrictive clothing
  - Seek help from community agencies and resources
  - Comply with medical follow-up

● Complications
- Hypovolemic shock
- Septicemia
- Acute respiratory failure
- Multiple-organ-dysfunction syndrome

● Surgical interventions
- Skin grafting
- Tissue debridement
- Escharotomy

SKIN CANCER

● Definition
- Malignant primary tumor of the epidermal layer of the skin
- Three types of skin cancer
  - Basal cell epithelioma
  - Melanoma
  - Squamous cell carcinoma

● Causes
- Prolonged exposure to UV rays

● Risk factors
- Heredity
- Chemical irritants
- Radiation
- Friction or chronic irritation
- Immunosuppressive drugs
- Precancerous lesions: leukoplakia, nevi, senile keratoses
- Infrared heat or light

● Pathophysiology
- Unregulated cell growth and uncontrolled cell division result in the development of a neoplasm
- Basal cell epithelioma: basal cell keratinization causes tumor growth in basal layer of the epidermis
- Melanoma: tumor arises from melanocytes of the epidermis
- Squamous cell carcinoma: tumor arises from keratinocytes

● **Assessment findings**
  - Basal cell epithelioma: waxy nodule with telangiectasis
  - Melanoma: irregular, circular bordered lesion with hues of tan, black, or blue
  - Squamous cell carcinoma: small, red, nodular lesion that begins as an erythematous macule or plaque with indistinct margins
  - Pruritus
  - Local soreness
  - Change in color, size, or shape of preexisting lesion
  - Oozing, bleeding, crusting lesion

● **Diagnostic test findings**
  - Skin biopsy: cytology positive for cancer cells

● **Medical management**
  - I.V. therapy: fluids as needed
  - Monitoring: graft viability (with dressing changes), pain control
  - Radiation therapy
  - Cryosurgery with liquid nitrogen (basal cell or squamous cell)
  - Chemosurgery with zinc chloride (basal cell)
  - Immunotherapy: bacille Calmette-Guérin (BCG) vaccine (melanoma); imiquimod cream (Aldara) (basal cell)
  - Antineoplastics: 5-fluorouracil (Efudex), dacarbazine (DTIC)
  - Analgesic: oxycodone (Tylox)
  - Antiemetics: prochlorperazine (Compazine), ondansetron (Zofran)
  - Wound care

● **Nursing interventions**
  - Monitor and record vital signs; assess for signs and symptoms of infection
  - Administer medications as prescribed
  - Encourage the patient to express his feelings about the disorder
  - Provide postchemotherapeutic and postradiation nursing care
    – Provide prophylactic skin, mouth, and perineal care
    – Monitor dietary intake
    – Administer antiemetics and antidiarrheals as prescribed
    – Monitor for bleeding, infection, and electrolyte imbalance
    – Provide rest periods
  - Assess lesions; provide appropriate wound care
  - Individualize home care instructions
    – Know about the disorder and its treatment
    – Follow instructions for medication use and be aware of possible adverse effects
    – Avoid contact with chemical irritants
    – Use sunblock when outdoors
    – Monitor self for lesions and moles that don't heal or that change characteristics
    – Have moles that are subject to chronic irritation removed
    – Contact the Skin Cancer Foundation
    – Seek help from community agencies and resources

Key signs and symptoms of skin cancer

- Basal cell epithelioma: waxy nodule with telangiectasis
- Melanoma: irregular, circular bordered lesion with hues of tan, black, or blue
- Squamous cell carcinoma: small, red, nodular lesion that begins as an erythematous macule or plaque with indistinct margins
- Change in color, size, or shape of preexisting lesion

Diagnosing skin cancer

- Skin biopsy: positive for cancer cells

Treating skin cancer

- Cryosurgery with liquid nitrogen
- Chemosurgery with zinc chloride
- Antineoplastics

Key nursing interventions for a patient with skin cancer

- Monitor and record vital signs. Assess for signs and symptoms of infection
- Administer medications as prescribed
- Assess lesions and provide approriate wound care

Key complications of skin cancer

- Metastasis
- Recurrence

Key facts about pressure ulcers

- Localized areas of tissue destruction
- Stages determined by amount of injury

Common causes of pressure ulcers

- Pressure and shearing forces
- Friction

Key signs and symptoms of pressure ulcers

- Suspected deep-tissue injury: purple or maroon areas of skin
- Stage I: nonblanchable erythema of intact skin
- Stage II: partial-thickness skin loss involving the epidermis and dermis
- Stage III: full-thickness skin loss involving damage or necrosis of subcutaneous tissue
- Stage IV: damage to muscle, bone, tendon, or joint; full-thickness skin loss with extensive destruction
- Unstageable: deep crater with slough or eschar at base

● **Complications**
- Metastasis (melanoma)
- Recurrence

● **Surgical interventions**
- Curettage and electrodesiccation (basal cell)
- Surgical excision of lesion
- Lymph node dissection

PRESSURE ULCERS

● **Definition**
- Localized areas of tissue destruction
- Stages determined by amount of injury: Suspected deep-tissue injury, stages I to IV, unstageable

● **Causes**
- Pressure, particularly over bony prominences
- Shearing forces
- Friction

● **Pathophysiology**
- Pressure interrupts circulation, producing tissue ischemia and increased capillary pressure (see *Pressure points: Common sites of pressure ulcers*)
- As capillaries collapse, thrombosis occurs, leading to edema and tissue necrosis
- Necrotic tissue predisposes to bacterial invasion and infection

● **Assessment findings**
- Visual inspection reveals pressure ulcer
- Suspected deep-tissue injury
  - Purple or maroon area on skin
  - Intact skin or blood-filled blister
- Stage I
  - Nonblanchable erythema of intact skin
  - Skin discoloration
  - Warmth and hardness
- Stage II
  - Abrasion
  - Blister
  - Partial-thickness skin loss involving the epidermis and dermis
  - Shallow crater
- Stage III
  - Deep crater with or without undermining of adjacent tissue
  - Full-thickness skin loss involving damage or necrosis of subcutaneous tissue that may extend down to, but not through, underlying fascia
- Stage IV
  - Damage to muscle, bone, tendon, or joint
  - Full-thickness skin loss with extensive destruction

Pressure points: Common sites of pressure ulcers

Pressure ulcers may develop in any of these 16 pressure points. To prevent ulcers, reposition the patient frequently, and check carefully for any change in the patient's skin tone.

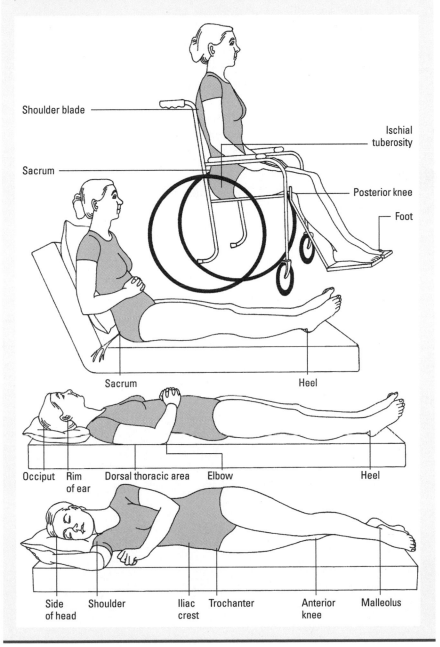

16 sites of pressure points

- Shoulder blade
- Sacrum
- Ischial tuberosity
- Posterior knee
- Foot
- Heel
- Occiput
- Rim of ear
- Dorsal thoracic area
- Elbow
- Side of head
- Shoulder
- Iliac crest
- Trochanter
- Anterior knee
- Malleolus

  – Tissue necrosis
- Unstageable
  – Deep crater with slough or eschar at base
  – Full-thickness skin loss

Diagnosing pressure ulcers

- Wound culture: positive

Treating pressure ulcers

- Foam, gel, or air mattress
- Wound care
- Debridement

Key nursing interventions for a patient with pressure ulcers

- Assess and document pressure ulcer.
- Provide wound care and dressing changes, as ordered.
- Reposition the patient every 2 hours and assess skin integrity.
- Assess for signs of infection.
- Use special mattress on bed.
- Maintain the patient's diet and encourage oral intake.

Key complications of pressure ulcers

- Progression of ulcer to more severe state
- Sepsis

● **Diagnostic test findings**
- Wound culture and sensitivity: identifies infecting organism

● **Medical management**
- Diet: high-protein, high-calorie diet in small frequent feedings; nutritional supplements, such as vitamin C and zinc
- I.V. therapy: hydration as needed
- Position: reposition patient every 2 hours, keeping pressure off ulcer site
- Treatments: foam, gel, or air mattress; wound care as ordered
- Activity: as tolerated, active or passive ROM exercises
- Monitoring: response of wound to treatment
- Laboratory studies: electrolytes, Hb, RBC, WBC, platelet, complete blood count, serum albumin, serum protein
- Nutritional support: parenteral or enteral feedings if the patient can't or won't take adequate nourishment orally

● **Nursing interventions**
- Assess stage and document pressure ulcer: measure size of wound and obtain photo per facility policy
- Provide wound care and dressing changes, as ordered
- Reposition the patient every 2 hours and assess skin integrity
- Provide meticulous skin care
- Monitor and record vital signs, I/O, laboratory studies, and daily weight
- Maintain the patient's diet and encourage fluid intake
- Assess for signs of infection
- Use special mattress on bed
- Individualize home care instructions
  - Know about the disorder and its treatment
  - Follow instructions for medication use and be aware of possible adverse effects
  - Perform wound and skin care
  - Institute prevention measures
  - Recognize signs and symptoms of complications
  - Eat a nutritious diet
  - Comply with medical follow-up

● **Complications**
- Progression of ulcer to more severe stage
- Sepsis

● **Surgical interventions**
- Debridement
- Tissue flap

NCLEX CHECKS

It's never too soon to begin your NCLEX preparation. Now that you've reviewed this chapter, carefully read each of the following questions and choose the best answer. Then compare your responses to the correct answers.

1. What key symptom would a second-degree burn wound show?

☐ **1.** Edema
☐ **2.** Blanching
☐ **3.** Eschar
☐ **4.** Fluid-filled vesicles

2. What's the best method for preventing hypovolemic shock in a client admitted with severe burns?

☐ **1.** Administering dopamine
☐ **2.** Applying medical antishock trousers
☐ **3.** Infusing I.V. fluids
☐ **4.** Infusing fresh frozen plasma

3. A client undergoes a biopsy to confirm a diagnosis of skin cancer. Immediately following the procedure, the nurse should observe the site for:

☐ **1.** skin color changes.
☐ **2.** dehiscence.
☐ **3.** hemorrhage.
☐ **4.** swelling.

4. The skin lesions evident in herpes zoster are similar to those seen in:

☐ **1.** impetigo.
☐ **2.** syphilis.
☐ **3.** varicella.
☐ **4.** rubella.

5. A client experiences problems in body temperature regulation associated with a skin impairment. Which gland is most likely involved?

☐ **1.** Eccrine
☐ **2.** Sebaceous
☐ **3.** Apocrine
☐ **4.** Endocrine

6. A nurse is caring for a client with a new skin donor site that was harvested to treat a burn. The nurse should position the client to: (Select all that apply.)

☐ **1.** allow ventilation of the site.
☐ **2.** make the site dependent.
☐ **3.** avoid pressure on the site.
☐ **4.** keep the site elevated.
☐ **5.** keep the donor site dry and open to air.
☐ **6.** be lying on the site.

7. A client is admitted with a suspected malignant melanoma on his left shoulder. When performing the physical assessment, the nurse should expect to find:

☐ **1.** a brown birthmark that has lightened in color.
☐ **2.** an area of petechiae.
☐ **3.** a brown or black mole with areas of blue and irregular borders.
☐ **4.** a red birthmark that has recently become darker.

TOP 10

Items to study for your next test on the integumentary system

1. Layers of the skin
2. Key signs and symptoms of an integumentary disorder
3. Nursing interventions before and after a skin graft
4. What causes herpes zoster
5. Classification of burns
6. Types of skin cancer
7. Four stages of pressure ulcers
8. Modifiable and nonmodifiable risk factors
9. Probable nursing diagnoses
10. Teaching topics for a patient with an integumentary disorder

8. When assessing the skin of a client, the nurse notes reddened, intact skin over the sacrum that doesn't blanch. The nurse determines that this client has which stage pressure ulcer?

- ☐ **1.** Stage I
- ☐ **2.** Stage II
- ☐ **3.** Stage III
- ☐ **4.** Stage IV

9. A client who was hospitalized for a third-degree burn is being prepared for discharge. Which statement by the client indicates an understanding of the nurse's instructions?

- ☐ **1.** "I should avoid wearing constrictive clothing over the burn site."
- ☐ **2.** "I should keep a pressure dressing over the burn site"
- ☐ **3.** "I no longer have to worry about infection because I was already treated with antibiotics."
- ☐ **4.** "I no longer have to worry about skin care."

10. A possible complication of skin cancer is:

- ☐ **1.** second-degree burn.
- ☐ **2.** recurrence of cancer.
- ☐ **3.** renal calculi.
- ☐ **4.** herpes zoster.

ANSWERS AND RATIONALES

1. CORRECT ANSWER: 4

Second-degree burn wounds show fluid-filled vesicles. Edema and blanching on pressure are characteristics of first-degree burns. Eschar is seen in third-degree burns.

2. CORRECT ANSWER: 3

During the early postburn period, large amounts of plasma fluid extravasates into interstitial spaces. Restoring the fluid loss is necessary to prevent hypovolemic shock. Fresh frozen plasma is expensive and carries a slight risk of disease transmission. Apply medical antishock trousers to treat—not prevent—shock. Dopamine causes vasoconstriction and elevates blood pressure but it doesn't prevent hypovolemia in burn patients.

3. CORRECT ANSWER: 3

The nurse's main concern following a skin biopsy procedure is bleeding. Infection is a later possible consequence of a biopsy. Dehiscence is more likely in larger wounds, such as surgical wounds of the abdomen or thorax. Skin color change and swelling are normal reactions associated with any event that traumatizes the skin.

4. CORRECT ANSWER: 3

Varicella (chickenpox) characteristically has vesicles as the hallmark lesion. Impetigo has pustules. In syphilis the primary lesion is the chancre, and in rubella the lesion is a maculopapular rash.

5. CORRECT ANSWER: 1

Eccrine glands are associated with body temperature regulation, sebaceous glands lubricate the skin and hair, and apocrine glands are involved in bacteria decomposition. Endocrine glands are a group of glands that secrete hormones responsible for the regulation of body processes, such as metabolism and glucose regulation.

6. CORRECT ANSWER: 1, 3, 4, 5

Allowing ventilation of the site, avoiding pressure on the site, elevating the site, and keeping the donor site dry and open to air are all appropriate interventions for this client. Elevating the site, rather than keeping it dependent, may reduce edema. If the client lies on the site, it will be exposed to pressure, which the client should avoid.

7. CORRECT ANSWER: 3

Melanomas have an irregular shape and lack uniformity in color. They may appear brown or black with red, white, or blue areas. The other assessment findings don't describe melanomas.

8. CORRECT ANSWER: 1

In a stage I pressure ulcer, the skin is intact with nonblanchable erythema. Intact, nonblanchable skin isn't characteristic of stage II, III, or IV ulcers.

9. CORRECT ANSWER: 1

The client being discharged after being treated for a third-degree burn should avoid wearing constrictive clothing over the burn site to avoid tissue compromise and promote healing.

10. CORRECT ANSWER: 2

Recurrence of skin cancer is a complication of any type of skin cancer, especially with prolonged exposure to ultraviolet light without effective sunblock.

Hematologic and lymphatic systems

PRETEST

1. A client has just been diagnosed with acquired immunodeficiency syndrome. What information should the nurse provide regarding transmission of human immunodeficiency virus (HIV)?

☐ 1. HIV is transmitted by saliva, semen, and blood.

☐ 2. HIV is transmitted by all body fluids and stools.

☒ 3. HIV is transmitted by blood, semen. and vaginal secretions.

☐ 4. HIV is transmitted only by blood.

CORRECT ANSWER: 3

2. A client who has undergone a bone marrow transplant is being prepared for discharge. Which statement by the client indicates an understanding of the nurse's instructions?

☒ 1. "I should avoid crowds and anyone with an infection."

☐ 2. "I should take antibiotics for at least 1 month."

☐ 3. "I no longer have to worry about infection because I have new bone marrow."

☐ 4. "I no longer have to take antibiotics because I have new bone marrow."

CORRECT ANSWER: 1

3. A possible complication of idiopathic thrombocytopenic purpura is:

☐ 1. pulmonary emboli.

☐ 2. sepsis.

☐ 3. renal calculi.

☒ 4. hemorrhage.

CORRECT ANSWER: 4

4. A probable nursing diagnosis for the client with leukemia is:

☐ 1. *Risk for imbalanced nutrition: More than body requirements*

☐ 2. *Energy field disturbance*

☐ 3. *Ineffective health maintenance*

☒ 4. *Risk for activity intolerance*

CORRECT ANSWER: 4

5. Which of these assessment findings may indicate iron deficiency anemia?

☒ 1. Pica

☐ 2. Right upper quadrant tenderness

☐ 3. Costovertebral tenderness

☐ 4. Butterfly rash

CORRECT ANSWER: 1

LEARNING OBJECTIVES

After studying this chapter, you should be able to:

● Describe the psychosocial impact of hematologic or lymphatic disorders.

● Differentiate between modifiable and nonmodifiable risk factors in the development of a hematologic or lymphatic disorder.

● List three probable and three possible nursing diagnoses for a patient with any hematologic or lymphatic disorder.

● Identify nursing interventions for a patient with a hematologic or lymphatic disorder.

● Identify three teaching topics for a patient with a hematologic or lymphatic disorder.

CHAPTER OVERVIEW

Caring for the patient with a hematologic or lymphatic disorder requires a sound understanding of cardiovascular and lymphatic anatomy and physiology, hemodynamics, and fluid balance. A thorough assessment is essential to planning and implementing appropriate care. The assessment includes a complete history, a physical examination, diagnostic testing, identification of modifiable and nonmodifiable risk factors, and information related to the psychosocial impact of the disorder on the patient.

Nursing diagnoses focus primarily on activity intolerance, impaired gas exchange, risk for infection, and anxiety. Nursing interventions are designed to monitor bleeding, prevent infection, and help the patient adjust to the effects of chronic illness. Patient teaching—a crucial nursing activity—involves providing the patient information about the disorder and its treatments, medication regimens, signs and symptoms of possible complications, reducing modifiable risk factors by adhering to infection control measures and by changing behaviors that lead to increased bleeding, and medical follow-up.

ANATOMY AND PHYSIOLOGY REVIEW

- **Lymphatic vessels**
  - Consist of capillary-like structures that are permeable to large molecules
  - Prevent edema by moving fluid and proteins from interstitial spaces to venous circulation
  - Reabsorb fats from the small intestine
- **Lymph nodes**
  - Tissue that filters out bacteria and other foreign cells
  - Regional grouping of lymph nodes: cervicofacial, supraclavicular, axillary, epitrochlear, inguinal, and femoral
- **Lymph**
  - Fluid found in interstitial spaces
  - Composition of lymph: water and end products of cell metabolism
- **Spleen**
  - The largest lymphatic organ
  - Filters blood
  - Traps formed particles
  - Destroys bacteria
  - Serves as blood reservoir
  - Forms lymphocytes and monocytes
- **Erythrocytes: red blood cells (RBCs)**
  - RBCs are formed in the bone marrow
  - RBCs contain hemoglobin (Hb)
  - Oxygen binds with Hb to form oxyhemoglobin
- **Thrombocytes (platelets)**
  - Formed in the bone marrow

WBC types and functions

White blood cells (WBCs), or leukocytes, protect the body against harmful bacteria and infection. WBCs are classified as granular leukocytes (basophils, neutrophils, and eosinophils) or nongranular leukocytes (lymphocytes, monocytes, and plasma cells). WBCs are usually produced in bone marrow; lymphocytes and plasma cells are produced in lymphoid tissue as well. Neutrophils have a circulating half-life of less than 6 hours, while some lymphocytes may survive for weeks or months. Normally, WBCs number between 5,000 and 10,000 µl. There are six types of WBCs:

- Neutrophils—The predominant form of granulocyte, neutrophils make up about 60% of WBCs and help devour invading organisms by phagocytosis.
- Eosinophils—Minor granulocytes, eosinophils may defend against parasites and lung and skin infections, and may act in allergic reactions. They account for 1% to 5% of the total WBC count.
- Basophils—Minor granulocytes, basophils may release heparin and histamine into the blood and participate in delayed hypersensitivity reactions. They account for up to 1% of the total WBC count.
- Monocytes—Along with neutrophils, monocytes help devour invading organisms by phagocytosis. Monocytes help process antigens for lymphocytes and form macrophages in the tissues. They account for 1% to 6% of total WBC count.
- Lymphocytes—These occur as B cells and T cells: B cells form lymphoid follicles, produce humoral antibodies, and help T-cell mediated delayed hypersensitivity reactions and the rejection of foreign cells or cell products. Lymphocytes account for 20% to 40% of the total WBC count.
- Plasma cells—Residing in tissue, plasma cells develop from lymphoblasts and produce antibodies.

Types of WBCs

- Neutrophils: predominant form; help devour invading organisms
- Eosinophils: minor granulocytes; defend against parasites and infections
- Basophils: minor granulocytes; participate in delayed hypersensitivity reactions
- Monocytes: help devour invading organisms; help process antigens
- Lymphocytes: occur as B cells and T cells
- Plasma cells: reside in tissue; produce antibodies

- Function in the coagulation of blood
- **Leukocytes: white blood cells (WBCs)**
  - WBCs are formed in the bone marrow and lymphatic tissue (see *WBC types and functions*)
  - WBCs include granulocytes and agranulocytes
  - Provide immunity and protection from infection by phagocytosis
- **Plasma**
  - Liquid portion of the blood
  - Composition of plasma: water, protein (albumin and globulin), glucose, and electrolytes
- **ABO blood groups**
  - System of antigens located on the surface of RBCs that determines blood type
  - Blood types: A antigen, B antigen, AB antigens, O (zero) antigens
  - Universal donor: blood type O
  - Universal recipient: blood type AB
- **Coagulation**
  - Blood clotting

Key facts about plasma

- Liquid portion of blood
- Contains water, protein, glucose, and electrolytes

Key facts about ABO blood groups

- Antigens that determine blood type
- Blood types: A antigen, B antigen, AB antigens, O antigens
- Blood type O: universal donor; blood type AB: universal recipient

Key facts about bone marrow

- Red: source of lymphocytes and macrophages; carries out hematopoiesis
- Yellow: red bone marrow that has changed to fat

Key functions of the liver

- Produces and conveys bile
- Metabolizes carbohydrates, fats, and proteins
- Stores vitamins
- Detoxifies chemicals
- Excretes bilirubin
- Produces and stores glycogen

Key history findings in hematologic and lymphatic disorders

- Enlarged glands
- Pain
- Fatigue and weakness
- Bleeding
- Activity intolerance

Key physical assessment findings in hematologic and lymphatic disorders

- Lymph node enlargement
- Ecchymosis
- Skin: pallor, cyanosis, jaundice, and petechiae

- Series of reactions involving the conversion of prothrombin to thrombin to fibrinogen to fibrin to form a clot

● **Bone marrow**
- Two types exist: red and yellow
- Hematopoiesis is carried out by red marrow
- Hematopoiesis produces erythrocytes, leukocytes, and thrombocytes
- Red bone marrow is a source of lymphocytes and macrophages
- Yellow bone marrow is red bone marrow that has changed to fat

● **Liver**
- The largest internal organ in the body
- Produces bile (main function), which emulsifies fats and stimulates peristalsis
- Conveys bile to the duodenum at the sphincter of Oddi through the common bile duct
- Metabolizes carbohydrates, fats, and proteins
- Synthesizes coagulation factors VII, IX, X, and prothrombin
- Stores vitamins A, D, B_{12}, and iron
- Detoxifies chemicals
- Excretes bilirubin
- Receives dual blood supply from portal vein and hepatic artery
- Produces and stores glycogen
- Promotes erythropoiesis when bone marrow production is insufficient

ASSESSMENT FINDINGS

● **History**
- Enlarged glands
- Pain
- Fatigue and weakness
- Bleeding
- Pallor
- Lassitude
- Shortness of breath
- Fainting
- Vertigo
- Jaundice
- Night sweats
- Fever
- Weight loss
- Tachycardia
- Activity intolerance
- Frequent infections
- Melena
- Headache

● **Physical examination**
- Lymph node enlargement

- Ecchymosis
- Skin: pallor, cyanosis, jaundice, and petechiae
- Gingivitis
- Ophthalmoscopic examination: bleeding fundi
- Sclera: jaundice, capillary hemorrhage
- Hepatomegaly
- Sternal tenderness
- Splenomegaly
- Dyspnea on exertion

DIAGNOSTIC TESTS AND PROCEDURES

● **Blood chemistry**
  - Definition and purpose
    – Laboratory test of a blood sample
    – Analysis for potassium, calcium, blood urea nitrogen (BUN), creatinine, protein, albumin, and bilirubin
  - Nursing interventions
    – Explain the procedure to the patient
    – Check the site for bleeding after the procedure

● **Hematologic studies**
  - Definition and purpose
    – Laboratory test of a blood sample
    – Analysis for WBCs, RBCs, erythrocyte sedimentation rate (ESR), Hb, hematocrit (HCT), and platelet count
  - Nursing interventions
    – Explain the procedure to the patient
    – Check the site for bleeding after the procedure

● **Coagulation studies**
  - Definition and purpose
    – Laboratory tests of a blood sample
    – Analysis for prothrombin time (PT), partial thromboplastin time (PTT), International Normalized Ratio, activated coagulation time (ACT), bleeding time, fibrinogen, and fibrin degradation products
  - Nursing interventions
    – Explain the procedure to the patient
    – Note current coagulation therapy
    – Check the site for bleeding after the procedure

● **Lymphangiography**
  - Definition and purpose
    – Procedure involving an injection of contrast media through a catheter into lymphatic vessels in the hands and feet
    – Radiographic picture of lymphatic system and dissection of lymph vessel taken at intervals after injection
  - Nursing interventions before the procedure
    – Explain the procedure to the patient

Key facts about blood chemistry

- Laboratory test of a blood sample
- Analysis for potassium, calcium, BUN, creatinine, protein, albumin, and bilirubin
- Intervention: check the site for bleeding after the procedure

Key facts about hematologic studies

- Laboratory test of a blood sample
- Analysis for WBCs, RBCs, ESR, Hb, HCT, and platelet count
- Intervention: note current drug therapy before the procedure

Key facts about coagulation studies

- Laboratory tests of blood sample
- Analysis for platelet function, platelet count, PT, PTT, ACT, and bleeding time
- Intervention: check the site for bleeding after the procedure

Key facts about lymphangiography

- Procedure involving an injection of contrast media into lymphatic vessels in the hands and feet
- Intervention: check catheter insertion site for bleeding after the procedure

Key facts about bone marrow examination

- Procedure that involves the percutaneous removal of bone marrow
- Examines erythrocytes, leukocytes, thrombocytes, and precursor cells
- Intervention: administer analgesics or anxiolytics, as ordered

Key facts about the Shilling test

- Administration of oral radioactive cyanocobalamin and I.M. cyanocobalamin
- Microscopic examination of 24-hour urine specimen for cyanocobalamin
- Intervention: withhold food and fluids after midnight

Key facts about erythrocyte life span determination

- Procedure involving reinjection of the patient's blood that has been tagged with chromium 51
- Measures life span of RBCs
- Intervention: inform the patient that frequent blood samples will be drawn over a 2-week period

---

- Note the patient's allergies to iodine, seafood, and radiopaque dyes
- Inform the patient of possible throat irritation and flushing of the face after injection of the dye
- Place obtained written informed consent in the patient's chart
- Withhold food and fluids, as directed
- Nursing interventions after the procedure
  - Assess vital signs and peripheral pulses
  - Check catheter insertion site for bleeding
  - Advise the patient that skin, stools, and urine will have a blue discoloration for 48 hours

Bone marrow examination (aspiration or biopsy)
- Definition and purpose
  - Procedure involving the percutaneous removal of bone marrow
  - Examination of erythrocytes, leukocytes, thrombocytes, and precursor cells
- Nursing interventions before the procedure
  - Explain the procedure to the patient
  - Place obtained written informed consent in the patient's chart
  - Administer analgesics or anxiolytics, as ordered
- Nursing interventions after the procedure
  - Maintain pressure dressing
  - Check the aspiration site for bleeding and infection

Schilling test
- Definition and purpose
  - Procedure involving administration of oral radioactive cyanocobalamin and I.M. cyanocobalamin
  - Microscopic examination of a 24-hour urine specimen for cyanocobalamin (vitamin B_{12})
- Nursing interventions before the procedure
  - Explain the procedure to the patient
  - Withhold food and fluids after midnight
  - Place obtained written informed consent in the patient's chart
- Nursing interventions after the procedure
  - Instruct the patient to save all voided urine for 24 hours
  - Keep urine at room temperature

Erythrocyte life span determination
- Definition and purpose
  - Procedure involving reinjection of the patient's blood that has been tagged with chromium 51
  - Measurement of the life span of circulating RBCs
- Nursing interventions
  - Explain the procedure to the patient
  - Inform the patient that frequent blood samples will be drawn over a 2-week period
  - Check the venipuncture site for bleeding

- **Bence Jones protein assay**
  - Definition and purpose
    - Procedure involving a 24-hour urine specimen
    - Microscopic examination for the Bence Jones protein
  - Nursing interventions
    - Explain the procedure to the patient
    - Withhold all medications for 48 hours before the test
    - Instruct the patient to void and note the time (collection of urine starts with the next voiding)
    - Place urine container on ice
    - Measure each voided urine
    - Instruct the patient to void at the end of the 24-hour period

- **Erythrocyte fragility test**
  - Definition and purpose
    - Laboratory test of a blood sample
    - Analysis to measure the rate at which RBCs burst in varied hypotonic solutions
  - Nursing interventions
    - Explain the procedure to the patient
    - Check the venipuncture site for bleeding

- **Bone scan**
  - Definition and purpose
    - Procedure using an I.V. injection of radioisotope
    - Visual imaging of bone metabolism
  - Nursing interventions before the procedure
    - Explain the procedure to the patient
    - Determine the patient's ability to lie still

PSYCHOSOCIAL IMPACT OF HEMATOLOGIC AND LYMPHATIC DISORDERS

- **Developmental impact**
  - Fear of dying
  - Decreased self-esteem

- **Economic impact**
  - Disruption or loss of employment
  - Cost of hospitalization
  - Cost of medications

- **Occupational and recreational impact**
  - Restrictions in work activity
  - Changes in leisure activity

- **Social impact**
  - Changes in role performance
  - Social isolation

Key facts about Bence Jones protein assay

- Involves 24-hour urine specimen
- Examines for Bence Jones protein
- Intervention: instruct the patient to void and note the time

Key facts about erythrocyte fragility test

- Laboratory test of blood sample
- Measures the rate at which RBCs burst in hypotonic solutions
- Intervention: check the site for bleeding after the procedure

Key facts about bone scan

- Procedure involving injection of radioisotope
- Visual imaging of bone metabolism
- Intervention: determine the patient's ability to lie still

Major impacts of hematologic and lymphatic system disorders

- Fear of dying
- Costs of loss of employment, hospitalizations, and medications
- Restrictions in activity
- Changes in role performance

Key modifiable risk factors for hematologic and lymphatic system disorders

- Exposure to pollutants
- Sexual activity patterns
- Aspirin use

Key nonmodifiable risk factors for hematologic and lymphatic system disorders

- Ethnic background
- History of liver disease

Probable nursing diagnoses for a patient with a hematologic and lymphatic system disorder

- Risk for activity intolerance
- Ineffective breathing pattern
- Chronic pain
- Impaired gas exchange

Possible nursing diagnoses for a patient with a hematologic and lymphatic system disorder

- Risk for infection
- Disturbed body image
- Social isolation

Key facts about splenectomy

- Surgical removal of the spleen

RISK FACTORS

- **Modifiable risk factors**
  - Exposure to chemical and environmental pollutants
  - Aspirin use
  - Alcohol consumption
  - Drug toxicity
  - Diet
  - Exposure to occupational radiation or radiation therapy
  - Sexual activity patterns

- **Nonmodifiable risk factors**
  - Ethnic background
  - Age
  - Malabsorption syndromes
  - History of liver disease
  - History of malignancy

NURSING DIAGNOSES

- **Probable nursing diagnoses**
  - Risk for activity intolerance
  - Ineffective breathing pattern
  - Chronic pain
  - Impaired gas exchange
  - Fatigue
  - Anxiety

- **Possible nursing diagnoses**
  - Risk for infection
  - Imbalanced nutrition: Less than body requirements
  - Impaired oral mucous membrane
  - Disturbed body image
  - Situational low self-esteem
  - Social isolation
  - Risk for impaired skin integrity

SPLENECTOMY

- **Description**
  - Surgical removal of the spleen

- **Preoperative nursing interventions**
  - Complete patient and family preoperative teaching
    - Explain the procedure to the patient
    - Describe the operating room, postanesthesia care unit (PACU), and preoperative and postoperative routines

    – Demonstrate postoperative turning, coughing, deep breathing, splinting, and incentive spirometry

    – Explain the postoperative need for drainage tubes, surgical dressings, oxygen therapy, I.V. therapy, and pain control

- Complete a preoperative checklist and make sure a signed informed consent is in the patient's chart
- Administer preoperative medications as prescribed
- Allay the patient's and his family's anxiety about surgery
- Document the patient's history and physical assessment database
- Monitor PT, PTT, HCT, Hb, and platelet count
- Verify inoculation with polyvalent pneumococcal vaccine 2 weeks before the procedure

● Postoperative nursing interventions

- Assess cardiac, respiratory, and neurologic status
- Assess pain level, administer postoperative analgesics as prescribed, and evaluate response
- Assess for return of peristalsis; advance diet as tolerated
- Administer I.V. fluids and transfusion therapy, as prescribed
- Provide wound care as directed
- Encourage turning, coughing, deep breathing, and use of incentive spirometry
- Increase activity as tolerated
- Monitor and record vital signs, intake and output (I/O), laboratory studies, and pulse oximetry
- Monitor and maintain position and patency of drainage tubes
- Monitor for signs and symptoms of infection
- Individualize home care instructions
    - Know about the surgery and recovery
    - Complete incision care daily
    - State the need for prophylactic use of antibiotics
    - Avoid contact sports

● Surgical complications

- Pneumococcal pneumonia
- Infection
- Hemorrhage
- Disseminated intravascular coagulation (DIC)
- Atelectasis
- Subphrenic abscess
- Thrombophlebitis

BONE MARROW TRANSPLANT

● Description

- Bone marrow is aspirated from multiple sites along the donor's iliac crest
- Donor bone marrow is infused I.V. into the recipient

Key nursing interventions before bone marrow transplant

- Administer preoperative medications.
- Administer chemotherapy or radiation therapy.
- Protect the patient from infection.

Key nursing interventions after bone marrow transplant

- Administer antibiotics as prescribed.
- Provide postchemotherapeutic and postradiation nursing care.
- Inspect for bruising and petechiae.
- Administer immunosuppressants as prescribed.

Key complications after bone marrow transplant

- Marrow graft rejection
- Graft versus host disease
- Hemorrhage

● Preoperative nursing interventions

- Complete patient and family preoperative teaching
  - Explain the procedure to the patient
  - Describe the operating room, PACU, and preoperative and postoperative routines
  - Demonstrate postoperative turning, coughing, deep breathing, splinting, and incentive spirometry
  - Explain the postoperative need for drainage tubes, surgical dressings, oxygen therapy, I.V. therapy, and pain control
- Complete a preoperative checklist and make sure a signed informed consent is in the patient's chart
- Administer preoperative medications as prescribed
- Allay the patient's and his family's anxiety about surgery
- Document the patient's history and physical assessment database
- Administer chemotherapy or radiation therapy, as directed
- Protect the patient from infection

● Postoperative nursing interventions

- Assess cardiac and respiratory status
- Administer I.V. fluids
- Allay the patient's anxiety
- Maintain activity as tolerated
- Monitor and record vital signs, I/O, central venous pressure (CVP), laboratory studies, daily weight, and pulse oximetry values
- Encourage the patient to express feelings about the procedure
- Administer antibiotics as prescribed, and monitor for signs and symptoms of infection
- Provide postchemotherapeutic and postradiation nursing care
  - Provide prophylactic skin, mouth, and perineal care
  - Monitor dietary intake
  - Administer antiemetics and antidiarrheals, as prescribed
  - Monitor for bleeding, infection, and electrolyte imbalance
  - Provide rest periods
- Inspect for bruising and petechiae
- Administer immunosuppressants as prescribed
- Individualize home care instructions
  - Know about the procedure and recovery
  - Avoid crowds and people with infection
  - Recognize the signs and symptoms of infection and bleeding

● Surgical complications

- Marrow graft rejection
- Graft-versus-host disease
- Cataracts
- Stomatitis
- Hemorrhage

LEUKEMIA

- **Definition**
  - Unregulated proliferation or accumulation of WBCs in the bone marrow
  - Three types
    - Acute myelogenous
    - Chronic lymphocytic
    - Chronic myelocytic

- **Causes**
  - Unknown
  - Genetic influence
  - Viral pathogenesis
  - Exposure to chemicals
  - Radiation
  - Altered immune system
  - Chemotherapy
  - History of hematologic disorder

- **Pathophysiology**
  - Normal hemopoietic cells are replaced by leukemic cells in bone marrow
  - Immature forms of WBCs circulate in the blood, infiltrating the liver, spleen, and lymph nodes, and invading nonhematologic organs, such as the meninges, GI tract, kidneys, and skin

- **Assessment findings**
  - Weakness and fatigue
  - Petechiae
  - Ecchymosis
  - Frequent infections
  - Elevated temperature
  - Enlarged lymph nodes, spleen, and liver
  - Joint, abdominal, and bone pain
  - Gingivitis, bleeding gums
  - Night sweats
  - Stomatitis
  - Prolonged menses
  - Hematemesis
  - Melena
  - Pallor or jaundice
  - Tachycardia
  - Hypotension
  - Epistaxis
  - Generalized pain

- **Diagnostic test findings**
  - Hematology: decreased HCT, Hb, RBCs, and platelets; increased ESR, immature WBCs, and bleeding time
  - Bone marrow biopsy: large number of immature leukocytes

Key facts about leukemia

- Unregulated proliferation or accumulation of WBCs in the bone marrow
- Three types: acute myelogenous, chronic lymphocytic, and chronic myelocytic

Common causes of leukemia

- Genetic influence
- Viral pathogenesis
- Exposure to chemicals

TOP 3

Signs and symptoms of leukemia

1. Frequent infections
2. Enlarged lymph nodes, spleen, and liver
3. Weakness and fatigue

Diagnosing leukemia

- Hematology: decreased HCT, Hb, RBCs, and platelets; increased ESR, immature WBCs, and bleeding time
- Bone marrow biopsy: large number of immature leukocytes

Treating leukemia

- Radiation therapy
- Antineoplastics
- Antibiotics
- Transfusion therapy

Key nursing interventions for a patient with leukemia

- Monitor and record vital signs, I/O, laboratory studies, and daily weight.
- Administer transfusion therapy as prescribed.
- Monitor for bleeding and infection.
- Maintain protective precautions.
- Avoid giving the patient I.M. injections and enemas and taking his temperature rectally.
- Provide postchemotherapeutic and postradiation nursing care.

● **Medical management**
- Diet: neutropenic (no raw meat, fruits, or vegetables)
- I.V. therapy: fluids as needed
- Oxygen therapy
- Activity: as tolerated
- Monitoring: vital signs, I/O, and laboratory studies
- Radiation therapy
- Transfusion therapy: platelets, packed RBCs, and whole blood
- Antibiotics: doxorubicin (Adriamycin), plicamycin (Mithracin)
- Antipyretic: acetaminophen (Tylenol)
- Analgesic: ibuprofen (Motrin)
- Antigout: allopurinol (Zyloprim)
- Cortocosteroids: prednisone (Deltasone)
- Antineoplastics: vincristine (Oncovin), methotrexate (MTX), daunorubicin (Cerubidine), cytarabine (Cytosar-U), cytosine arabinoside (ARA-U)
- Enzyme: Asparaginase (Elspar)
- Interferon alfa-2b (Intron A)
- Tyrosine kinase inhibitor: imatinib mesylate (Gleevec)
- Stem cell transplant
- Leukapheresis
- Granulocyte colony–stimulating factor: filgrastim (Neupogen)

● **Nursing interventions**
- Monitor the patient's diet for restrictions
- Administer I.V. fluids
- Administer oxygen
- Promote turning, coughing, and deep breathing
- Assess cardiovascular, neurologic, respiratory, and renal status and fluid balance
- Monitor and record vital signs, I/O, laboratory studies, and daily weight
- Administer transfusion therapy as prescribed
- Administer medications as prescribed
- Encourage the patient to express feelings about his diagnosis
- Allay the patient's anxiety and provide emotional support
- **Monitor for bleeding and infection**
- Maintain protective precautions
- Provide mouth and skin care
- **Avoid giving the patient I.M. injections and enemas and taking his temperature rectally**
- Provide postchemotherapeutic and postradiation nursing care
  - Provide prophylactic skin, mouth, and perineal care
  - Monitor dietary intake
  - Administer antiemetics and antidiarrheals, as prescribed
  - Monitor for bleeding, infection, and electrolyte imbalance
  - Provide rest periods
- Individualize home care instructions (for teaching tips, see *Patients with hematologic or lymphatic disorders*)
  - Know about the disorder and its treatment

TIME-OUT FOR TEACHING

Patients with hematologic or lymphatic disorders

Be sure to include the following topics in your teaching plan when caring for patients with hematologic or lymphatic disorders.

- Medication therapy, including the action, adverse effects, and scheduling of medications
- Infection control measures
- Signs and symptoms of infection and bleeding
- Daily skin, mouth, and foot care
- Dietary recommendations and restrictions
- Avoidance of over-the-counter medications
- Prevention of constipation
- Medical identification jewelry
- Safe environment
- Independence in activities of daily living (ADLs)
- Reactions to limitation on lifestyle and ADLs
- Rest and activity patterns, including any limitations or restrictions
- Community agencies and resources for supportive services
- Smoking cessation
- Follow-up appointments

– Follow instructions for medication use and be aware of possible adverse effects
– Follow dietary restrictions
– Contact the American Cancer Society
– Recognize the signs and symptoms of bleeding and infection
– Comply with medical follow-up

● **Complications**
- Gross systemic hemorrhage
- Acute renal failure
- Stroke
- Thrombocytopenia
- Perirectal abscess
- GI bleeding
- Fungal and bacterial infection
- Meningitis

● **Surgical intervention**
- Splenectomy

LYMPHOMAS

● **Definition**
- Neoplastic cells of lymphoid origin
- Hodgkin's disease: proliferation of malignant Reed-Sternberg cells within lymph nodes
- Non-Hodgkin's lymphoma: malignant tumors of lymph nodes and lymphatic tissues that can't be classified as Hodgkin's disease

---

Key teaching topics for a patient with a hematologic or lymphatic disorder

- Infection control measures
- Signs and symptoms of infection and bleeding
- Medication therapy
- Daily skin, mouth, and foot care
- Medical identification jewelry

Key complications of leukemia

- Gross systemic hemorrhage
- Fungal and bacterial infection

Key facts about lymphomas

- Neoplastic cells of lymphoid origin
- Hodgkin's disease: proliferation of malignant Reed-Sternberg cells within lymph nodes
- Non-Hodgkin's lymphoma: malignant tumors of lymph nodes and lymphatic tissues that can't be classified as Hodgkin's disease
- Classes of non-Hodgkin's lymphoma: B-lymphocyte malignancies, T-lymphocyte malignancies, and histiocyte malignancies

Common causes of lymphomas

- Unknown

Key risk factors for lymphomas

- Genetic
- Environmental
- Immunologic

Key signs and symptoms of lymphomas

Hodgkin's disease
- Fatigue
- Dyspnea
- Recurrent intermittent fever

Non-Hodgkin's lymphoma
- Enlarged, nontender, firm, and movable lymph nodes in lower cervical regions
- Anorexia
- Weight loss
- Severe pruritus

Diagnosing lymphomas

- Bone marrow aspiration and biopsy: small, diffuse lymphocytic or large, follicular-type cells (non-Hodgkin's lymphoma)
- Lymph node biopsy: positive for Reed-Sternberg cells (Hodgkin's disease)

- Classes of non-Hodgkin's lymphoma: B-lymphocyte malignancies, T-lymphocyte malignancies, and histiocyte malignancies

● **Causes**
- Unknown

● **Risk factors**
- Viral
- Genetic (Hodgkin's disease)
- Environmental (Hodgkin's disease)
- Immunologic disorder

● **Pathophysiology**
- Reed-Sternberg cells proliferate in a single lymph node and travel contiguously through the lymphatic system to other lymphatic nodes and organs (Hodgkin's disease)
- Immune system cell tumors occur throughout lymph nodes and lymphatic organs in unpredictable patterns (non-Hodgkin's lymphoma)

● **Assessment findings**
- Enlarged, nontender, firm, and movable lymph nodes (non-Hodgkin's lymphoma)
- Recurrent, intermittent fever
- Fatigue
- Weight loss
- Malaise
- Severe pruritus (non-Hodgkin's lymphoma)
- Dyspnea (Hodgkin's disease)
- Anorexia (non-Hodgkin's lymphoma)
- Bone pain (Hodgkin's disease)
- Cough
- Weight loss (non-Hodgkin's lymphoma)
- Recurrent infection
- Hepatomegaly
- Splenomegaly
- Dysphagia (Hodgkin's disease)
- Edema and cyanosis of face and neck (Hodgkin's disease)

● **Diagnostic test findings**
- Bone marrow aspiration and biopsy: small, diffuse lymphocytic or large, follicular-type cells (non-Hodgkin's lymphoma)
- Hematology: decreased Hb, HCT, and platelets (non-Hodgkin's lymphoma and Hodgkin's disease); increased ESR (Hodgkin's disease and non-Hodgkin's lymphoma); increased leukocytes and gamma globulin (Hodgkin's disease)
- Lymphangiogram: positive lymph node involvement (Hodgkin's disease)
- Lymph node biopsy: positive for Reed-Sternberg cells (Hodgkin's disease), malignant cells (non-Hodgkin's lymphoma)
- Chest X-ray: lymphadenopathy (Hodgkin's disease)

- Positron-emission tomography: positive for malignant tumor cells (non-Hodgkin's lymphoma)

Medical management

- Diet: neutropenic if WBC count is low
- I.V. therapy: fluids as needed
- Oxygen therapy
- Activity: as tolerated
- Monitoring: vital signs, I/O, and laboratory studies
- Radiation therapy
- Transfusion therapy: packed RBCs
- Combined chemotherapy
  - MOPP chemotherapy protocol (Hodgkin's disease): mechlorethamine (Mustargen), vincristine (Oncovin), procarbazine (Matulane), and prednisone (Deltasone)
  - ABVD chemotherapy protocol (Hodgkin's disease): doxorubicin (Adriamycin), bleomycin (Blenoxane), vinblastine (Velban), and dacarbazine (DTIC-Dome)
  - CVP chemotherapy protocol (non-Hodgkin's lymphoma): cyclophosphamide (Cytoxan), vincristine (Oncovin), and prednisone (Deltasone)
  - CHOP chemotherapy protocol (non-Hodgkin's lymphoma): cyclophosphamide (Cytoxan), hydroxydaunorubicin (Adriamycin), vincristine (Oncovin), and prednisone (Deltasone)
- Analgesic: meperidine (Demerol)
- Immunotherapy: rituximab (Rituxan) (non-Hodgkin's lymphoma)
- Radioimmunotherapy: ibritumomab tiuxetan (Zevalin) (non-Hodgkin's lymphoma)
- Antipruritic: diphenhydramine (Benadryl)
- Antiemetic: ondansetron (Zofran)
- Bone marrow or stem cell transplant

Nursing interventions

- Encourage fluids
- Administer I.V. fluids as needed
- Administer oxygen
- Promote turning, coughing, and deep breathing
- Assess respiratory, cardiovascular, and neurologic status and fluid balance
- Monitor and record vital signs, I/O, and laboratory studies
- Administer medications as prescribed
- Encourage the patient to express feelings about his diagnosis
- Encourage activity as tolerated, with frequent rest periods
- Provide mouth and skin care
- Administer transfusion therapy as prescribed
- Allay the patient's anxiety and provide emotional support
- Provide postchemotherapeutic and postradiation nursing care
  - Provide prophylactic skin, mouth, and perineal care
  - Monitor dietary intake

- – Administer antiemetics and antidiarrheals, as prescribed
- – Monitor for bleeding, infection, and electrolyte imbalance
- – Provide rest periods
- Individualize home care instructions
  - – Know about the disorder and its treatment
  - – Follow instructions for medication use and be aware of possible adverse effects
  - – Follow dietary restrictions if neutropenic
  - – Avoid crowds and people with infections
  - – Contact the American Cancer Society
  - – Recognize the signs and symptoms of complications
  - – Avoid taking aspirin
  - – Comply with medical follow-up

● **Complications**
- Metastasis (Hodgkin's disease)
- Hypersplenism
- Pleural effusion (Hodgkin's disease)
- Herpes zoster (Hodgkin's disease)
- Depression
- Pancytopenia (Hodgkin's disease)
- Hypothyroidism (Hodgkin's disease)
- Neuralgia (Hodgkin's disease)
- Obstructive jaundice (Hodgkin's disease)
- Infections: viral, bacterial, fungal
- Intestinal obstruction (non-Hodgkin's lymphoma)
- Leukemia (non-Hodgkin's lymphoma)
- Superior vena cava obstruction (non-Hodgkin's lymphoma)

● **Surgical interventions**
- Splenectomy

ACQUIRED IMMUNODEFICIENCY SYNDROME (AIDS)

● **Definition**
- Defect in T-cell mediated immunity that allows the development of fatal opportunistic infections
- An illness characterized by laboratory evidence of human immunodeficiency virus (HIV) infection coexisting with one or more indicator diseases, such as herpes simplex virus, cytomegalovirus, mycobacteria, candidal infection, *Pneumocystis carinii,* Kaposi's sarcoma, wasting syndrome, or dementia

● **Causes**
- Exposure to blood containing HIV: transfusions, contaminated needles, handling of blood, or in utero
- Exposure to semen and vaginal secretions containing HIV: unprotected sexual intercourse or handling of semen and vaginal secretions

---

Key complications of lymphomas

- Metastasis
- Infections
- Leukemia (non-Hodgkin's lymphoma)

Key facts about AIDS

- Defect in T-cell mediated immunity that allows the development of fatal opportunistic infections

Common causes of AIDS

- Exposure to blood containing HIV
- Exposure to semen or vaginal secretions containing HIV

Pathophysiology

- HIV is transmitted by contact with infected blood or body fluids
  - HIV-infected lymphocytes are carried in semen, vaginal secretions, and blood
  - Infected lymphocytes in semen and vaginal secretions are transferred through minute breaks in the skin and mucosa
  - Infected lymphocytes in blood are transferred via transfusion, fetal circulation, and minute breaks in the skin and mucosa
- HIV, a retrovirus, selectively infects human cells containing CD4+ antigen on their surface, the majority of which are T4 lymphocytes
- HIV virus reproduces within the T4 lymphocytes and destroys them
- The destruction of the T4 lymphocytes diminishes resistance to disease

Assessment findings

- Fatigue
- Weakness
- Anorexia
- Weight loss
- Recurrent diarrhea
- Fever
- Lymphadenopathy
- Pallor
- Night sweats
- Malnutrition
- Disorientation, confusion, dementia
- Opportunistic infections

Diagnostic test findings

- Enzyme linked immunosorbent assay (ELISA): positive HIV antibody titer
- Western blot: positive
- CD4+ level: less than 200 cells/mm^3

Medical management

- I.V. therapy: hydration, electrolyte replacement, and saline lock
- Oxygen therapy
- Activity: as tolerated, active and passive ROM exercises
- Monitoring: vital signs, I/O, pulse oximetry, daily weight, and laboratory studies
- Nutritional support: total parenteral nutrition (TPN) if the patient can't take food by mouth
- Treatments: chest physiotherapy, postural drainage, and incentive spirometry
- Transfusion therapy: fresh frozen plasma, platelets, and packed RBCs
- Antibiotics: pentamidine (Pentam), trimethoprim/sulfamethoxazole (Bactrim)
- Highly active antiretroviral therapy (HAART)
  - Nucleoside reverse transcriptase inhibitors: zidovudine (Retrovir, AZT), zalcitabine (Dideoxycytidine, ddC), lamivudine (Epivir), abacavir (Ziagen), and stavudine (Zerit)

Key signs and symptoms of AIDS

- Anorexia
- Weight loss
- Recurrent diarrhea
- Night sweats
- Disorientation, confusion, dementia
- Opportunistic infections

Diagnosing AIDS

- ELISA: positive HIV antibody titer
- Western blot: positive
- CD4+ level: less than 200 cells/mm^3

Treating AIDS

- Transfusion therapy: fresh frozen plasma, platelets, and packed RBCs
- HAART
- Antibiotics

– Protease inhibitors: lopinavir/ritonavir (Kaletra), indinavir (Crixivan), nelfinavir (Viracept), amprenavir (Agenerase), and saquinavir (Invi-rase)
– Nonnucleoside reverse transcriptase inhibitors: nevirapine (Vira-mune), efavirenz (Sustiva), and delavirdine (Rescriptor)
● Fusion inhibitor: enfuvirtide (Fuzeon)
● Antifungals: fluconazole (Diflucan) and amphotericin B (Fungizone)
● Glucocorticoid: prednisone (Deltasone) (*Pneumocystis carinii* pneumonia)

● **Nursing interventions**
● Administer I.V. fluids as ordered
● Administer oxygen
● Encourage turning, coughing, deep breathing, and use of incentive spirometry
● Assess respiratory and neurologic status and fluid balance
● Monitor and record vital signs, I/O, laboratory studies, daily weight, and pulse oximetry
● Administer TPN as ordered
● Administer medications as prescribed
● Encourage the patient to express his feelings about his diagnosis
● Maintain activity as tolerated, and provide rest periods
● Allay the patient's anxiety and provide emotional support
● Provide skin and mouth care
● Monitor for opportunistic infections
● Individualize home care instructions
    – Know about the disorder and its treatment
    – Follow instructions for medication use and be aware of possible ad-verse effects
    – Refrain from donating blood
    – Avoid using alcohol and recreational drugs
    – Use condoms during sexual intercourse
    – Contact community resources
    – Comply with medical follow-up

● **Complications**
● *Pneumocystis carinii* pneumonia
● Cryptococcal meningitis
● Burkitt's lymphoma
● Encephalopathy
● Depression
● Herpes simplex virus
● Cytomegalovirus infection
● Epstein-Barr virus
● Oral and esophageal candidiasis
● Kaposi's sarcoma
● Toxoplasmosis
● *Mycobacterium avium* intracellular infection
● Neuropathies

- Myopathies
- **Surgical intervention**
  - None

IRON DEFICIENCY ANEMIA

- **Definition**
  - Chronic, slowly progressive decrease in circulating RBCs
  - Iron deficiency caused by inadequate absorption or excessive loss of iron; decreased iron affects formation of Hb and RBCs
- **Causes**
  - Acute and chronic bleeding
  - Inadequate intake of iron-rich foods
  - Malabsorption syndrome
  - Pregnancy
  - Lead poisoning
  - Mechanical erythrocyte trauma caused by prosthetic heart valve or vena cava filter
- **Pathophysiology**
  - Iron deficiency is caused by inadequate absorption or excessive loss of iron
  - Decreased iron affects formation of Hb and RBCs
  - Decreased Hb and RBCs reduce the capacity of the blood to transport oxygen to cells
- **Assessment findings**
  - Weakness and fatigue
  - History of bleeding
  - Palpitations, tachycardia
  - Leg cramps
  - Inability to concentrate
  - Stomatitis
  - Dyspnea on exertion
  - Pale, dry mucous membranes
  - Red, swollen, smooth, shiny, and tender tongue
  - Cheilosis (inflammation and cracking of the corners of the mouth)
  - Pica
  - Pallor
  - Koilonychia (spoon-shaped nails)
- **Diagnostic test findings**
  - Hematology: decreased Hb, HCT, iron, ferritin, reticulocytes, red cell indices, transferrin saturation; absent hemosiderin; increased total iron-binding capacity
  - Peripheral blood smear: microcytic and hypochromic RBCs
  - Bone marrow aspiration: absence of stainable iron

Key facts about iron deficiency anemia

- Chronic, slowly progressive decrease in circulating RBCs
- Iron deficiency caused by inadequate absorption or excessive loss of iron
- Decreased iron affects formation of Hb and RBCs

Common causes of iron deficiency anemia

- Acute and chronic bleeding
- Malabsorption syndrome
- Pregnancy

Key signs and symptoms of iron deficiency anemia

- Weakness and fatigue
- Pallor
- History of bleeding

Diagnosing iron deficiency anemia

- Decreased Hb, HCT, and iron levels
- Increased total iron-binding capacity

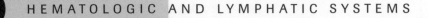

Treating iron deficiency anemia

- High-iron, high-roughage, high-protein, high-ascorbic acid, high-vitamin diet with increased fluids; avoid teas
- Transfusion therapy
- Mineral supplements

Key nursing interventions for a patient with iron deficiency anemia

- Assess cardiovascular and respiratory status.
- Monitor stools, urine, and emesis for occult blood.
- Provide mouth, skin, and foot care.
- Provide rest periods as needed.

Key complications of iron deficiency anemia

- Angina pectoris
- Heart failure

Key facts about pernicious anemia

- Chronic, progressive megaloblastic anemia
- Results in impaired absorption of vitamin B_{12}

Common causes of pernicious anemia

- Deficiency of intrinsic factor
- Inadequate dietary intake (vegetarian diet)
- Gastric mucosal inflammation
- Genetics
- Bacterial or parasitic infections

● Medical management

- Diet: high-iron, high-roughage, high-protein, high-ascorbic acid, high-vitamin with increased fluids; avoid teas and bread
- Oxygen therapy
- Activity: as tolerated
- Monitoring: vital signs and laboratory studies (arterial blood gas [ABG] analysis, Hb, HCT, iron, iron-binding capacity)
- Transfusion therapy: packed RBCs
- Mineral supplements: ferrous sulfate (Feosol), iron dextran (INFeD)
- Vitamins: pyridoxine (vitamin B_6), ascorbic acid (vitamin C)

● Nursing interventions

- Assist the patient with dietary choices
- Administer oxygen as needed
- Assess cardiovascular and respiratory status
- Monitor and record vital signs, and laboratory studies
- Administer medications as prescribed
- Monitor stools, urine, and emesis for occult blood
- Provide rest periods as needed
- Provide mouth, skin, and foot care
- Individualize home care instructions
  - Know about the disorder and its treatment
  - Follow instructions for medication use and be aware of possible adverse effects
  - Follow dietary recommendations
  - Recognize the signs and symptoms of bleeding
  - Monitor stools for occult blood
  - Comply with medical follow-up

● Complications

- Plummer-Vinson syndrome
- Angina pectoris
- Heart failure

● Surgical intervention

- Correction of hemorrhage

PERNICIOUS ANEMIA

● Definition

- Chronic, progressive megaloblastic anemia caused by a deficiency of intrinsic factor, which results in impaired absorption of vitamin B_{12}

● Causes

- Inadequate dietary intake (vegetarian diet)
- Gastric mucosal inflammation
- Genetics
- Lack of administration of vitamin B_{12} after small-bowel resection or total gastrectomy

- Insufficient pancreatic protease
- Bacterial or parasitic infections

● **Pathophysiology**
- Without intrinsic factor, dietary vitamin B_{12} can't be absorbed by the ileum
- Normal deoxyribonucleic acid synthesis is inhibited, resulting in defective maturation of RBCs

● **Assessment findings**
- Weakness, fatigue
- Beefy, smooth, red, sore tongue
- Tingling and paresthesia of hands and feet
- Pallor
- Palpitations, tachycardia
- Sore mouth
- Weight loss and anorexia
- Dyspepsia
- Constipation or diarrhea
- Mild jaundice of sclera
- Positive Romberg test
- Memory loss
- Gait disturbances

● **Diagnostic test findings**
- Schilling test: urine excretion of less than 3% in 24 hours
- Gastric analysis: hypochlorhydria
- Peripheral blood smear: oval, macrocytic, hyperchromic erythrocytes
- Bone marrow: increased megaloblasts; few maturing erythrocytes; defective leukocyte maturation
- Blood chemistry: increased bilirubin and lactate dehydrogenase
- Hematology: decreased HCT and Hb levels

● **Medical management**
- Diet: well-balanced, with increased intake of foods containing vitamin B_{12}
- Activity: as tolerated
- Monitoring: laboratory studies (Hb, HCT, and bilirubin)
- Transfusion therapy: packed RBCs (rare)
- Vitamins: cyanocobalamin (vitamin B_{12}), multivitamins

● **Nursing interventions**
- Assist the patient with dietary choices
- Assess neurologic, cardiovascular, and respiratory status
- Monitor laboratory studies
- Administer medications as prescribed
- Provide mouth care before and after meals
- Prevent the patient from falling
- Individualize home care instructions
  - Know about the disorder and its treatment

TOP 3

Signs and symptoms of pernicious anemia

1. Weakness, fatigue
2. Sore mouth
3. Tingling and paresthesia of hands and feet

Diagnosing pernicious anemia

- Peripheral blood smear results: oval, macrocytic, hyperchromic erythrocytes
- Bone marrow: increased megaloblasts; few maturing erythrocytes; defective leukocyte maturation

Treating pernicious anemia

- Transfusion therapy
- Vitamins
- Well-balanced diet with increased vitamin B_{12}

Key nursing interventions for a patient with pernicious anemia

- Assist with dietary choices.
- Provide mouth care before and after meals.
- Prevent the patient from falling.

– Follow instructions for medication use and be aware of possible adverse effects
– Follow dietary recommendations
– Alter activities of daily living to compensate for paresthesia
– Comply with medical follow-up

● **Complications**
  • Neurologic deficits
  • Gastric cancer
  • Heart failure
  • Angina

● **Surgical intervention**
  • None

APLASTIC ANEMIA (PANCYTOPENIA)

● **Definition**
  • Failure of bone marrow to produce adequate amounts of erythrocytes, leukocytes, and platelets

● **Causes**
  • Idiopathic
  • Congenital or inherited
  • Exposure to chemicals or radiation
  • Drug induced
  • Transfusional graft-versus-host disease
  • Pregnancy
  • Viral infection

● **Pathophysiology**
  • Bone marrow suppression, destruction, or aplasia results in failure of bone marrow to produce an adequate number of stem cells
  • Without an adequate number of stem cells, sufficient amounts of erythrocytes, leukocytes, and platelets can't be produced
  • Pancytopenia includes leukopenia, thrombocytopenia, and anemia

● **Assessment findings**
  • Weakness and fatigue
  • Dyspnea, tachypnea
  • Multiple infections
  • Elevated temperature
  • Headache
  • Anorexia
  • Gingivitis
  • Epistaxis
  • Purpura, petechiae, or ecchymosis
  • Pallor
  • Palpitations, tachycardia
  • Melena

● Diagnostic test findings
- Peripheral blood smear: pancytopenia
- Hematology: decreased granulocytes, thrombocytes, RBCs
- Bone marrow biopsy: fatty marrow with reduction of stem cells

● Medical management
- Transfusion therapy: platelets and packed RBCs
- Diet: well-balanced
- I.V. therapy: hydration
- Oxygen therapy: as needed
- Activity: as tolerated, with frequent rest periods
- Monitoring: vital signs, I/O, and laboratory studies (RBCs, WBCs, platelets, and stools for occult blood)
- Antibiotics: penicillin G (Pfizerpen), ticarcillin (Ticar), and tobramycin (Nebcin)
- Analgesics: ibuprofen (Motrin) and acetaminophen (Tylenol)
- Immunosuppressants: antithymocyte globulin (Atgam), cyclosporine (Sandimmune), methylprednisolone (Solu-Medrol)
- Androgenic steroids: fluoxymesterone (Halotestin) and oxymetholone (Anadrol)
- Granulocyte colony–stimulating factor: filgrastim (Neupogen)
- Hematopoietic growth factor: epoetin alfa (Epogen)

● Nursing interventions
- Administer transfusion therapy as prescribed
- Administer I.V. fluids
- Administer oxygen
- Encourage turning, coughing, and deep breathing
- Assess cardiovascular and respiratory status and fluid balance
- Monitor and record vital signs; I/O; laboratory studies; and stools, urine, and emesis for occult blood
- Administer medications as prescribed
- Allay the patient's anxiety and provide emotional support
- Alternate rest periods with activity
- Provide mouth care before and after meals
- Provide skin care
- **Avoid giving the patient I.M. injections**
- Monitor for infection, bleeding, and bruising
- Individualize home care instructions
  - Know about the disorder and its treatment
  - Follow instructions for medication use and be aware of possible adverse effects
  - Recognize the signs and symptoms of bleeding
  - Avoid contact sports
  - Wear medical identification jewelry
  - Monitor stools for occult blood
  - Avoid taking aspirin
  - Comply with medical follow-up

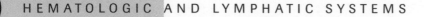

Key complications of aplastic anemia

- Hemorrhage
- Infection

Key facts about ITP

- Decreased amount of circulating platelets, which causes bleeding
- Classified as acute (with normal bone marrow) or chronic (without a known cause of thrombocytopenia)
- Acute ITP affects children; chronic ITP affects adults

Common causes of ITP

- Autoimmune disease
- Viral infection

Key signs and symptoms of ITP

- Petechiae, purpura, and ecchymosis
- Epistaxis
- Recent viral infection

Diagnosing ITP

- Hematology: decreased Hb, HCT, and platelets; normal PT and PTT; prolonged bleeding time
- Bone marrow biopsy: increased and abnormal megakaryocytes

Treating ITP

- IgG antibody: immune globulin I.V.
- Corticosteroids

- **Complications**
  - Hemorrhage
  - Infection
- **Surgical interventions**
  - Bone marrow transplant
  - Splenectomy

IDIOPATHIC THROMBOCYTOPENIC PURPURA (ITP)

- **Definition**
  - Decreased amount of circulating platelets, with normal bone marrow (acute ITP) and without a known cause of thrombocytopenia (chronic ITP)
  - Acute ITP affects children; chronic ITP affects adults
- **Causes**
  - Unknown
  - Autoimmune disease
  - Viral infection
- **Pathophysiology**
  - Antibody-coated platelets are removed from circulation by reticuloendothelial cells of the spleen and liver
  - Decreased number of circulating platelets causes bleeding
- **Assessment findings**
  - Petechiae, purpura, and ecchymosis
  - Epistaxis
  - Gingivitis and bleeding
  - Vision disturbances
  - Menorrhagia
  - Hematomas
  - GI bleeding
  - Positive Rumpel-Leede capillary fragility tourniquet test, with increased capillary fragility
  - Recent viral infection
- **Diagnostic test findings**
  - Hematology: decreased Hb, HCT, and platelets; normal PT and PTT; prolonged bleeding time
  - Blood chemistry: increased immunoglobulins, complement fixation
  - Bone marrow biopsy: increased and abnormal megakaryocytes
- **Medical management**
  - Transfusion therapy: fresh frozen plasma, platelets, packed RBCs, and plasma
  - I.V. therapy: fluids as needed
  - Activity: as tolerated, with frequent rest periods

- Monitoring: vital signs, daily weight, stools for occult blood, and laboratory studies (Hb, HCT, and platelets)
- Immune globulin (Ig) G antibody: immune globulin I.V. (Gammagard)
- Immunosuppressants: azathioprine (Imuran), cyclophosphamide (Cytoxan), vincristine (Oncovin)
- Anabolic steroid: danazol (Danocrine)
- Corticosteroid: prednisone (Deltasone), methylprednisolone (Solu-Medrol)

● **Nursing interventions**
- Maintain airway, breathing, and circulation if patient is acutely bleeding
- Administer I.V. fluids and transfusion therapy, as ordered
- Assess for bruising, bleeding, and infection
- Monitor and record vital signs; I/O; laboratory studies; daily weight; and stools, urine, and emesis for occult blood
- Administer medications, as prescribed
- Allay the patient's anxiety and provide emotional support
- Provide mouth and skin care
- Protect the patient from falls
- Avoid giving the patient I.M. injections, aspirin, enemas, and rectal temperatures
- Alternate rest periods with activity
- Rotate extremities for blood pressure monitoring
- Individualize home care instructions
  - Know about the disorder and its treatment
  - Follow instructions for medication use and be aware of possible adverse affects
  - Recognize the signs and symptoms of bleeding
  - Avoid contact sports
  - Wear medical identification jewelry
  - Avoid sneezing, coughing, nose blowing, straining while defecating, and heavy lifting
  - Avoid aspirin and ibuprofen
  - Comply with medical follow-up

● **Complications**
- Hemorrhage
- Hypersplenism
- Shock
- Peripheral paralysis and paresthesia

● **Surgical intervention**
- Splenectomy

POLYCYTHEMIA VERA

● **Definition**
- Myeloproliferative disorder that results in the increased production of erythrocytes, Hb, myelocytes, and thrombocytes

---

Key nursing interventions for a patient with ITP

- Assess for bruising, bleeding, and infection.
- Monitor and record vital signs; I/O; laboratory studies; daily weight; stool, urine, and emesis for occult blood.
- Protect the patient from falls.
- Rotate extremities for blood pressure monitoring.

Key complications of ITP

- Hemorrhage
- Shock

Key facts about polycythemia vera

- Myeloproliferative disorder
- Results in the increased production of erythrocytes, Hb, myelocytes, and thrombocytes
- Overproduction causes increased blood viscosity, increased total blood volume, and severe congestion of all tissues and organs

Common causes of polycythemia vera

- Unknown

Key signs and symptoms of polycythemia vera

- Ruddy complexion
- Headaches
- Dizziness
- Dyspnea and orthopnea

Diagnosing polycythemia vera

- RBC mass greater than or equal to 36 ml/kg (males) or 32 ml/kg (females),
- Blood chemistry: alkaline phosphatase greater than 100 units/L
- Serum vitamin B_{12} concentration: greater than 900 pg/ml
- Hematology: increased WBCs, HCT, and Hb; platelet count greater than 400,000/mm³
- Bone marrow biopsy: increased number of immature cell forms and decreased iron in marrow

Treating polycythemia vera

- Phlebotomy
- Antimetabolite
- Imidazole quinazoline
- Interferon
- Myelosuppressants

● **Causes**
- Unknown

● **Pathophysiology**
- Hyperplasia of bone marrow results in increased production of erythrocytes, Hb, granulocytes, and platelets
- Overproduction results in increased blood viscosity, increased total blood volume, and severe congestion of all tissues and organs

● **Assessment findings**
- Ruddy complexion
- Dusky mucosa
- Hypertension
- Vertigo
- Headaches
- Dizziness
- Dyspnea and orthopnea
- Tachycardia
- Ecchymosis
- Hepatomegaly and splenomegaly
- Weakness and fatigue
- Pruritus
- Epistaxis
- GI bleeding
- Angina

● **Diagnostic test findings**
- Blood chemistry: alkaline phosphatase greater than 100 units/L
- Serum vitamin B_{12} concentration: greater than 900 pg/ml
- RBC mass greater than or equal to 36 ml/kg (males) or 32 ml/kg (females)
- Hematology: WBC count greater than 12,000/µl, increased HCT and Hb, platelet count greater than 400,000/mm³
- Bone marrow biopsy: increased number of immature cell forms and decreased iron in marrow
- ABG analysis: normal partial pressure of arterial oxygen

● **Medical management**
- Phlebotomy
- I.V. therapy: fluids as needed
- Activity: as tolerated
- Monitoring: vital signs, CVP, I/O, and laboratory studies (Hb, HCT, WBCs, RBCs, platelets, and unconjugated bilirubin)
- Analgesic: acetaminophen (Tylenol)
- Antimetabolite: hydroxyurea (Hydrea)
- Imidazole quinazoline: anagrelide (Agrylin)
- Interferon (Roferon A)
- Antigouts: colchicine (Colchicine) and allopurinol (Zyloprim) (for hyperuricemia)
- Radioactive phosphorus

- Myelosuppressants: busulfan (Myleran), chlorambucil (Leukeran), and cyclophosphamide (Cytoxan)

● **Nursing interventions**
- Encourage fluids; administer I.V. fluids as ordered
- Assess cardiovascular and respiratory status
- Monitor and record vital signs, I/O, laboratory studies, CVP, and fecal occult blood
- Administer medications as prescribed
- Allay the patient's anxiety and provide emotional support
- Protect the patient from falls
- Apply sequential compression stockings while in bed
- Provide postchemotherapeutic and postradiation nursing care
  - Provide prophylactic skin, mouth, and perineal care
  - Monitor dietary intake
  - Administer antiemetics and antidiarrheals, as prescribed
  - Monitor for bleeding, infection, and electrolyte imbalance
  - Provide rest periods
- Individualize home care instructions
  - Know about the disorder and its treatment
  - Follow instructions for medication use and be aware of possible adverse effects
  - Recognize the signs and symptoms of heart failure, thrombophlebitis, and bleeding
  - Comply with medical follow-up

● **Complications**
- Stroke
- Pulmonary emboli
- Deep vein thrombosis (DVT)
- Hemorrhage
- Peptic ulcer
- Gout
- Acute leukemia

● **Surgical intervention**
- Splenectomy

DISSEMINATED INTRAVASCULAR COAGULATION (DIC)

● **Definition**
- Syndrome of activated coagulation, which causes widespread clotting in small vessels and obstructs blood supply of organs
- Coagulation factors are consumed, resulting in bleeding

● **Causes**
- Unknown
- Frequent, rapid transfusions

Key nursing interventions for a patient with polycythemia vera

- Encourage fluids and administer I.V. fluids, as ordered.
- Assess cardiovascular and respiratory status.
- Monitor and record vital signs, I/O, laboratory studies, CVP, and fecal occult blood.

Key complications of polycythemia vera

- Pulmonary emboli
- DVT

Key facts about DIC

- Syndrome of activated coagulation
- causes widespread clotting in small vessels
- obstructs blood supply of organs
- Coagulation factors are consumed, resulting in bleeding

Common causes of DIC

- Unknown
- Frequent, rapid transfusions
- Infection

What happens in DIC

- Activation of coagulation
- Circulating thrombin
- Blood vessel blockage by microthrombi
- Organ failure
- Clot destruction by fibrinolysis
- Hemorrhage
- Consumption of platelets and factors

TOP 4

Signs and symptoms of DIC

1. Abnormal bleeding
2. Petechiae
3. Ecchymosis
4. Hematuria

GO WITH THE FLOW

Three mechanisms of DIC

However disseminated intravascular coagulation (DIC) begins, accelerated clotting (characteristic of DIC) usually results in excess thrombin, which in turn causes fibrinolysis with excess fibrin formation and fibrin degradation products (FDP), activation of fibrin-stabilizing factor (factor XIII), consumption of platelet and clotting factors, and, eventually, hemorrhage.

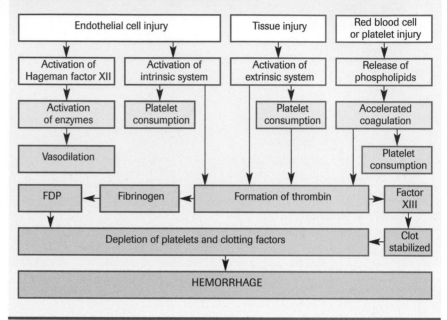

- Infection
- Obstetric complications
- Neoplastic disease
- Massive burns
- Massive trauma
- Anaphylaxis
- Chronic disease

Pathophysiology

- Underlying disease causes release of thromboplastic substances that promote the deposition of fibrin throughout the microcirculation (see *Three mechanisms of DIC*)
- RBCs are trapped in fibrin strands and are hemolyzed
- Platelets, prothrombin, and other clotting factors are destroyed, leading to bleeding
- Excessive clotting activates the fibrinolytic system that inhibits platelet function, causing further bleeding
- Acute activation of clotting mechanism results in consumption of plasma-clotting factors that the liver can't replenish quickly enough

- Activation of the thrombin and fibrinolytic system results in simultaneous bleeding and thrombosis

● **Assessment findings**
- Abnormal bleeding without a history of a serious hemorrhagic disorder
- Petechiae, ecchymosis, purpura
- Hematuria
- Anxiety, restlessness
- Acrocyanosis
- Muscle, back and abdominal pain
- Dyspnea
- Hemoptysis

● **Diagnostic test findings**
- Hematology: decreased platelets, RBCs, fibrinogen, and factor assay (II, V, VII); increased fibrin split products, thrombin, PT, and PTT; positive protamine sulfate test
- Urine chemistry: hematuria
- ABG analysis: metabolic acidosis
- Ophthalmoscopic exam: retinal hemorrhage
- Fecal occult blood: positive

● **Medical management**
- Treatment of the underlying cause
- Oxygen therapy with possible intubation and mechanical ventilation
- Transfusion therapy: platelets, packed RBCs, fresh frozen plasma, whole blood, volume expanders, and cryoprecipitates
- I.V. therapy: hydration and electrolyte replacement, as needed
- Activity: as tolerated
- Monitoring: vital signs, I/O, cardiac rhythm, pulse oximetry, and laboratory studies (PT, PTT, platelets, fibrinogen, and fibrin split products)
- Anticoagulant: heparin

● **Nursing interventions**
- Monitor for signs of bleeding
- Administer I.V. fluids and blood products, as ordered
- Administer oxygen; monitor pulse oximetry and respiratory status
- Assess cardiovascular status and fluid balance
- Monitor and record vital signs, I/O, laboratory studies, cardiac rhythm, and pulse oximetry
- Administer medications as prescribed
- Allay the patient's anxiety and provide emotional support
- Maintain activity as tolerated
- Provide gentle mouth and skin care
- Avoid giving the patient I.M. injections, enemas, and rectal temperatures
- Individualize home care instructions
  - Know about the disorder and its treatment
  - Follow instructions for medication use and be aware of possible adverse effects

Diagnosing DIC
- Hematology: decreased platelets, RBCs, fibrinogen, and factor assay (II, V, VII); increased fibrin split products, thrombin, PT, and PTT; positive protamine sulfate test
- Urine chemistry: hematuria

Treating DIC
- Treatment of underlying cause
- Transfusion therapy: platelets, packed RBCs, fresh frozen plasma, whole blood, volume expanders, and cryoprecipitates
- Anticoagulant

Key nursing interventions for a patient with DIC
- Monitor for signs of bleeding
- Assess cardiovascular status and fluid balance.
- Monitor and record vital signs, I/O, laboratory studies, cardiac rhythm, and pulse oximetry.
- Provide gentle mouth and skin care.

Key complications of DIC

- Organ dysfunction
- Hemorrhage
- Respiratory failure

Key facts about multiple myeloma

- Abnormal proliferation of plasma cells in the bone marrow
- Plasma cells produce abnormal amounts of immunoglobulins, which triggers osteoblastic activity

Common causes of multiple myeloma

- Unknown

Key risk factors for multiple myeloma

- Genetic
- Environmental

Key signs and symptoms of multiple myeloma

- Constant, severe bone pain
- Pain on movement
- Peripheral paresthesia

Diagnosing multiple myeloma

- X-ray: diffuse, round, punched out bone lesions; osteoporosis; osteolytic lesions of the skull; widespread demineralization
- Bence Jones protein assay: positive

– Comply with medical follow-up

- **Complications**
  - Organ dysfunction
  - Hemorrhage
  - Shock
  - Stroke
  - Hepatic damage
  - Respiratory failure

- **Surgical intervention**
  - None

MULTIPLE MYELOMA

- **Definition**
  - Abnormal proliferation of plasma cells in the bone marrow

- **Causes**
  - Unknown

- **Risk factors**
  - Genetic
  - Environmental

- **Pathophysiology**
  - Single tumor in bone marrow disseminates into lymph nodes, liver, spleen, kidneys, and bone
  - Plasma cell tumors produce abnormal amounts of immunoglobulins
  - Tumor cells trigger osteoblastic activity, leading to bone destruction throughout the body

- **Assessment findings**
  - Constant, severe bone pain
  - Peripheral paresthesia
  - Skeletal deformities of sternum and ribs
  - Pain on movement
  - Arthritic symptoms
  - Loss of height

- **Diagnostic test findings**
  - X-ray: diffuse, round, punched out bone lesions; osteoporosis; osteolytic lesions of the skull; and widespread demineralization
  - Bone marrow biopsy: increased number of immature plasma cells
  - Hematology: decreased HCT, WBCs, and platelets; increased ESR
  - Serum electrophoresis: abnormal globulin spike
  - Urine chemistry: increased calcium and uric acid
  - Bence Jones protein assay: positive

- **Medical management**
  - Radiation therapy
  - I.V. therapy: hydration and electrolyte replacement, as needed

- Activity: as tolerated
- Monitoring: vital signs, I/O, and laboratory studies (HCT, calcium, BUN, creatinine, uric acid, WBCs, protein, platelets, and surveillance cultures)
- Transfusion therapy: packed RBCs
- Antibiotic: trimethoprim/sulfamethoxazole (Bactrim DS)
- Antineoplastics: bortezomib (Velcade), melphalan (Alkeran), doxorubicin (Adriamycin)
- Analgesic: meperidine (Demerol)
- Glucocorticoids: prednisone (Deltasone), dexamethasone (Decadron)
- Immunosuppressant: thalidomide (Thalomid)
- Interferon: interferon alfa-2a (Roferon-A)
- Bisphosphonates: pamidronate (Aredia), zoledronic acid (Zometa)
- Colony-stimulating factor: erythropoietin (Epogen)
- Orthopedic devices: braces, splints, and casts
- Peritoneal and hemodialysis (with renal failure)

● **Nursing interventions**
- Administer I.V. fluids and blood products, as ordered
- Assess renal, cardiovascular, and respiratory status and fluid balance
- Monitor and record vital signs, I/O, and laboratory studies
- Administer transfusion therapy as prescribed
- Administer medications as prescribed
- Allay the patient's anxiety and provide emotional support
- Provide skin and mouth care
- Alternate rest periods with activity
- Monitor for infection and bruising
- Provide postchemotherapeutic and postradiation nursing care
  - Provide prophylactic skin, mouth, and perineal care
  - Monitor dietary intake
  - Administer antiemetics and antidiarrheals, as prescribed
  - Monitor for bleeding, infection, and electrolyte imbalance
  - Provide rest periods
- Assess pain level, administer analgesics as prescribed, and evaluate response
- Apply and maintain braces, splints, and casts
- Individualize home care instructions
  - Know about the disorder and its treatment
  - Follow instructions for medication use and be aware of possible adverse effects
  - Contact the American Cancer Society
  - Exercise regularly, with particular attention to muscle-strengthening exercises
  - Recognize the signs and symptoms of complications
  - Use braces, splints, and casts as appropriate
  - Comply with medical follow-up

● **Complications**
- Infection

Treating multiple myeloma

- Antineoplastics
- Glucocorticoids
- Immunosuppressant
- Bisphosphonates
- Radiation therapy

Key nursing interventions for a patient with multiple myeloma

- Administer I.V. fluids and blood products, as ordered.
- Assess renal, cardiovascular, and respiratory status and fluid balance.
- Monitor for infection and bruising.
- Provide postchemotherapeutic and postradiation nursing care.
- Assess pain level, administer analgesics as prescribed, and evaluate response.

Key complications of multiple myeloma

- Acute renal failure
- Infection
- Hematologic imbalances
- Carpal tunnel syndrome

- Acute renal failure
- Hematologic imbalances
- Urolithiasis
- Pathologic fractures
- Seizures
- Carpal tunnel syndrome

● **Surgical intervention**
- Laminectomy (with vertebral compression)

HEMOPHILIA

● **Definition**
- Hereditary bleeding disorder
- Two types
  - Hemophilia A—most common type caused by deficiency of factor VIII
  - Hemophilia B—deficiency of factor IX

● **Causes**
- Inherited as X-linked recessive trait, primarily by males
- Asymptomatic mothers and sisters as carriers

● **Pathophysiology**
- Hemophilia A: deficiency of factor VIII causes extended clotting time
- Hemophilia B: deficiency of factor IX causes extended clotting time

● **Assessment findings**
- Large spreading bruises
- Prolonged or spontaneous bleeding episodes
- Bleeding into muscles, joints, and soft tissues after minimal trauma
- Pain in joints
- Joint swelling and limited ROM
- Recurrent joint hemorrhages
- Spontaneous hematuria
- Spontaneous GI bleeding

● **Diagnostic test findings**
- Hemophilia A
  - Factor VIII: 25% or less of normal
  - PTT: prolonged
  - Platelet count and function, bleeding time, PT: normal
- Hemophilia B
  - Factor IX: deficient
  - Coagulation factors: similar to hemophilia A
  - Factor VIII: normal

● **Medical management**
- Stop the bleeding by administering clotting factors, applying pressure to the bleeding site (if possible), and using cold compresses
- Hemostatic: cryoprecipitated antihemophilic factor (Hemophilia A) or factor IX concentrate (Hemophilia B)

- Activity: guided by degree of factor deficiency
- Monitoring: vital signs, I/O, and laboratory studies (HCT, Hb, and coagulation time)
- I.V. therapy: whole blood, blood components, and I.V. fluids
- Antifibrinolytics: aminocaproic acid (Amicar), tranexamic acid (Cyklokapron)
- Vasopressor: desmopressin (DDAVP) (hemophilia A)
- Analgesics: acetaminophen (Tylenol), oxycodone (OxyContin)

● **Nursing interventions**
- Assess the patient for internal bleeding, hematuria, melena, hematemesis, joint space hemorrhages, and muscle hematomas
- Assess cardiac, renal, and respiratory status
- Monitor and record vital signs, I/O, and laboratory studies
- Administer medications as prescribed
- Allay the patient's anxiety and provide emotional support
- Provide skin and mouth care
- Administer I.V. fluids, blood, and blood components, as prescribed
- Assess the location and intensity of pain, and medicate, as necessary
- Avoid aspirin and I.M. injections
- Apply gentle pressure and cold compresses to external bleeding sites
- Individualize home care instructions
  - Know about the disorder and its treatment
  - Follow instructions for medication use and be aware of possible adverse effects
  - Take measures to avoid bleeding episodes
  - Comply with activity restrictions
  - Observe for signs and symptoms of complications
  - Administer factor VIII or factor IX at first sign of bleeding
  - Wear joint and muscle splints and orthopedics, as prescribed
  - Comply with medical follow-up

● **Complications**
- Infection
- Shock
- Hemorrhage
- Sensitization to antihemolytic factor

● **Surgical intervention**
- None

SICKLE CELL ANEMIA

● **Definition**
- Congenital hemolytic anemia resulting from a defective Hb molecule (Hb S) that causes RBCs to roughen and become sickle-shaped

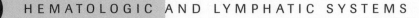

Common cause of sickle cell anemia

- Inheritance of autosomal recessive gene that produces a defective HB molecule

Key signs and symptoms of sickle cell anemia

- Aching bones
- Jaundice or pallor
- Spiderlike body build in adult

Sickle-cell crisis
- Hematuria
- Pale lips, tongue, and nail beds
- Severe pain

Painful crisis
- Severe abdominal, thoracic, muscle, or bone pain
- Worsening jaundice
- Dark urine

Aplastic crisis
- Dyspnea
- Lethargy
- Possible coma

Acute sequestration crisis
- Hypovolemic shock
- Liver congestion and enlargement
- Worsened chronic jaundice

● Causes
- Homozygous inheritance of an autosomal recessive gene that produces a defective Hb molecule
- Occurs primarily in persons of African and Mediterranean descent, but it also affects other populations

● Pathophysiology
- A change in the gene that encodes the beta chain of Hb results in a defect in Hb (Hb S)
- When hypoxia occurs, Hb S in the RBCs becomes insoluble
- The cells become rigid and rough, forming an elongated sickle shape and impairing circulation
- Infection, stress, dehydration, and conditions that provoke hypoxia may lead to periodic crisis
- Crises can occur in different forms, including painful crisis, aplastic crisis, and acute sequestration crisis

● Assessment findings
- Sickle cell anemia
  - Aching bones
  - Chronic fatigue
  - Frequent infections
  - Jaundice or pallor
  - Joint swelling
  - Leg ulcers (especially on ankles)
  - Delayed growth and puberty
  - Spiderlike body build in adult
- Sickle-cell crisis
  - Hematuria
  - Pale lips, tongue, and nail beds
  - Severe pain
- Painful crisis (vaso-occlusive crisis, which appears periodically after age 5)
  - Severe abdominal, thoracic, muscle, or bone pain
  - Dark urine
  - Low-grade fever
  - Worsening jaundice
- Aplastic crisis (generally associated with viral infection)
  - Dyspnea
  - Lethargy and sleepiness
  - Markedly decreased bone marrow activity
  - Pallor
  - Possible coma
  - RBC hemolysis
- Acute sequestration crisis (rare; occurs in infants ages 8 months to 2 years)
  - Lethargy
  - Pallor

– Hypovolemic shock
  – Liver congestion and enlargement
  – Worsened chronic jaundice

● **Diagnostic test findings**
  • Hb electrophoresis: Hb S
  • Stained blood smear: shows sickle cells
  • Hematologic studies: low RBCs, elevated WBCs and platelets, decreased ESR, increased serum iron levels, decreased RBC survival, and reticulocytosis
  • Hb levels: low or normal
  • Lateral chest X-ray: "Lincoln log" deformity in the vertebrae

● **Medical management**
  • Oxygen therapy as needed
  • Activity: bed rest during a crisis
  • Diet: high in iron and folic acid; increased fluid intake
  • Monitoring: vital signs, I/O, and laboratory studies (HCT, Hb, RBC, WBC, platelets, ESR, and serum iron levels)
  • I.V. therapy: hydration as ordered
  • Warm compresses to painful joints
  • Blood transfusions as indicated
  • Analgesics: morphine, ketorolac (Toradol)
  • Antimetabolite: hydroxyurea (Hydrea)
  • Vitamin: folic acid (Folate)
  • Antibiotic: cefuroxime (Ceftin)
  • Genetic counseling
  • Allogeneic bone marrow transplant
  • Transcutaneous electrical nerve stimulation
  • Plasmaphoresis

● **Nursing interventions**
  • Assess cardiovascular, respiratory, neurologic, GI, and renal status
  • **Assess pain level, administer analgesics as prescribed, and evaluate response**
  • Monitor and record vital signs, I/O, and laboratory studies
  • Encourage increased oral fluid intake
  • Administer medications as prescribed
  • Apply warm compresses as prescribed
  • Allay the patient's anxiety and provide emotional support
  • Individualize home care instructions
    – Know about the disorder and its treatment
    – Follow instructions for medication use and be aware of possible adverse effects
    – Avoid restricting circulation
    – Receive childhood immunizations
    – Recognize and promptly treat infections
    – **Increase fluid intake**

Diagnosing sickle cell anemia

● Hematologic studies: low RBCs, elevated WBCs and platelets, decreased ESR, increased serum iron levels, decreased RBC survival, and reticulocytosis
● Hb electrophoresis: Hb S

Treating sickle cell anemia

● Analgesics
● Oxygen therapy
● Antimetabolite
● Vitamin: folic acid

Key nursing interventions for a patient with sickle cell anemia

● Encourage increased oral fluid intake.
● Assess pain level, administer analgesics as prescribed, and evaluate response.
● Apply warm compresses as prescribed.

– Avoid strenuous exercise, vasoconstricting medications, cold temperatures, unpressurized aircraft, high altitude, and other conditions that provoke hypoxia

– Comply with medical follow-up

● **Complications**
- Bacterial infection
- Organ dysfunction
- Cerebral vessel occlusion
- Death

● **Surgical intervention**
- None

NCLEX CHECKS

It's never too soon to begin your NCLEX preparation. Now that you've reviewed this chapter, carefully read each of the following questions and choose the best answer. Then compare your responses to the correct answers.

1. A nurse is caring for a client with non-Hodgkin's lymphoma. What symptom is typical of non-Hodgkin's lymphoma?

- ☐ **1.** Small, hard, irregular, and tender mass
- ☒ **2.** Enlarged, nontender lymph nodes
- ☐ **3.** Pain and swelling at the site
- ☐ **4.** Cat's eye reflex

2. Which of the following is the least important area of home care instruction to include in discussions with a client with multiple myeloma?

- ☐ **1.** Skeletal system symptoms
- ☐ **2.** Renal system symptoms
- ☐ **3.** Nervous system symptoms
- ☒ **4.** Cardiovascular system symptoms

3. Which substance helps control bleeding when given to a client with hemophilia B?

- ☐ **1.** Protamine sulfate
- ☐ **2.** Platelet transfusions
- ☒ **3.** Factor IX concentrate
- ☐ **4.** Vitamin K (AquaMEPHYTON)

4. A nurse is reviewing the laboratory report for a client who underwent a bone marrow biopsy. The finding that would most strongly support a diagnosis of leukemia is the existence of a large number of immature:

- ☐ **1.** lymphocytes.
- ☐ **2.** thrombocytes.
- ☐ **3.** reticulocytes.
- ☒ **4.** leukocytes.

Key complications of sickle cell anemia

- Bacterial infection
- Organ dysfunction
- Cerebral vessel occlusion

TOP 10

Items to study for your next test on the hematologic and lymphatic systems

1. Facts about RBCs and WBCs
2. ABO blood groups
3. Possible complications after a splenectomy
4. Nursing interventions before and after bone marrow transplant
5. Assessment findings in leukemia
6. Types of lymphomas
7. Diagnostic test findings and medications for treating AIDS
8. How DIC happens
9. Types of hemophilia and their treatments
10. Difference between normal RBCs and sickled RBCs

5. A nurse suspects DIC in a client who sustained a pelvic fracture in a motor vehicle accident. Which laboratory test result helps diagnose DIC?

- [ ] **1.** Elevated platelet count
- [x] **2.** Decreased fibrinogen level
- [ ] **3.** Low fibrin split product level
- [ ] **4.** Decreased PTT

6. A nurse is planning care for a client with hemophilia A. A client with hemophilia A is deficient in which clotting factor?

- [ ] **1.** VII
- [x] **2.** VIII
- [ ] **3.** IX
- [ ] **4.** X

7. Which nursing intervention is appropriate when caring for a client diagnosed with sickle cell anemia?

- [ ] **1.** Keep the client flat in bed and logroll every 2 hours.
- [x] **2.** Assess pain level and administer analgesics, as prescribed.
- [ ] **3.** Restrict fluid intake and maintain strict intake and output.
- [ ] **4.** Perform active and passive ROM exercises every 2 hours.

8. A nurse is administering cyanocobalamin (vitamin B_{12}) to a client with pernicious anemia, secondary to gastrectomy. Which route should the nurse use to most effectively administer the vitamin?

- [ ] **1.** Topical
- [ ] **2.** Transdermal
- [ ] **3.** Enteral
- [x] **4.** Parenteral

9. A nurse is teaching a community group about sickle cell anemia. Sickle cell anemia is most common in clients of which ethnic background?

- [ ] **1.** Asian
- [x] **2.** Black
- [ ] **3.** Hispanic
- [ ] **4.** White

10. A client with sickle cell anemia is ordered morphine 4 mg I.V. The concentration of the vial is 10 mg/ml of solution. How many milliliters should the nurse administer? Record your answer using one decimal place. _____ milliliters

ANSWERS AND RATIONALES

1. CORRECT ANSWER: 2
Enlarged, nontender, firm, and painless lymph nodes in the supraclavicular area are the main symptoms of non-Hodgkin's lymphoma. A small, hard, tender mass and localized pain and swelling aren't typical symptoms of non-Hodgkin's lymphoma. A white spot, or cat's eye reflex, is a symptom of retinoblastoma.

2. CORRECT ANSWER: 4

Multiple myeloma usually doesn't have a direct effect on the heart. Multiple myeloma usually affects the skeletal, renal, and nervous systems.

3. CORRECT ANSWER: 3

Hemophilia B, a congenital bleeding disorder, is caused by a deficiency of factor IX. The treatment for hemophilia B is the administration of factor IX. Vitamin K, protamine sulfate, and platelets are used to stop bleeding, but they aren't specific treatments for hemophilia B.

4. CORRECT ANSWER: 4

Leukemia is manifested by an abnormal overproduction of immature leukocytes in the bone marrow. Large numbers of lymphocytes, thrombocytes, and reticulocytes aren't characteristic of leukemia.

5. CORRECT ANSWER: 2

DIC involves depletion of such clotting substances as fibrinogen and platelets, which are used for widespread clotting within the vessels. As a result, the client's fibrinogen level and platelet count are abnormally low. Fibrin split product levels, a by-product of clot lysis, are elevated in DIC. The PTT is elevated because of clotting factor depletion.

6. CORRECT ANSWER: 2

Hemophilia A, which affects more than 80% of all hemophilia clients, is caused by a deficiency of clotting factor VIII. A deficiency of the other factors doesn't cause hemophilia A. Hemophilia B results from a deficiency of factor IX.

7. CORRECT ANSWER: 2

The nurse should evaluate the client with sickle cell anemia for his pain level, administer analgesics as prescribed, and evaluate response to medication. The client with sickle cell anemia doesn't need to be kept flat or logrolled. Fluid intake should be increased with clients having sickle cell disease. ROM exercises aren't needed every 2 hours and physical activity would need to be recommended according to joint involvement.

8. CORRECT ANSWER: 4

Following a gastrectomy, the client no longer has the intrinsic factor available to provide vitamin B_{12} in his GI tract. Vitamin B_{12} is administered parenterally (I.M. or deep subcutaneous). Topical and transdermal administration aren't available, and the enteral route is inappropriate after a gastrectomy.

9. CORRECT ANSWER: 2

Sickle cell anemia, a genetically determined hemolytic anemia, is most common in Blacks. It also occurs in people of Mediterranean descent and, infrequently, in Whites.

10. CORRECT ANSWER: 0.4

The nurse should calculate the volume to be given using this equation:
4 mg/X ml = 1 mg/1 ml; 10x = 4; X = 0.4 ml

Glossary
Selected references
Index

Glossary

accessory muscles: thoracic and abdominal muscles used during respiratory distress to help expand and contract the chest so the patient can inhale and exhale

anemia: reduction in the number and volume of red blood cells, the amount of hemoglobin, or the volume of packed red cells

aneurysm: sac formed by the dilation of the wall of an artery, a vein, or the heart

angiography: radiographic visualization of blood vessels after injection of radiopaque contrast material

anorexia: lack or loss of appetite

antigen: foreign substance that evokes an immune response

ascites: fluid in the peritoneal cavity

ataxia: lack of muscular coordination

atelectasis: failure of a portion of the lung to expand, preventing respiratory exchange in that area

auscultation: physical assessment technique by which the examiner listens (usually with a stethoscope) for sounds coming from the heart, lungs, abdomen, or other organs

autoimmune disorder: disorder in which the body launches an immunologic response against itself

bruit: abnormal sound heard over peripheral vessels on auscultation that indicates turbulent blood flow

cancer: multiple and varying alterations in cell function resulting from overproduction of immature and nonfunctional cells or tissue enlargement for no physiologic reason

cardiac output: volume of blood ejected from the heart per minute

chemotherapy: medical treatment with highly toxic doses of medication aimed at interfering with the miotic division of cancerous cells

crepitation: grating or crackling sound produced by bone rubbing against bone

disease: pathologic condition that occurs when the body can't maintain homeostasis

distal: farthest away

dysphagia: difficulty swallowing

dyspnea: difficult, labored breathing

ecchymosis: bruise

embolism: sudden obstruction of a blood vessel by foreign substances or a blood clot

exacerbation: increase in the severity of a disease

fasciculation: involuntary twitching or contraction of the muscle

hematuria: blood in the urine

hemoglobin: iron-containing pigment in red blood cells that carries oxygen from the lungs to the tissues

hemoptysis: expectoration of bloody sputum

hemorrhage: escape of blood from a ruptured vessel

hirsutism: excessive hair growth or unusual distribution of hair

hormone: chemical substance produced in the body that has a specific regulatory effect on the activity of specific cells or organs

hypertension: high arterial blood pressure

hypotension: abnormally low blood pressure

hypoxia: reduction of oxygen in body tissues to below normal levels

idiopathic: disease with no known cause

immunotherapy: use of specially treated white blood cell immunoprotectors to replace immunocompetent lymphoid tissue, such as bone marrow and thymus

inspection: critical observation of the patient during which the examiner may use sight, hearing, or smell to make informed observations

insulin: hormone secreted into the blood by the islets of Langerhans of the pancreas; promotes the storage of glucose, among other functions

ischemia: decreased blood supply to a body organ or tissue

jugular vein distention: distended neck veins that may indicate increased central venous pressure

lethargy: slowed responses, sluggish speech, and slowed mental and motor processes in a person oriented to time, place, and person

lichenification: thickening and hardening of the epidermis

lymphadenopathy: enlargement of the lymph nodes

melena: black, tarry stools

metastasize: growth and spread of malignant cells from the primary site to other tissues

murmur: abnormal sound heard on auscultation of the heart; caused by abnormal blood flow through a valve

necrosis: tissue death

oliguria: urine output of less than 30 ml/hour

orthopnea: respiratory distress that's relieved by sitting upright

palpation: physical assessment technique by which the examiner uses the sense of touch to feel pulsations and vibrations or to locate body structures and assess their texture, size, consistency, mobility, and tenderness

pathogen: disease producing agent or microorganism

percussion: physical assessment technique by which the examiner taps on the skin surface with his fingers to assess the size, border, and consistency of internal organs, and to detect and evaluate fluid in a body cavity

peristalsis: intestinal contractions, or waves, that propel food toward the stomach and into and through the intestine

petechiae: multiple, small, hemorrhagic areas on the skin

plasma: liquid part of the blood that carries antibodies and nutrients to tissues and carries wastes away from tissues

platelet: disk-shaped structure in blood that plays a crucial role in blood coagulation

polydipsia: excessive thirst

polyphagia: excessive eating

polyuria: excessive urination

proximal: nearest to

pruritus: severe itching

ptosis: drooping of the eyelid

renal colic: flank pain that radiates to the groin

subluxation: partial dislocation of a joint

thrombosis: development of a thrombus (blood clot)

tophi: clusters of urate crystals surrounded by inflamed tissue; occur in gout

vasopressor: drug that stimulates contraction of the muscular tissue of the capillaries and arteries

virus: microscopic, infectious parasite that contains genetic material and needs a host cell to replicate

Selected references

Bickley, L.S., and Szilagyi, P.G. *Bates' Guide to Physical Examination and History Taking,* 9th ed. Philadelphia: Lippincott Williams & Wilkins, 2007.

Black, J.M., et al. *Medical-Surgical Nursing: Clinical Management for Positive Outcomes,* 7th ed. Philadelphia: W.B. Saunders Co., 2005.

Bray, A. "Preoperative Nursing Assessment of the Surgical Patient," *Nursing Clinics of North America* 41(2):135-50, June 2006.

Burns, N., and Grove, S.K. *Understanding Nursing Research: Building an Evidence-based Practice,* 4th ed. Philadelphia: W.B. Saunders Co., 2007.

Chitty, K., and Perry Black, B. *Professional Nursing: Concepts and Challenges.* Philadelphia: W.B. Saunders, 2007.

Craven, R.F., and Hirnle, C.J. *Fundamentals of Nursing: Human Health and Function,* 5th ed. Philadelphia: Lippincott Williams & Wilkins, 2006.

Dellinger, E.P. "Prophylactic Antibiotics: Administration and Timing Before Operation are More Important Than Administration After Operation," *Clinical Infectious Diseases* 44(7): 928-30, April 2007.

Frye, C. *Frye's 3300 Nursing Bullets for NCLEX-RN,* 6th ed. Philadelphia: Lippincott Williams & Wilkins, 2006.

Gregory, D.M. et al. "Patient Safety: Where is Nursing Education?" *Journal of Nursing Education* 46(2): 79-82, February 2007.

Gulanik, M., and Myers, J. *Nursing Care Plans,* 6th ed. Philadelphia: Mosby, 2007.

Ignatavicius, D.D., and Workman, M.L. *Medical-Surgical Nursing: Critical Thinking for Collaborative Care,* 5th ed. Philadelphia: W.B. Saunders Co., 2006.

Klug Redman, B. *The Practice of Patient Education: A Case Study Approach.* Philadelphia: Mosby, 2007.

Medical-Surgical Nursing: Lippincott Manual of Nursing Practice Pocket Guide. Philadelphia: Lippincott Williams & Wilkins, 2006.

Medical-Surgical Nursing Made Incredibly Easy, 2nd ed. Philadelphia: Lippincott Williams & Wilkins, 2007.

NCLEX-RN Review Made Incredibly Easy, 4th ed. Philadelphia: Lippincott Williams & Wilkins, 2008.

Nurse's 3 Minute Clinical Reference, 2nd ed. Philadelphia: Lippincott Williams & Wilkins, 2007.

Nursing2008 Drug Handbook, 28th ed. Philadelphia: Lippincott Williams & Wilkins, 2008.

Nursing: Deciphering Diagnostic Tests. Philadelphia: Lippincott Williams & Wilkins, 2008.

Peterson, A.M., and Walker, P.H. "Hospital-Acquired Infections as Patient Safety Indicators," *Annual Review of Nursing Research* 24:75-99, 2006.

Portable RN: The All-in-One Nursing Reference, 3rd ed. Philadelphia: Lippincott Williams & Wilkins, 2006.

Porth, C.M. *Essentials of Pathophysiology: Concepts of Altered Health,* 2nd ed. Philadelphia: Lippincott Williams & Wilkins, 2006.

Professional Guide to Pathophysiology, 2nd ed. Philadelphia: Lippincott Williams & Wilkins, 2006.

Russell, S.S. "Continuing Education Changes Affect Medsurg Nursing," *Medsurg Nursing* 15(5): 313-14, October 2006.

Smeltzer, S.C., and Bare, B.G., eds. *Brunner and Suddarth's Textbook of Medical-Surgical Nursing,* 11th ed. Philadelphia: Lippincott Williams & Wilkins, 2006.

Springhouse Review for Medical-Surgical Nursing Certification: An Indispensable Study Guide for the A.N.A. Exam, 4th ed. Philadelphia: Lippincott Williams & Wilkins, 2006.

Wagner, D., et al. "Effects of Comfort Warming on Preoperative Patients," *AORN Journal* 84(3): 427-48, September, 2006.

Index

i refers to an illustration; t refers to a table.

i refers to an illustration; t refers to a table.

i refers to an illustration; t refers to a table.

i refers to an illustration; t refers to a table.

i refers to an illustration; t refers to a table.

i refers to an illustration; t refers to a table.

i refers to an illustration; t refers to a table.

ABOUT THE CD-ROM

The enclosed CD-ROM is just one more reason why the *Straight A's* series is at the head of its class. The more than 250 additional NCLEX-style questions contained on the CD provide you with another opportunity to review the material and gauge your knowledge. The program allows you to:

- take tests of varying lengths on subject areas of your choice
- learn the rationales for correct and incorrect answers
- print the results of your tests to measure progress over time.

Minimum system requirements

To operate the *Straight A's* CD-ROM, we recommend that you have the following computer equipment:

- Windows XP-Home edition
- Pentium 4
- 512 MB RAM
- 10 MB of free hard-disk space
- SVGA monitor with high color (16-bit)
- CD-ROM drive
- mouse.

Installation

Before installing the CD-ROM, make sure that your monitor is set to High Color (16-bit) and your display area is set to 800 × 600. If it isn't, consult your monitor's user's manual for instructions about changing the display settings. (The display settings are typically found in Start/Settings/Control Panel/Display/Settings tab.)

To run this program, you must install it onto the hard drive of your computer, following these three steps:

1. Start Windows XP-Home edition (minimum).
2. Place the CD in your CD-ROM drive. After a few moments, the install process will automatically begin. *Note:* If the install process doesn't automatically begin, click the Start menu and select Run. Type *D:\setup.exe* (where *D:* is the letter of your CD-ROM drive) and then click OK.
3. Follow the on-screen instructions for installation.

Technical support

For technical support, call toll-free 1-800-638-3030, Monday through Friday, 8:30 a.m. to 5 p.m. Eastern Time. You may also write to Lippincott Williams & Wilkins Technical Support, 351 W. Camden Street, Baltimore, MD 21201-2436, or e-mail us at *wkhealth-support@wolterskluwer.com*.
